T0074341

Thornicroft · Tansella (Eds.) Mental Health Outcome Measures

Springer
Berlin
Heidelberg
New York
Barcelona
Budapest
Hong Kong
London
Milan
Paris
Santa Clara
Singapore
Tokyo

Graham Thornicroft · Michele Tansella
(Eds.)

Mental Health Outcome Measures

With 6 Figures and 30 Tables

 Springer

Editors

Professor GRAHAM THORNICROFT
PRiSM, Institute of Psychiatry
De Crespigny Park
Denmark Hill
London SE5 8AF, UK

Professor MICHELE TANSELLA
Servizio di Psicologica Medica
Istituto di Psichiatria
Università di Verona
Ospedale Policlinico
I-37134 Verona, Italy

ISBN-13: 978-3-642-80204-1

Cip-Data applied for
Die Deutsche Bibliothek – CIP-Einheitsaufnahme
Mental Health Outcome Measures/G. Thornicroft; M. Tansella (eds.) –
Berlin; Heidelberg; New York; Barcelona; Budapest; Hong Kong; London; Milan; Paris; Tokyo: Springer, 1996
   ISBN-13: 978-3-642-80204-1   e-ISBN-13: 978-3-642-80202-7
   DOI: 10.1007/978-3-642-80202-7
NE: Thornicroft, Graham [Hrsg.]

This work is subject to copyright. All rights are reserved, whether the whole or part of the material is concerned, specifically the rights of translation, reprinting, reuse of illustrations, recitation, broadcasting, reproduction on microfilm or in any other way, and storage in data banks. Duplication of this publication or parts thereof is permitted only under the provisions of the German Copyright Law of September 9, 1965, in its current version, and permission for use must always be obtained from Springer-Verlag. Violations are liable for prosecution under the German Copyright Law.

© Springer-Verlag Berlin Heidelberg 1996
Softcover reprint of the hardcover 1st edition 1996

The use of general descriptive names, registered names, trademarks, etc. in this publication does not imply, even in the absence of a specific statement, that such names are exempt from the relevant protective laws and regulations and therefore free for general use.
Product liability: The publishers cannot guarantee the accuracy of any information about dosage and application contained in this book. In every individual case the user must check such information by consulting the relevant literature.

SPIN: 10534027   25/3134 – 5 4 3 2 1 0 – Printed on acid-free paper

We are very pleased to acknowledge the continuing encouragement of JOHN and RHODA THORNICROFT and CHRISTA and CAROLE TANSELLA in realising this book.

Foreword

Mental health services across Europe are in a state of ferment. It is essential that researchers use replicable measures to assess those developments that are desirable, as well as those forms of service that can be shown to be cost-effective. The appearance of this book is timely since it brings together a set of influential papers on the measurement of outcome. There is therefore a chance that investigators in different countries can use measures and procedures which are comparable with one another. At present we do not have a single set of measures which can be confidently recommended; however, the various contributions should allow researchers to make an informed choice.

This book brings together two sets of articles recently written for special issues of *Social Psychiatry and Psychiatric Epidemiology* (Vol. 29 no. 5; vol. 31 no. 2) with five articles especially written for this volume. A useful paper by Taylor and Thornicroft considers the limitations of randomized controlled trials (RCTs) in the evaluation of mental health services, which are numerous and real, despite the obvious theoretical appeal of such designs. All of the famous RCTs excluded patients who were homicidal, and many excluded patients who had no home to go to. This is important since planners of services have tended to generalize the results of such studies, with the result that, in England at least, too many beds have been closed in the name of community care. It may be concluded that other, naturalistic designs should be used in the evaluation of complex services. The RCT should be reserved for situations in which prospective randomization is feasible, and in which specifiable outcomes are likely to follow the treatment to which subjects are being randomized. However, naturalistic studies also have their shortcomings, so that investigators tend to use unsatisfactory compromises between the two designs. An alternative approach is to use multi-dimensional assessments of outcome, as described by Biggeri and others in this volume. At present such approaches are in their early stages, and serve to generate hypotheses about possible relationships between variables.

A consensus is beginning to emerge on methods of evaluation; this would indicate that progress has been made. We hope that this book will contribute to the understanding which is developing between investigators working in very different settings. In the conclusion of this volume, Rachel Jenkins emphasizes the preoccupation of previous studies with input and process variables, and welcomes the present emphasis on outcome variables. At present, investigators tend to use separate measures of symptom loss, user and carer satisfaction with services, quality of life, and various measures of need which are reviewed in this book. It is evident that we are still picking our way across a minefield. The chapters which follow offer the reader a state-of-the-art map of the territory and point out the various hazards which lie ahead.

London   Professor DAVID GOLDBERG

Institute of Psychiatry, De Crespigny Park, Denmark Hill, London SE5 8AF, UK

Contents

List of Contributors

You will find the addresses at the beginning of the respective contribution

CHAPTER 1

Introduction

GRAHAM THORNICROFT and MICHELE TANSELLA

This book focuses on the methods used in psychiatric research for mental health service evaluation. Whilst an airline pilot would not consider flying without an altimeter that had been very carefully calibrated, assessments without established psychometric properties are still common in psychiatric research. The contributions in this book therefore aim to assess the psychometric adequacy of commonly used measures, as discussed by Salvador, and to propose how they should be further developed. To this end we shall address three overlapping themes. Firstly, the full evaluation of mental health services requires the measurement of a wide array of social, clinical and economic variables. Secondly, considerable progress has been made in most of these aspects of evaluation over the last decade. Thirdly, reports on the use and translation of measures of known psychometric adequacy are not yet widespread in the research literature.

Until recently the outcome of mental health service research has been directed almost entirely towards two issues: psychopathology (e.g., symptom severity) and service utilization (e.g., number of admissions, time to readmission or length of stay). Those involved in community-orientated research increasingly recognise the limitations of this approach, and indeed very few innovative services in the field of community mental health have yielded benefits in terms of symptom improvement and/or reduced bed usage.

Since 1990 a wider perspective is being adopted in relation to research design, data analysis and the outcome measures which are important and may yield improvements in patient care. With respect to research design, for example, Taylor et al. have set out the advantages of randomised controlled trials for medical research, in addition to the possible limitations in their application to mental health services. The difficulties inherent in the interpretation of data in complex human service systems and the need for refined and innovative statistical methods are outlined by Dunn, Biggeri, Tansella and colleagues.

In terms of domains of measurement that go beyond symptoms, Phelan et al. demonstrate that global rating scales are conceptually attractive but extremely difficult to operate well. There is also a lack of conceptual clarity about the subjective per-

G. Thornicroft
PRiSM, Institute of Psychiatry, De Crespigny Park, Denmark Hill, London SE5 8AF, UK

M. Tansella
Servizio di Psicologia Medica, Istituto di Psichiatria, Università di Verona, Ospedale Policlinico, I-37134 Verona, Italy

spective of users on outcome. Patient satisfaction is a case in point, and as Ruggieri makes clear, satisfaction must be considered both in relation to expectations and in relation to the wider cultural context of health practices and beliefs. Moreover, in order to be valid, the measure of satisfaction must be sufficiently detailed and comprehensive and cannot rely on only a few general questions. Furthermore, as the need for mental health service research extends into community settings, the importance of the mutual effects of patients and their families gains prominence, as discussed by Schene et al.

The contributions in this book also demonstrate that care is needed in establishing new measurement scales. As detailed by Wing, both Present State Examination (PSE) 9 and Schedules for Clinical Assessment in Neuropsychiatry (SCAN) were developed over 10-year period and are part of the wider family of scales developed within the framework of the WHO, which are discussed in detail by Sartorius and Janca. A further example of the careful development of a scale suitable for widespread international use is the Composite International Diagnostic Interview (CIDI), described here by Wittchen.

In addition to the recent emphasis on community-orientated mental health services, there is an increasing interest in three further research areas. With respect to therapeutic, planning and political aspects, cost evaluation has become of paramount interest, as detailed by McCrone and Weich. Indeed cost analyses have revealed that service use is more often associated with disability than symptom levels. Wiersma's review considers both the conceptual and the operational aspects of social disability. Finally, as Lehman argues, the quality of patients' lives and the quality of care they receive are important considerations in that differences are often detected in comparing treatment settings and service models, and because they are seen as important by people who use mental health services.

Research instruments are the basic tools of health service evaluation. These tools must be well designed to suit their purpose and only used by well trained people. The recurring themes in this book are the time-consuming and costly development of health service evaluation methods, the importance of standardising their use in different reference groups and the stringent requirements for their use in different languages. This work is now beginning under the auspices of European Network for Mental Health Service Evaluation[1] (ENMESH). These are exacting conditions, but optimal results such precise instruments and rigorous methods now need to be developed.

---

[1] ENMESH. Details from A. Schene, Secretary of the ENMESH Executive Committee, Academisch Medisch Centrum, Polikliniek Psychiatrie, 9, 1105 AZ, Amsterdam, (ZO), The Netherlands, (tel + 31 20 05 66 20 01, fax + 31 20 56 64 40).

CHAPTER 2

Statistical Methods for Measuring Outcomes

GRAHAM DUNN

Introduction

This book concerns promotion of the routine use of outcome measures in clinical practice; the purpose of this chapter, however, is to warn care providers to think *very very* carefully before routinely using such measures. Just what are the benefits of their use? What are the outcome measures intended to demonstrate? In order to try to convince the reader that there might be real difficulties in the interpretation of the results, the main body of the paper concentrates on the difficulties in the interpretation of data from a structured research project that has been specifically designed to evaluate an innovation in mental health care provision. The difficulties of interpreting haphazardly collected data as part of routine clinical or administrative practice will be far greater. One of the main purposes of an evaluative exercise is comparison: which approach to service provision is the better? If care providers really want to be involved in mental health service evaluation then their time would be much better spent in taking part in a large multicentre trial.

Outcome Measures in Routine Clinical Practice

The title of this chapter might have been better formulated as "Statistical problems in the interpretation of outcomes". The main aim of the chapter is to point out the great difficulties in the analysis and interpretation of routinely collected but unstructured clinical outcome data. But it will make this point by discussing the design and analysis of research programmes, on the assumption that if the reader is convinced of the difficulties of doing worthwhile research then he or she might realize how difficult it might be to make sense of data collected as part of routine clinical practice. The collection of outcome data has a cost, however well hidden that cost might be. In the context of a research study, there are staff specifically employed to collect the data. It is a very time-consuming and expensive activity. Given the cost of collecting, recording and analysing the resulting data, one must ask if the benefits of the exercise are worthwhile. Just what are the intended benefits? What are the data meant to show, and to whom?

It is not the intention of the present author to try to prevent the introduction of outcome measures into routine clinical practice, but to stop clinicians and other care providers from enthusiastically rushing to collect data without giving very care-

Department of Biostatistics and Computing, Institute of Psychiatry, De Crespigny Park, Denmark Hill, London SE5 8AF, UK ful thought to the costs and the potential benefits of the exercise. Much routinely collected data will be unanalysable because it is unstructured, full of holes (missing values) and laden with subjective biases. The letter are likely to arise because the outcomes are likely to be measured by the clinicians themselves rather than by neutral observers. It is for the same reasons that much data collected as part of the exercise of medical audit also has such limited value.

The author's conclusion is that anyone really wishing to evaluate the clinical services he or she is instrumental in providing should get involved in some sort of formal and appropriately planned evaluation exercise, that is, some sort of controlled health care trial. The rest of this chapter will be concerned with statistical approaches to the design and analysis of such a trial, partly to underline the enormous difficulties in drawing inferences from outcome data, and partly to convince him or her of the benefits of multicentred evaluations involving cluster randomization. We start by explaining what is meant by a health care trial.

What is a Health Care Trial?

We will assume that all clinicians are familiar with the concept of a controlled clinical trial in which the investigator assesses the relative effectiveness of competing treatments (typically, chemotherapies). Arguments in favour of the controlled trial will not be rehearsed here. According to Spitzer et al. (1975): "The research strategy of the controlled clinical trial has been a powerful scientific tool that can avoid or minimize the errors produced either by the fashions of authoritarian pronouncement or by the oversimplifications of sociopolitical zealotry" (p. 161). The randomized controlled trial is the 'gold standard' (in terms of methodological rigour) against which other forms of evaluation are to be assessed. In a traditional clinical trial the experimental conditions are usually competing therapies and the experimental subjects are individual patients. In a health care trial the experimental conditions are competing ways of providing a health care service and the experimental subjects may be patients, but are not necessarily so. They might, for example, be care providers, managers or units of health care provision (clinics, wards or hospitals, for example). Spitzer et al. (1975) distinguish two types of health care trial: a *health service trial*, in which one assesses the mechanisms (or records) of health care provision and a *patient care trial*, in which one assesses conventional therapies but the clinical outcome variables are augmented by sociopersonal data. The patient care trial is distinguished from the traditional clinical trial through the use of the non-clinical outcome measures. The latter may include use of medical and other services, administrative problems, family burden, days of confinement to bed and absence from work or school. They might also include estimates of cost. The health service trial may include sociopersonal data among the variables under assessment, but not always.

Experiment, Quasi-Experiment or Survey?

In his discussion on the methodology of clinical trials in psychiatry, Johnson (1989) starts with a quotation from one of the founders of clinical trial methodology, Sir Austin Bradford Hill. He describes a clinical trial as a carefully, and ethically, designed experiment with the aim of answering some precisely framed question. In its most rigorous form it demands equivalent groups of patients concurrently treated in different ways. These groups are constructed by the random allocation of patients to one or other treatment. In some instances patients may form their own controls, different treatment being applied to them in random order and the effect compared. In principle the method is applicable with any disease and any treatment. (Hill, 1955).

The key component of a trial of this type is *random allocation of patients (or clusters of patients) to treatments*. Randomization serves three important roles. First, it is an impartial method of allocation of patients to the competing treatments. Second, it will tend to balance the treatment groups in terms of the effects of extraneous variables that might influence the outcome of treatment. One might argue that it would be more effective to match or stratify on the basis of the extraneous variables. Stratification can be an important component of trial design, but it cannot cope with the extraneous variable(s) that no one has thought of. A stratified trial should still have random allocation within the strata. The third role for randomization is that it guarantees the validity of a subsequent statistical test of significance. If there are no treatment effects (i.e. the null hypothesis is true) then, apart from unforeseen or uncontrolled biases, the observed treatment differences must be the result of randomization (chance). One can simply ask 'What is the probability that the results have arisen solely as a result of randomization?' and decide whether the data are consistent with the null hypothesis accordingly.

Returning to the problem of health care evaluation, randomized controlled trials of the type described by Johnson (1989) and Hill (1955) cannot always be conducted for a variety of reasons including logistics, ethics, cost or public opinion (Spitzer et al. 1975). The allocation of services to patients is often beyond the control of the evaluator. He or she simply has to act as a neutral observer of someone else's innovation. That someone else might be an clinician, a health service administrator or manager, or a politician. This does not preclude evaluation, but it does considerably weaken the validity of any conclusions arising from it.

The type of evaluative experiment that, for whatever reason, cannot include random allocation of experimental subjects to the competing treatments or services has often been called a *quasi-experiment* (Cook and Campbell 1979). Spitzer et al. (1975) talk of *health care surveys*. Cochran (1983) uses the term *observational study*. This last phrase will be used here. We illustrate the idea of an observational study by reference to two simple alternative designs, one using historical controls and the other using concurrent ones. In the first type of observational study we first assess the outcome of care for a cohort of patients prior to the introduction of the innovation. We then introduce the innovation (a reorganization of the clinical services or the introduction of a case-management service, for example) and then monitor the outcome for a new cohort of patients receiving the new or reorganized clinical service. Comparison of the outcomes for these two cohorts will, we hope, given us an estimate of the effect of the innovation. In the second example of an observational study we might be planning to introduce a new service in one particular clinic, hospital or health district. Prior to its introduction, however, we search for another clinic, hospital or district that is as similar as possible to ours – except that there are no immediate plans to change its health care services. The latter centre provides us with a concurrent control. Observation of the outcomes for a cohort of patients exposed to the innovation in one centre can be compared with the outcomes for another cohort in the centre in which the innovation has not been introduced. Again, comparison of the outcomes for the two cohorts of patients will, we hope, give us an estimate of the impact of the introduction of the innovation.

The weaknesses in both of the above designs are the very weaknesses that randomization helps to rectify. First, there may be differences between the patients in the two arms of the study. Referral patterns may have inadvertently changed at about the same time as the introduction of the innovation, for example. There may be other differences between the innovative and the control arms of the trial. Innovation is usually managed by a newly appointed enthusiast (or even an evangelist) with commitment, drive and lots of energy. In the control situation there may be a run-down service managed by an ageing sceptic who is just looking forward to early retirement. As Buck and Donner (1982) point out, in many health care experiments the placebo effect falls upon the providers rather than the recipients of care. The estimate of the effectiveness is likely to be biased – that is, usually over-optimistic: the effect of the innovation per se is likely to be confounded with inherent patient differences, environmental and staff differences and non-specific effects of the introduction of an innovative service (the Hawthorne effect). Finally, we have more subtle problems of statistical inference. In the absence of randomization we have to build in more assumptions for our significance tests, and so on. We usually pretend, quite unrealistically, for example, that the innovative and control groups have been randomly selected from a much larger population of potential treatment groups. We then ask 'What is the probability of selecting by chance two groups that are as different as these two?'

Now, the above weaknesses of observational studies have not been pointed out in an attempt to stop people carrying them out, but to point out the care that is needed in drawing valid inferences from the results. We have to try to avoid biases by carefully matching centres, for example, or by ensuring that the care staff are equally well organized or motivated, with equal access to appropriate facilities in both arms of the trial. We also have to think more carefully about the use of various methods of statistical analysis (covariate adjustment, for example) to attempt to eliminate or reduce the impact of potential sources of bias. Cochran (1983) gives the following advice:

Control can usually be attempted on only a few of many variables that influence outcome; that control is likely to be only partially effective on these variables. Thus the investigator might do well to suppose that, in general, estimates from an observational study are likely to be biased. It is therefore worthwhile to think hard about what biases are most likely, and to think seriously about their sources, directions, and even their plausible magnitudes. (p.14)

In the following section we continue to discuss potential problems in the interpretation of the results of an evaluation, and return again to randomization of experimental units to the different arms of a trial. We suggest that the experimental unit should be a group (cluster) of patients, however, rather than the individuals themselves.

What are the Experimental Units?

In the interpretation of the outcome of an innovation, we are concerned with two possible threats to the validity of our inferences. These are threats to the *internal validity* of our evaluation (has the change we've seen really arisen as the result of the innovation or via some other unintended mechanism?) and to the *external validity* (can we generalize our findings to other settings or services?). Interesting analogies can be drawn with the outcome of the clinical psychologist's well-controlled single-case study and with that of a controlled clinical trial. In the single-case study the quality of the design of the experiment might be such that it is very safe to conclude that the therapy or management given was indeed the cause of the resulting changes to the patient. But what about other patients? One cannot safely use statistical inference to predict the behaviour of future patients from this one, possibly very atypical patient, however well-controlled the study was demonstrated to be. We need an evaluation involving several patients to find out how patients respond to treatment or management in general. The single-case study may have near perfect internal validity, but we cannot safely generalize from it – it has very limited or even no external validity.

The above arguments apply equally cogently to the evaluation of, say, a new clinic or clinical service. Can we infer anything about clinics in general from our knowledge of this one? Do we want to? We may simply want to demonstrate that our unique clinic works very effectively and are quite happy to leave others to evaluate their own services. If, however, we wish to generalize from our evaluation to other clinics then we either have to acknowledge that statistical inference does not play a part in this generalization or that we need to observe the behaviour of several similar clinics and compare it with that of a control group of services. It is vital that the correct unit of observation is identified at all stages of the evaluation: in the design, in the analysis of the results and in the interpretation of the findings.

Now consider a related but slightly more subtle problem. In both qualitative and quantitative approaches to evaluation one has to be very wary of the pitfalls of what Manly (1992), after Hurlbert (1984), calls 'pseudoreplication'. This arises when the units of measurement (patients, clinics, districts) are not independent replicates. Patients within a clinic will tend to have similar experiences of service provision, they share facilities and care staff, and may talk to each other and influence each other's views; they will have relatively similar outcomes (as compared with patients from different clinics), and so on. Patients, to some extent, will exhibit within-clinic or within-group correlations and they will thus not provide statistically independent items of information. The data obtained, whether qualitative or quantitative, should not be treated as if they had been obtained from a group of completely independent patients. The evaluator is not obtaining as much information as he or she might naively think! The problem is particularly acute in group-based therapies or activities. The group as a whole might do well, or it might fail. In either case the experience of the patients within the group is likely to exhibit fairly high within-group correlation. Often evaluators treat the individual patient as the unit for their analysis when, in fact, it should be the group, clinic, and so on. What is needed is replication of groups, not replication of individual units within the group.

The above provides reasons why we might wish to summarize and interpret the outcomes at the level of groups or, in a more sophisticated analysis, simultaneously analyse variation at the level of the group, as well as at the level of the individual. There are also reasons why one might wish to *allocate clusters of patients*, rather than individual patients, to the competing arms of a health care trial; that is, to change the design of the trial. One reason is the rather obvious administrative and managerial one: it is often impossible to introduce an innovative service or change in administration to only part of a service and leave the rest as it is. These changes are usually all-or-nothing. The cost of having two competing services within a single district, for example, might be prohibitive. Sometimes it would simply the impossible not to introduce the changes at the level of the cluster rather than the individual. Outside the mental health field one simply needs to think of the evaluation of the fluoridation of drinking water or the introduction of car seat-belt legislation to realize that there are often overriding practical difficulties concerning the introduction of change at the level of the individual patient. Another powerful argument in favour of cluster allocation is the fact that patients within a cluster are not isolated individuals (see the immediately preceding paragraph on pseudoreplication). However, as well as correlation within groups receiving the same service, there may also be contamination between the competing arms of the trial if they were both present within a cluster. If a trial invovles the evaluation of some sort of educational activity (either at the level of the patient or that of the service providers or clinicians) then there will be contamination through 'cross-talk'. Patients might try to compensate for the perceived deficiencies in their service and might even attempt to change sides. Patient knownledge (lack of 'blindness') is likely to contribute to a placebo effect, and there is also the possibility of patient resentment if one of the competing services is perceived to be better than the other. If the innovations occur at the level of clinic, hospital or district, on the other hand, all the patients within the same cluster get the same service. They do not necessarily know that there is an alternative service being offered in a different location – there will usually be no need to inform the patients that they are part of a trial, nor might there be a need to seek informed consent. The problem of informed consent, however, does need careful thought. If a trial adds an active ingredient to the traditional service, personal counselling or case management, for example would it be necessary to consider whether it is unethical for the control groups to know what they are missing? Is it ethically justified to randomly allocate this extra service at the level of the individual patient? Buck and Donner (1982) consider this problem and decide that the situation should not be regarded as analogous to the traditional drug trial. They conclude that "if group unawareness is ethically permissible in certain kinds of intervention and health care trials, it offers a means of achieving subject blindness which is attractively congruent with the method of randomization".

The literature on trials involving randomization of clusters has been reviewed by Donner et al. (1990). Let us assume that we are to allocate clusters of patients (clinics, districts, and so on) randomly to the alternative services, rather than randomly allocating the individual patients themselves. One of the major concerns of the clinical trial designer is that of statistical power: how many patients are required to have a sufficiently high probability of finding a statistically significant effect? This requires a knowledge of patient variability and a fairly clear idea of the likely difference between the effects of the competing therapies (including expert judgement on what would constitute a *clinically* significant differences between the groups). Readers who are unfamiliar with power calculations are referred to Lachin (1981), Pocock (1983) or to Day and Graham (1991). Once we acknowledge that the cluster is the unit of randomization, rather than the individual patient, we then have to take this into account in our power calculations. The total number of patients entering the trial is the product of the number of clusters and the number of patients within each cluster (assuming for simplicity that the latter is constant). Cornfield (1978) provides a method for estimating sample size when large clusters, such as districts or hospitals, are being randomized, whilst Donner et al. (1981) deal primarily with the case of small clusters, such as families. The design of a trial involving cluster randomization can involve completely randomized clusters, stratification of clusters prior to randomization or, as a special case of stratification, matched-pairs of clusters. Outcome might be assessed by an interval-scaled measurement, or it might be binary (well versus ill, for example). Sample size formulae for intervention studies involving all these possibilities are provided by Hsieh (1988). Shipley et al. (1989) also discuss power considerations for matched-pair studies. One of the aims of stratification of clusters prior to randomization is to reduce the probability of lack of comparability of patients in the two (or more) arms of the trial. Stratification can be based on the demographic characteristics of the clusters' patients, geographical and social differences between the areas within which the clusters are embedded, various administrative characteristics of the clusters, and so on. Further issues concerning cluster randomization in large public health trials are discussed by Duffy et al. (1992).

Returning to power calculations for trials involving complete randomization (i. e. no stratification or matching), what is the effect of randomizing at the level of the cluster rather than the individual patient on required sample sizes? It should be obvious from the discussion of the problem of pseudoreplication that we need more patients in the trial, but how many more? Basically, the size of the trial (number of patients in each arm of the trial) should be increased by the factor

$$[1 + (m-1)\,\varrho] \tag{1}$$

where ϱ is the *intra-class correlation* (the within-cluster or within-group correlation or dependence) and m the number of patients per cluster (Buck and Donner 1982), to achieve the same statistical power as would be obtained under a design with no clustering. The intra-class correlation would typically be estimated from pilot data in which several patients from a sample of clusters were assessed and the results subjected to a one-way analysis of variance (i. e. outcome measure by cluster membership) – see, for example, Dunn (1989). This analysis of variance will yield a between-cluster mean square (BMS) and a within-cluster mean square (WMS). The required estimate of the intra-class correlation is then given by

$$\hat{\varrho} = (BMS - WMS)/[BMS + (m-1)WMS] \tag{2}$$

where, as before, m is the number of patients per cluster. The estimation of intra-class correlation coefficients will also be discussed in the section on the evaluation of outcome measures below.

Evaluation of Outcome Measures

Before we proceed to evaluate outcome, we need to assess the quality of the outcome measures themselves. We need to be assured that we have adequate tools for the job in hand. The discussion will not include the development of outcome measures –

for this the reader is referred to Streiner and Norman (1989) and Wright and Feinstein (1992) – nor will we be concerned with validity, this being more of a substantive problem than a statistical one. Instead, we will primarily be concerned with *reliability* estimation and even then with the most simple of situations. More complex examples can be found elsewhere (Dunn 1989, 1992).

Perhaps the most important need in the planning of a health care trial is to check the consistency of the raters or interviewers who are to assess the outcome of the innovation(s). Typically, two or more raters will be asked to co-rate the problems or symptoms of a pilot sample of patients. We assume that all raters have assessed each of the sample of patients once and we wish to estimate a measure of agreement between these raters. For both quantitative and binary (yes/no) assessments we can carry out a two-way analysis of variance (outcome by rater and subject) and use the resulting mean squares from the ANVOA table to estimate a form of the intra-class correlation coefficient:

$$\hat{\varrho} = n(\text{PMS} - \text{EMS})/[\text{n.PMS} + \text{m.RMS} + (\text{nm} - \text{n} - \text{m})\text{EMS}] \tag{3}$$

where n is the number of patients and m the number of raters. PMS is the patient mean square, RMS is the rater mean square and EMS is the error or residual mean square. The dots (.) in this expression indicate multiplication. The derivation of this expression is beyond the scope of this article, but is based on the assumption that we are looking at the performance of a random selection of raters selected from a potentially much larger population of potential raters (the so-called random effects model) – see, for example, Fleiss (1987), Dunn (1989) or Streiner and Norman (1989). This intra-class correlation is a measure of reliability. In the case of a binary assessment it is also equivalent to the well-known *kappa coefficient;* in the case of an ordinal measure of outcome it is equivalent to the form of a weighted kappa coefficient (using quadratic weights) – see, for example, Dunn (1989) or Streiner and Norman (1989).

If the reliability exercise involved, say, the use of only one rater who replicated his or her assessment of each patient m times (a simple replication study with m usually equal to 2), then the appropriate analysis would be a one-way analysis of variance followed by an estimation of an intra-class correlation using Eq. 2 – but in this case BMS would be the between-patient mean square and WMS the within-patient mean square. Again this intra-class correlation provides an estimate of reliability.

Be wary of relying on reliability coefficients provided in the literature or test manuals. They are only estimates (often based on inadequate sample sizes) and *they are not fixed characteristics of a particular outcome measure.* They are a measure of the proportion of the variability in the outcome measure that is explained by differences amongst the patients. They will vary as the heterogeneity of the patients changes and also as the heterogeneity (inconsistency) of the raters varies. That is, the reliability will depend on raters using the outcome measure and on the population of patients being assessed.

What is good reliability? Basically, the higher the better, but there is no magic threshold for reliability above which you can relax. The key problem in the context of a health care trial is the power of the trial. Power can be increased by increasing the number of subjects or by decreasing the variability of the measures (i.e. by increasing their reliability or by using a more homogeneous group of patients), or both. The reliability of the outcome measures will be improved by multiple assessment of each patient, but then the investigator needs to ask whether this is feasible and more cost-effective than simply increasing the number of patients in the trial. The final answer is bound to be a balance between the two.

Analysis of Outcomes

This section will be very brief. The statistical analysis of large health care trials is no more the province of amateurs than the analysis of clinical trial data. We will briefly illustrate, however, the problems that the analysis needs to address. Typically, there will be a need to adjust for potentially confounding variables. This will involve some sort of analysis of covariance (either for quantitative outcome measures or for binary ones). This will be particularly true for observational studies in which we are trying to convince the sceptic that we have allowed for sources of bias (Cook and Campbell 1979; Cochran 1983). It may also be true for randomized trials. Here the aim is usually to improve precision although covariate adjustment may also cope with lack of balance that has arisen by chance in the randomization. In the analysis of a randomized clinical trial it is an illogical and pointless exercise to carry out significance tests for differences between baseline measures. Unless someone has been cheating, you *know* that the results have arisen by chance. Important prognostic factors should be included as covariates whether or not there are statistically significant differences on these variables across groups. If the analysis is being carried out on data arising from cluster randomization then the covariates can be measured either at the level of the individual patient, or at the level of the cluster, or both, and the analysis will need to take this into account (Goldstein 1987).

In recent years there has been considerable stress laid on the reporting of confidence intervals in the medical literature (Gardner and Altman 1989). Confidence interval construction for effect measures arising from cluster randomization trials is described by Donner and Klar (1993). More complex statistical analyses of cluster-randomized trials will involve modelling of outcome data in which it is explicitly acknowledged that there are different levels of random variation in the measurements. There will be random variation of measurement errors amongst replications within patients, random variation between patients within clusters and random variations between clusters. Some form of random effects model will be needed for the data. Readers are referred to Goldstein (1987) for a general discussion, and to Collett (1991; pp. 279–280) for a description of random effects models for binary outcome measures.

Conclusions

It should be clear from the above that the author has a lot of misgivings about the design of many research studies to demonstrate the impact of innovations in the provision of health care. What about the use of outcome measures in routine clinical practice? It would be clearly much more difficult to defend any particular interpretation put on the results. If it is so difficult to interpret the results of a carefully designed research study, of what possible use could they be in the haphazard world of routine clinical practice? The present author is clearly putting himself in the position of the devil's advocate and is accordingly putting forward a particularly strong view against the clinician routinely collecting outcome data. Nevertheless, it would be prudent of the clinician to convincingly answer this question before committing valuable resources to such an exercise.

Lest the reader is inclined to dismiss the author as a sceptical armchair theorist, he has been involved over the last 6 years in a trial to evaluate the effects of case management after severe head injury (Greenwood et al. 1994). It was a trial that exhibited many of the problems detailed in this article and also illustrates some of the technical solutions. The trial involved the comparison of the outcomes of care of patients from six hospitals in North London. Three of these hospitals were provided with the services of a case manager, three acted as controls. The whole point of the evaluation was *comparison*. The case managers were convinced that they were doing a good job and none of the outcome measures would have led them to doubt their beliefs. If there had been no control group of hospitals there would have been no reason to doubt the effectiveness of their service. Comparison of the outcomes for case-managed patients with those of the controls, however, failed to demonstrate any benefits of case management. Case management led to an increase in rates of referrals to specialist clinical services, but this did not appear to lead to any demonstrable benefits to the patients. Note that it is not the collection of outcome data as such that is important to the evaluation of a clinical service. On its own it is of very limited use. Only when it is used for comparison, and only then if that comparison is suitably controlled, does outcome data really become useful.

In conclusion, the present author has serious doubts about the benefits of routinely collected outcome data but is convinced that there is a need for large multicentred evaluations of mental health care services, possibly using cluster randomization as described by Donner et al. (1990). In this way care providers who wish to evaluate their services can do so within the context of a carefully controlled and properly resourced research study. Unfortunately, none of the trials reviewed by Donner et al. concern mental health care services (although one or two involve patients from mental hospitals and others are concerned with health education), and it is, therefore, difficult to direct the reader to successful examples!

References

Buck C, Donner A (1982) The design of controlled experiments in the evaluation of non-therapeutic interventions. J Chronic Dis 35: 531–538
Cochran WG (1983) Planning and analysis of observational studies. Wiley, Chichester New York
Collett D (1991) Modelling binary data. Chapman & Hall, London
Cook TD, Campbell TD (1979) Quasi-experimentation: design and analysiss issues for field settings. Houghton-Mifflin, Boston
Cornfield J (1978) Randomization by group: a formal analysis. Am J Epidemiol 108: 100–102
Day SJ, Graham DF (1991) Sample size estimation for comparing two or more treatment groups in clinical trials. Stat Med 10: 33–43
Donner A, Klar N (1993) Confidence interval construction for effect measures arising from cluster randomization trials. J Clin Epidemiol 46: 123–131
Donner A, Brown KS, Brasher P (1990) A methodological review of non-therapeutic intervention trials employing cluster randomization, 1979–1989. Int J Epidemiol 19: 795–800
Duffy SW, South MC, Day NE (1992) Cluster randomization in large public health trials: the importance of antecedent data. Stat Med 11: 307–316

Dunn G (1989) Design and analysis of reliability studies: the statistical evaluation of measurement errors. Edward Arnold, London

Dunn G (1992) Design and analysis of reliability studies. Stat Methods Med Res 1: 123–157

Fleiss JL (1987) Design and analysis of clinical experiments. Wiley, Chichester New York

Gardner MJ, Altman DG (1989) Statistics with confidence. BMJ, London

Goldstein H (1987) Multilevel models in educational and social research. Griffin, London

Greenwood RJ, McMillan TM, Brooks DN, Dunn G, Brock D, Dinsdale S, Murphy LD, Price JR (1994) An investigation into the effects of case management after severe head injury. BMJ 308: 1199–1205

Hill AB (1955) Introduction to medical statistics, 5th edn. (Monograph) Lancet London

Hsieh FY (1988) Sample size formulae for intervention studies with the cluster as unit of randomization. Stat Med 8: 1195–1201

Hurlbert SH (1984) Pseudoreplication in the design of ecological field experiments. Ecol Monogr 54: 187–211

Johnson AL (1989) Methodology of clinical trials in psychiatry. In: Freeman C, Tyrer P (eds) Research methods in psychiatry. Royal College of Psychiatrists, London, pp 12–45

Lachin JM (1981) Introduction to sample size determination and power analysis for clinical trials. Controlled Clin Trials 2: 93–113

Manly BFJ (1992) The design and analysis of research studies. Cambridge University Press, Cambridge

Pocock S (1983) Clinical trials: a practical approach. Wiley, Winchester New York

Shipley MJ, Smith PG, Dramaix M (1989) Calculation of power for matched pair studies when randomization is by group. Int J Epidemiol 18: 457–461

Spitzer WO, Feinstein AR, Sackett DL (1975) What is a health care trial? J Am Med Assoc 233: 161–163

Streiner DL, Norman GR (1989) Health measurement scales: a practical guide to their development and use. Oxford University Press, Oxford

Wright JG, Feinstein AR (1992) A comparative contrast of clinimetric and psychometric methods for constructing indexes and rating scales. J Clin Epidemiol 45: 1201–1218

CHAPTER 3

Global Function Scales

MICHAEL PHELAN, TIL WYKES and HOWARD GOLDMAN

Introduction

There is a close relationship between impairment of global functioning and mental illness. However valid measurement of global functioning is difficult, and there is no perfect scale. The instruments reviewed in this paper illustrate a range of different approaches. Despite the inherent difficulties the measurement of functioning is a critical domain in mental health evaluative research.

Functioning is an abstract concept, incorporating a range of abilities from being able to interact with other people to finding enough to eat. Because the notion of global functioning covers all these abilities there is little consensus about the precise meaning of the term. In this paper assessment schedules that attempt to provide a measure of a person's level of functioning in all or nearly all areas of his/her life are reviewed. The schedules vary in their approaches. Instrumental behaviours, which encompass the various activities prerequisite to an independent social life, feature strongly, along with impaired performance in major social roles, living skills and overall level of disability (Wykes 1992). There is a close and complex relationship between mental illness and impairment of global functioning. At times, impaired functioning such as poor self-care will be the only visible sign of mental illness, and may well be the most distressing feature for the sufferer. The level of support and care needed by a person is likely to be closely correlated with their level of functioning. Although impairment of functioning is usually viewed as a consequence of mental illness, it may at times be a significant causal or maintaining factor in specific disorders.

The use of schedules measuring level of function in mental health research and practice has been reviewed by Kane et al. (1985). They suggest three divisions; epidemiological studies that compare levels of functioning among those with and without mental disorders and within similar diagnostic groups, longitudinal studies that examine the effects of mental illness on levels of functioning and case finding studies, especially in primary care settings. In addition, a measure of global functioning is a useful outcome measure for mental health clinicians. Such measures are im-

M. Phelan and T. Wykes
PRiSM, Institute of Psychiatry, De Crespigny Park, Denmark Hill, London SE5 8AF, UK

H. Goldman
Department of Psychiatry, University of Maryland, School of Medicine, 645 West Redwood Street, Baltimore, MD 21201, USA

portant predictors of service utilisation and provide vital information for service planners.

Before examining individual schedules, it is important to consider the difficulties inherent in trying to measure global functioning. The majority of the scales reviewed in this paper are concerned with measuring levels of functioning that are below normal, and in general ignore higher than average levels of functioning. Underpinning this practical approach there is often an assumption that "normal" functioning can be defined as scoring no problems on a schedule. Clearly, any such norms may be dependent on individual factors such as age and culture, and may vary over time. In terms of social roles, normality is particularly difficult to define, with, for example, the changing role of women in Western societies, and the different roles given to older people in Western and non-Western cultures.

A second difficulty facing those designing measures of functioning is whether to include psychiatric symptoms. The distinction between impairments of functioning and psychiatric symptoms is often blurred. Some impairments of functioning, such as poor concentration, may be viewed as psychiatric symptoms in their own right. It is also important to distinguish between overt and covert symptoms, and their relationship to impairment of functioning. Overt symptoms, such as pressure of speech, will usually impinge on functioning. In contrast, covert symptoms, such as a fixed delusional belief, may not directly affect functioning, but may have an indirect effect, for instance if the person talks to others about his abnormal belief. Authors vary in their approach to this dilemma, although in most of the scales described here there is at least some reference to overt symptomatology.

The third area of difficulty is the establishment of validity. It is a complex task to demonstrate that any psychological or psychiatric schedule measures what is intended. To ensure content validity for a schedule measuring a concept as broad as global functioning requires that a large number of areas be included, but this has to be matched against the need to keep the schedule to a practical length. The lack of any "gold standard" measure of functioning poses problems in determining concurrent validity. Authors frequently compare scores with levels of service utilisation as a broad confirmation of validity. The danger behind this approach is that the level of service utilisation may have been one of the factors considered by the original rater when deciding the final score. Finally, when considering the construct validity of global functioning it is important to consider the interactions between the many diverse factors that contribute to the concept, e.g. personality, intelligence, physical abilities, social environment, the level of support received from others, the perception of potential abilities by others and rewards obtained.

The characteristics of the *ideal* scale for measuring functioning are similar to any other scale in the field of mental health: applicable to patients with disabilities of differing severity and aetiology, as well as to patients from a wide range of cultural backgrounds; reliable, valid and sensitive to change; usable by staff during the course of routine work. In addition, the perfect global functioning scale would produce a total rating that would accurately and equally reflect all aspects of a patient's functioning. Not surprisingly, such a scale does not exist, and there is always compromise. The schedules reviewed here, and summarised in Table 1, come from three areas. First, we have described the small number of schedules that attempt to summarise all aspects of a patient's functioning with a single rating. Second, the axis V

Table 1. Summary of schedules suitable for the assessment of global functioning

Schedule	Description	Strengths/weaknesses	Uses
Global Assessment Scale (GAS), Endicott et al. (1976)	Single rating on 0–100 scale Modified version used for DSM-III-R	Quick and easy to administer, and widely used; combines symptoms and functioning in single scale; limited reliability amongst practising clinicians	Clinical and research
Disabilities Assessment Schedule (DAS), WHO (1988)	11 item scale, covering social roles and disabilities; used for axis V of ICD 10	Appears to be valid reliable, but only a few published studies describing its use; difficult for untrained staff	Clinical and research; but users need training
Katz Adjustment Scale Katz and Lyerly (1963)	Separate versions for informant (205 items) and patient (138 items)	Specifically designed for people with serious mental illness; extensive coverage of psychopathology and behaviour; unsuitable for less disabled patients	Too long for routine clinical use, suitable for research
Denver Community Mental Health Questionnaire, Ciarlo and Riehman (1977)	61 item schedule, with emphasis on substance abuse and patient satisfaction	Suitable for wide range of patients; limited coverage of specific behaviours	Only of use in specific situations due to limited coverage
Psychiatric Status Schedule (PSS), Spitzer et al. (1970); Psychiatric Evaluation Form (PEF), Endicott and Spitzer (1972a); Current and Past Pathology Scale (CAPPS), Endicott and Spitzer (1972b)	Developed in tandem; PSS (321 items) administered to patient, PEF (28 items), and CAPPS (130 items) completed by clinician	Suitable for wide range of patients; limited coverage of social roles	Too long for routine clinical use, suitable for research
Morningside Rehabilitation Status Scale (MRSS), Affleck and McGuire (1984)	4 individual areas rated on 8-point scale	Easy to use for staff who know patient well; established reliability but validity unclear	More suitable for clinical use than research
Social Behaviour Schedule (SBS), Wykes and Sturt (1986)	21-item schedule; emphasis on observable behaviours	Easy to use, no training; good reliability and validity; suitable for more severely ill patients	Clinical and research
REHAB Baker and Hall (1988)	23-item schedule, covering general and deviant behaviour	Easy to use; impressive psychometric properties; only suitable for patients in residential or hospital setting	Clinical and research
Life Skills Profile (LSP) Rosen et al. (1989)	39-item schedule covering disability and functioning	Easy to use; free of jargon; currently few published studies	Clinical and research
Social Functioning Schedule (SFS), Remmington and Tyrer (1979); Social Maladjustment Schedule (SMS), Clare and Cairns (1978)	12 (SFS) and 48 (SMS) item schedules; designed specifically for people with non-psychotic illness	Few published studies; only limited psychometric data for both scales	Due to length SMS suitable for research, SFS suitable for both

scales of DSM-III, DSM-III-R and ICD-10 are described. Finally, a number of "social functioning" scales are reviewed, which are broad enough in their coverage to be considered, in some respects, as global measures of functioning.

Global Rating Scales

The earliest-published global rating scale is the Health Sickness Rating Scale (HSRS; Luborsky 1962). It was intended as a simple measure of change over time in the condition of psychotherapy patients. During the development of this scale the authors concluded that there are seven key factors that should be incorporated into a global rating of health: ability to function autonomously, symptom severity, degree of discomfort, effect upon the environment, utilisation of abilities, quality of interpersonal relationships, and breadth and depth of interests. A 0–100 scale was used, with eight anchor points ranging from "an ideal state of complete functioning integration, resiliency in the face of stress, and social effectiveness" to "any condition which, if unattended, would quickly result in the patient's death, but not necessarily by his own hand". In addition, 30 pre-rated case vignettes are provided for extra guidance.

Twelve years after the HSRS was first published, a review of 18 published studies conducted on a wide range of patient groups concluded that when used by experienced clinicians the scale is a reliable measure of mental health and correlates with a variety of more time-consuming scales (Luborsky and Bachrach 1974). The authors have concluded that reliability is correlated with the comprehensiveness of the information available to the raters, and have interpreted the finding that patients within any diagnostic category have a range of scores as indicating that the score is important additional information for the clinician. However, this latter finding can alternatively be interpreted as indicating weak validity of the diagnostic or functioning measure.

Attempts to improve upon the HSRS have resulted in the development of the Global Assessment Scale (GAS; Endicott et al., 1976). Whilst maintaining the same basic structure, the authors introduced a number of changes in an attempt to simplify the scale. The number of anchor points was increased from eight to ten. Any reference to diagnostic categories was removed; instead the anchor points rely on a combination of specific behavioural characteristics and symptoms. In addition, the authors did not believe it necessary to provide case vignettes, used when completing the HSRS, but did provide guidelines on difficult rating decisions, such as when the level of functioning varies during the evaluation period. The authors have demonstrated that low GAS scores are positively correlated with readmission rates in former in-patients. In five separate studies, the interrater reliability ranged from 0.61 to 0.91. The lowest reliability was amongst practising clinicians, as opposed to researchers, a worrying finding that has been described by others (Clark and Friedman 1983; Plakun et al. 1987). Systematic training with periodic refresher courses appears to improve reliability amongst clinical staff (Dworkin et al. 1990).

Axis V Measures

DSM-III

As part of the multiaxial approach of DSM-III, axis V was introduced as a global measure of "adaptive functioning". A seven-point scale ranging from superior to grossly impaired was used. During DSM-III field trials of axis V ratings, intraclass correlation coefficients for interrater and test re-test reliability were 0.80 and 0.69, respectively (Spitzer and Forman 1979). However, when the scale was used by a group of multidisciplinary clinical workers, reliability was as low as 0.49 (Fernando et al. 1986). When case summaries of adolescents were rated, a slightly higher reliability of 0.57 has been reported (Rey et al. 1988). Overall, the published studies are limited, and although reliability for axis V has been found to be higher than for axis IV, the reliability demonstrated has not been especially good (Rey et al. 1987).

A variety of approaches have been taken to examine the validity of DSM-III axis V ratings. A number of studies have compared the ratings between people in different diagnostic groups (Skodol et al. 1988; Mezzich et al. 1987; Westermeyer 1988). Together these findings indicate that people with a psychotic disorder score lower than those with a neurotic disorder, who in turn score lower than those with no diagnosis. One published study (Schrader et al. 1986), however, found no difference between psychotic, organic and non-psychotic patient groups. Concurrent validity has been examined by comparing ratings with other measures of adaptive functioning. Low ratings have been found to be positively correlated with low social and occupational functioning scores on the Psychiatric Epidemiology Research Interview (Skodol et al. 1988), and negatively correlated with ratings of social networks (Westermeyer and Neider 1988).

DSM-III-R

With the advent of DSM-III-R, the Global Assessment of Functioning Scale (GAF) was introduced to replace the 7-point scale of DSM-III, with the hope that it would increase the usefulness of the axis. The stated aim is that axis V is to be a measure of "a person's psychological, social, and occupational functioning", and that ratings will generally reflect the current need for treatment or care (APA 1987). The GAF itself is a modified version of the GAS (see above), with a reduction in the number of anchor points to nine, the scale ranging from 0–90 rather than 1–100 and minor changes in the wording of the anchor points. The other significant change is that both the highest level of functioning during the previous year and the current level of functioning are recorded, whereas the GAS only rates the lowest level of functioning during the previous week.

The major limitation of all of the above scales is that symptoms and functioning are combined to produce a single rating. There are proposals that these two factor should be rated separately for DSM-IV (Goldman et al. 1992). Unpublished work by Rey has examined interrater agreement between the proposed amended scale and the CGAS (Children's Global Assessment of Functioning Scale) and found similar reliabilities.

ICD-10

A multiaxial version of the *10th International classification of mental and behavioural disorders* (ICD-10) is currently under preparation. Axis V will be similar to that of DSM-III-R in that it will focus on the level of disability, and the Disabilities Assessment Schedule (DAS; Schubert et al. 1986; WHO 1988) will be used. Ratings for the DAS are based on information from the person who has had the most contact with the patient over the previous month. There are 11 items, mostly rated on an 8-point scale. Seven of the items are specifically concerned with roles, the other items cover social withdrawal, self-care, social contacts and interests and information. In contrast to the GAF, symptoms are not directly included. Interrater reliability appears to be high, with Kappa coefficients ranging from 0.82 to 0.85 for the different items. Some degree of validity has been established by demonstrating a correlation of 0.79 between the scale's global assessment score and the independent ratings of psychiatrists. However, the schedule has been criticised for being ambiguous in phrasing and being liable to cause difficulty for untrained raters (Rosen et al. 1989).

Social Functioning Scales

Social functioning scales are concerned with three broad areas of human life: social attainment, social role performance and instrumental behaviour (Wykes and Hurry 1991; Wykes 1992). In this review, scales that assess only social attainment, such as the Psychiatric Epidemiology Research Interview (Dohrenwend et al. 1981), have been excluded. Such scales have the advantage of being easily completed, and are suited to large-scale epidemiological studies. However, social attainment is greatly influenced by social conditions and local culture, and does not provide an accurate guide to individual global functioning. Similar limitations apply to schedules that are limited to assessing social roles, such as The MRC Social Role Performance Schedule (Hurry and Sturt 1981). Although greater precision is possible when assessing roles rather than attainments, again, cultural differences mean that individual functioning cannot be accurately gauged from role performance alone, Thus, we have only considered social functioning scales that measure instrumental behaviour either alone or in combination with social attainment and roles. Additionally, we have only included schedules that are sufficiently broad to be considered as global measures, are reasonably quick and easy to administer and have robust psychometric properties. For more detailed surveys of social functioning scales the comprehensive reviews by Weissman et al. (1981) and Wallace (1986) are recommended.

Katz Adjustment Scale

The Katz Adjustment Scale (KAS; Katz and Lyerly, 1963) was designed to assess people with serious mental health problems either prior to hospital admission or in the community after discharge. There are two versions, the 205-item KAS-R, to be completed by someone who knows the patient well, and the 138-item KAS-S to be completed by the patient. The KAS-R takes 25–40 min to administer, and assesses psychopathology, interpersonal behaviours and social performance (including actual and desired frequency of a range of behaviours) at length. The KAS-S is similar in its coverage, but also asks about the level of distress experienced by the patient. The time frame is "last few weeks". Internal consistency reliabilities for the KAS-R are reported to be between 0.41 and 0.81. Total scores discriminate between patients and community residents (Hogarty and Katz 1971) and different types of depressed patients (Paykel 1972). Despite the large number of items it is relatively easy to administer and score. It appears to be a useful instrument for the assessment of people with significant disability due to mental illness, but less appropriate for the assessment of those with transient or minor mental disorders.

Denver Community Mental Health Questionnaire

The Denver Community Mental Health Questionnaire (DCMHQ; Ciarlo and Riehman, 1977) was designed to assess the wide range of people presenting at a community mental health centre, and is suitable for people with a wide range of mental health disorders. The questionnaire comprises 61 items, and takes between 30 and 60 min to administer. The 12 areas covered are: psychological distress, interpersonal isolation from friends, productivity at work, productivity at home, dependency on public agencies, alcohol abuse, soft drug use, hard drug use, client satisfaction with services interpersonal aggression with friends, and legal difficulties. The time frame is between 24 h and last month. Reported interrater reliabilities range from 0.85 to 1.0 for 10 of the 12 areas (2 were not tested). Internal consistency reliabilities range from 0.52 to 0.96. Significant differences in all the areas, except interpersonal aggression, have been demonstrated between patients and a random sample of Denver residents. The schedule is distinctive for its emphasis on substance abuse (32 of the items) and the inclusion of service satisfaction. However, as a consequence it is rather limited in its coverage of instrumental behaviours.

Psychiatric Status Schedule

The Psychiatric Status Schedule (PSS; Spitzer et al. 1970) is a 321-item schedule that covers 15 areas of psychopathology and five social roles (wage earner, housekeeper, student or trainee, spouse and parent). The interview takes between 30 and 50 min. The time frame is the last week for psychopathology items and the last month for role items. Interrater reliability coefficients range from 0.57 to 0.99. Scores discriminate between in-patients, out-patients and non-patients, and are correlated with other measures of psychopathology such as the Brief Psychiatric Rating Scale and the Beck Depression Inventory. The roles in this schedule will not be relevant to more disabled patients.

Psychiatric Evaluation Form

The Psychiatric Evaluation Form (PEF; Endicott and Spitzer 1972a) is a 28-item schedule that was designed in tandem with the PSS, and there is considerable overlap in the content of these two schedules. The PEF is designed to be completed by experienced clinicians using information from a variety of sources, rather than from a direct patient interview. Ratings are on a 6-point scale, and overall scores for the severity of illness and role performance are obtained. The Current and Past Psychopathol-

ogy Scale (CAPPS; Endicott and Spitzer 1972b) is a longer version of the PEF and includes an additional 13 psychopathology items and 130 items concerning previous
social adjustment, psychopathology and personality characteristics from the age
12 years to 1 month prior to completion. Interrater reliabilities range from 0.68 to
1.0 for individual items, and total scores discriminate between different diagnostic
groups of patients. As with the PSS, these schedules are more appropriate for less
disabled patients.

The Morningside Rehabilitation Status Scale

This is a brief scale designed to measure the "main areas of change relevant to the
rehabilitation of psychiatric patients" (Affeck and McGuire 1984). Four areas (dependency, occupation and leisure activity, social isolation, and current symptoms) are
measured on an 8-point scale. The time taken will vary from a few minutes to
30 min, depending on how well the rater knows the patient. The time frame is the
last month. Interrater reliability for the four areas ranges from 0.68 to 0.90.

Social Behaviour Scale

The Social Behaviour Scale (SBS; Wykes and Sturt 1986) is designed to measure the
functioning of people with severe and long-lasting disabilities, and in particular to
identify behaviours that result in dependence on psychiatric care. It is based on the
Wing Ward Behaviour Scale, which was published over 30 years ago. It is a 21-item
schedule, with most items rated on a 5-point scale. The scores discriminate between
patients living in accomodation with differing levels of support. Reliability studies
have provided data on interrater and test-retest reliability for different settings and
informants, with Kappa coefficients ranging from 0.67 to 0.94. Internal consistency
for the two total problem scores is 0.71 and 0.75. It has been used in numerous studies on patients in institutions and in the community, as well as across different cultures.

REHAB

REHAB is a schedule specifically designed to assess people with long-term or disabling psychiatric handicap who at the time of assessment are "living in, or attending, a residential or day care institutional setting" (Baker and Hall 1988). One of
the aims of the authors was to design a scale that could correctly identify patients
who have the potential for living outside hospital. There are 23 items, 7 covering de-
viant behaviour and 16 covering general behaviour. Each item is measured along a
visual analogue scale. The psychometric properties have been extensively studied,
and norms for over 800 patients are available. Interrater reliability of the individual
items ranges from 0.61 to 0.92, and total scores discriminate day hospital patients,
long-stay in-patients and in-patients selected for a predischarge training programme
(Baker and Hall 1983). The REHAB is an easy to use scale, is suitable for patients
with a high level of disability, and provides a broad measure of behaviour. It is particularly suitable for repeated measures during the routine evaluation of a treatment
plan. A users' guide and other training material are available.

Life Skills Profile

The Life Skills Profile (LSP; Rosen et al. 1989) is a measure of disability and function designed specifically for people with schizophrenia. Five areas are addressed (self-care, non-turbulance, social contact, communication and responsibility), with 39 individual items that are rated on a 4-point scale. It does not contain any functioning measures directly related to symptoms. Reported internal consistency ranges from 0.67 to 0.88, and the mean interrater reliability coefficient is 0.68. Lower levels of functioning have been found in patients with higher degrees of mobility. This is a carefully developed schedule, which, although specifically designed for people with schizophrenia, can be used in a range of serious psychiatric disorders. It is suitable for routine use by a range of professional staff.

Instruments for Non-psychotic Patients

Social Functioning Schedule

The Social Functioning Schedule (SFS; Remington and Tyrer 1979) is primarily designed to measure the level of social functioning in people with a non-psychotic psychiatric disorder. Twelve main areas of functioning are included in the scale, which is measured along a 10-cm visual analogue scale. Symptoms are not included. Time frame is the last month. Interrater reliability for the different sections ranges from 0.45 to 0.81 (mean 0.62) when audiotape interviews are used, and from 0.5 to 0.8 with independent interviews. The scale discriminates between people with personality disorders and those with other psychiatric disorders.

Social Maladjustment Schedule

The Social Maladjustment Schedule (SMS; Clare and Cairns 1978) was designed to assess the social maladjustment and dysfunction in six main areas: housing, occupation and social role, economic situation, leisure and social activities, family and domestic relationships, and marital relationships. Answers are rated on a 4-point response scale, and total scores for objective conditions, instrumental performance, satisfaction and overall maladjustment are produced. It was designed for use with patients with chronic neurotic disorders. A 45-min structured interview is required with either the patient or informant. The authors have reported interrater reliability data for 17 of the 48 items, with weighted kappas ranging from 0.62 to 0.94 (there was insufficient data for other items).

Conclusions

The scales reviewed in this paper illustrate the difficulties in trying to measure global functioning in people with serious mental illness, and the different approaches to the problem. During the development of these instruments psychometric properties are often not fully explored. Reliability studies are often limited in their scope, and unsophisticated statistics, such as correlations, used for analysis. Validity studies are often limited to examining associations with diagnosis and service utilisation. A tendency for ratings to be influenced by the type of care received, for instance attendance at a day hospital, may, in particular, reduce sensitivity to change in the most disabled patients. In this same group many of the social roles incorporated into some of the scales will be inappropriate, and undue weight may be given to the patients' behaviour and symptoms.

Despite these reservations, global functioning scales can play an important role in mental health service evaluative research, as well as routine clinical work. Although outcome assessments clearly need to focus on a wide range of areas, functioning should be identified as a critical domain within batteries of outcome measures. The actual functioning measure that is selected will depend on the precise situation. For instance, for large population based surveys a quick measures such as the GAF may be suitable. Research studies aimed at specific groups of patients can select more comprehensive measures suitable for the population studied and the resources available.

Within routine clinical work there is a great demand for simple measures of functioning, and it is essential that the limitations of such measures are appreciated. The common finding that reliability improves with rater training indicates the need for regular training. In addition, staff must be encouraged to interpret the results with caution, and not view them in isolation from other outcome measures.

References

Affleck JW, McGuire RJ (1984) The measurement of psychiatric rehabilitation status: a review of the needs and a new scale. Br J Psychiatry 145: 517–525

American Psychiatric Association (1987) Diagnostic and statistical manual of mental disorders, 3rd edn revised. American Psychiatric Association, Washington, DC

Baker R, Hall JN (1983) Rehabilitation evaluation of Hall and Baker (REHAB). Vine Publishing Ltd, Aberdeen, Scotland

Baker R, Hall JN (1988) REHAB: a new assessment instrument for chronic psychiatric patients. Schizophr Bull 14: 95–113

Ciarlo JA, Riehman J (1977) The Denver Community Mental Health Questionnaire: development of a multidimensional program evaluation. In: Coursey RD, Specter GA, Murrell SA, Hunt B (eds) Program evaluation for mental health: methods, strategies and participants. Grune & Stratton, New York

Clare AW, Cairns VE (1978) Design, development and use of a standardized interview to assess social maladjustment and dysfunction in community studies. Psychol Med 8: 589–604

Clark A, Fiedman MJ (1983) Nine standardized scales for evaluating treatment outcomes in a mental health clinic. J Clin Psychol 39: 939–950

Dohrenwend BS, Cook D, Dohrenwend BP (1981) Measurement of social functioning in community populations. In: Wing JK, Bebbington P, Robbins L (eds) What is a case? Grant McIntyre, London

Dworkin RJ, Friedman LC, Telschow RL, Grant KD, Moffic HS, Sloan VJ (1990) The longitudinal use of the Global Assessment Scale in multiple-rater situations. Community Ment Health J 26: 335–344

Endicott J, Spitzer RL (1972a) What another rating scale? The Psychiatric Evaluation Form. J Nerv Ment Disord 154: 88–104

Endicott J, Spitzer RL (1972b) Current and Past Psychopathology Scales (CAPPS): rationale, reliability, and validity. Arch Gen Psychiatry 27: 678–687

Endicott J, Spitzer RL, Fleiss JL, Cohen J (1976) The Global Assessment Scale. Arch Gen Psychiatry 33: 766–771

Fernando T, Mellsop G, Nelson K, Peace K, Wilson J (1986) The reliability of axis V of DSM-III. Am J Psychiatry 143: 752–755

Goldman HH, Skodol AE, Lave TR (1992) Revising axis V for DSM-IV: a review of measures of social functioning. Am J Psychiatry 149: 1148–1156

Hogarty GE, Katz MM (1971) Norms of adjustment and social behaviour. Arch Gen Psychiatry 25: 470–480

Hurry J, Sturt E (1981) Social performance in a population sample: relation to psychiatric symptoms. In Wing JK, Bebbington P, Robbins L (eds) What is a case? Grant McIntyre, London

Kane RA, Kane RL, Arnold S (1985) Measuring social functioning in mental health studies: concepts and instruments. Mental Health Service System Reports, Series DN No. 5 NIMH

Katz MM, Lyerly SB (1963) Methods for measuring adjustment and social behaviour in the community: 1. rationale, description, discriminative validity and scale development. Psychol Rep 13: 503–535

Luborsky L (1962) Clinicians' judgements of mental health. A proposed scale. Arch Gen Psychiatry 7: 407–417

Luborsky L, Bachrach H (1974) Factors influencing clinician's judgements of mental health. Arch Gen Psychiatry 31: 292–299

Mezzich JE, Fabrega H Jr, Coffman GA (1987) Multiaxial characterization of depressive patients. J Nerv Ment Disord 175: 339–346

Paykel ES (1972) Correlates of a depressive typology. Arch Gen Psychiatry 27: 203–210

Plakun EM, Muller JP, Burkhardt PE (1987) The significance of borderline and schizotypal overlap. Hillside J Clin Psychiatry 9: 47–54

Remington M, Tyrer P (1979) The social functioning schedule – a brief semistructured interview. Soc Psychiatry 14: 151–157

Rey JM, Plapp JM, Stewart GW, Richards IN, Bashir MR (1987) Reliability of the psychosocial axes of DSM-III in an adolescent population. Br J Psychiatry 150: 228–234

Rey JM, Stewart GW, Plapp JM, Bashir MR, Richards IN (1988) Validity of axis V of DSM-III and other measures of adaptive functioning. Acta Psychiatr Scand 77: 534–542

Rosen A, Hadzi-Pavlovic D, Parker G (1989) The Life Skills Profile: a measure assessing function and disability in schizophrenia. Schizophr Bull 15: 325–337

Schrader G, Gordon M, Harcourt R (1986) The usefulness of DSM-III axis IV and V assessments. Am J Psychiatry 143: 904–907

Schubert C, Krumm B, Biehl H, Schwarz R (1986) Measurement of social disability in a schizophrenic patient group: definition, assessment and outcome over two years in a cohort of schizophrenic patients of recent onset. Soc Psychiatry 21: 1–9

Skodol AE, Link BG, Shrout PE, Horwath E (1988) Toward construct validity for DSM III axis V. Psychiatry Res 24: 13–23

Spitzer RL, Forman JBW (1979) DSM-III field trials, II: initial experience with the multiaxial system. Am J Psychiatry 136: 818–820

Spitzer RL, Endicott J, Fleiss JL, Cohen J (1970) The Psychiatric Status Schedule: a technique for evaluating psychopathology and impairment in role functioning. Arch Gen Psychiatry 23: 41–55

Wallace CJ (1986) Functional assessment in rehabilitation. Schizophr Bull 12: 604–624

Weissman MM, Sholomskas D, John K (1981) The assessment of social adjustment: an update. Arch Gen Psychiatry 38: 1250–1258

Westermeyer J (1988) DSM-III psychiatric disorders among Hmong refugees in the United States: a point prevalence study. Am J Psychiatry 145: 197–202

Westermeyer J, Neider J (1988) Social networks and psychopathology among substance abusers. Am J Psychiatry 145: 1265–1269

World Health Organisation (1988) WHO Psychiatric Disability Assessment Scale (WHO/DAS). WHO, Geneva

Wykes T, Sturt E (1986) The measurement of social behaviour in psychiatric patients: an assessment of the reliability and validity of the SBS schedule. Br J Psychiatry 148: 1–11

Wykes T (1992) The assessment of severely disabled psychiatric patients for rehabilitation. In: Kavanagh D (ed) Schizophrenia: an overview and practical handbook. Chapman Hall, London

Wykes T, Hurry J (1991) Social behaviour and psychiatric disorder. In: Bebbington P (ed) Social psychiatry: theory, methodology and practice. Transactional Publishers, New Brunswick

CHAPTER 4

Satisfaction with Psychiatric Services

MIRELLA RUGGERI

Abstract

Despite reservations made about its use as a means for evaluating interventions, various findings in the recent literature point to patients' and relatives' satisfaction with psychiatric services as a particularly salient and appropriate measure of outcome and quality. Even though substantial improvements have occurred in the last decade, research in the field suffers various methodological limitations regarding the study design, the instruments' construction and the lack of attention to their psychometric properties. In the last few years the need for research that develops and refines measures of client satisfaction and establishes their psychometric properties has been considered a priority in service evaluation by a growing number of authors. In spite of this, in the mental health field very few validated instruments for the measurement of satisfaction are currently available. The aims of the present paper are: (1) to update work done in the field of satisfaction with mental health services in the last decade; (2) to describe the main instruments currently available to measure patients' and relatives' satisfaction with mental health services; (3) to provide guidelines for the future development of instruments and their use in mental health settings. The author concludes by emphasizing that, in order to make further progress, considerable effort is needed in developing and spreading the use of validated instruments and discouraging the use of ad hoc measures. Comparability between studies should be pursued more vigorously in order allow both the refinement of existing instruments and a better understanding of the theoretical and substantive meaning of satisfaction with psychiatric services.

Introduction

As early as 1966, Donabedian stated that "... the effectiveness of care in achieving and producing health and satisfaction, as defined for its individual members by a particular society or subculture, is the ultimate validator of the quality of care" (Donabedian 1966). Later, Locker and Dunt (1978) suggested that, particularly in long-term care, "... quality of care can become synonymous with quality of life and satisfaction with care an important component of life satisfaction". Patient's and relative's satisfaction with services thus seems to be particularly salient and appropriate as outcome and quality measures; in service evaluation satisfaction may be viewed

Servizio di Psicologia Medica, Istituto di Psichiatria, Università di Verona, Ospedale Policlinico, I-37134 Verona, Italy

both as a *measure of outcome and quality per se* and/or as a *factor* in the process of care. Similarly, clients' satisfaction with services can be considered an independent or a dependent variable. As a *dependent* variable, satisfaction may be the effect of various factors such as subjects' expectations with services, subjects' attitudes toward life, self-esteem, illness, behaviour and previous experience with services, besides depending on the structure, the process and the outcome of care. However conflicting results have been obtained with regard to the characteristics of patients that correlate with satisfaction. No clear relationship has been found between patient satisfaction and age, education, family size, income, marital status, occupation, race, religion, sex, social class, and diagnosis (Lebow 1983a; Like and Zyzanski 1987). Lehman and Zastowny (1983), in a meta-analysis of the literature on satisfaction with mental health services between 1955 and 1983, have found that chronically ill patients tend to express less satisfaction with their treatment compared to non-chronically ill patients. Some characteristics of the intervention seem to be correlated with satisfaction. For example, Lehman and Zastowny in their meta-analysis have found that innovative programmes tend to be viewed more positively than conventional ones; no differences were found in rates of patient satisfaction between inpatient and outpatient programmes. A significant association between the level of patient satisfaction and treatment outcome has been found in a few studies, although this has been less well documented for mental health than for primary health care services.

As an *independent* variable, satisfaction can influence the efficacy of interventions and various behaviours of consumers such as compliance and service utilization. According to Ware and Davies (1983), satisfaction can influence *care-seeking behaviour* (for example, whether consumers seek care during an illness episode and the number of visits), *adherence behaviour* (whether patients do the things they are supposed to do while under care, for example adherence to regimes, compliance with follow-up visits and referrals) and *reactive behaviour* (actions initiated by consumers specifically to express their satisfaction or dissatisfaction, such as, for example, recommendations in favour or against a particular provider or facility, changing providers, registering formal complaints). They have found that differences in patient satisfaction are significant predictor of both changes in doctors and disenrollments from health plans, and that relatively small differences in satisfaction rating scores have noteworthy consequences for patient behaviour.

Despite these considerations, consumers' views have not been regarded until recently as a relevant contribution to service evaluation. This happened for a series of reasons. Sheppard (1993) summarizes in six points reservations about the use of client satisfaction as a means for evaluating interventions: (1) the concept of satisfaction is too general to provide a meaningful guide to the way clients think; (2) satisfaction may be related to the way a service is given rather than the outcome (positive or negative) of the intervention; (3) some clients may pronounce themselves satisfied, knowing little of the alternatives available; (4) in some cases, merely asking people to rate something can produce a favourable evaluation and cause bias in the measurement; (5) individuals' comments are the prisoner of the moment; what they say on one occasion may be different from another occasion; (6) the degree of satisfaction may owe more to the clients' cultural background and expectations than their actual experience of intervention. The prejudice that mental illness can completely deprive an individual of the capacity to make considered and rational judgements and the fact that patients' statements are often considered useful only as a basis for making and confirming a diagnosis have certainly played a major role in generating such scepticism (Brandon 1981). Empirical data disconfirm this prejudice. Various studies, in fact, have found that patients are sensitive to verbal and nonverbal elements of the health care process, that they are fairly accurate in distinguishing the quality of provider behaviours, such as courtesy and competence and that they base their satisfaction ratings on these discriminations. The satisfaction ratings of patients have also been found to correspond to criteria for physician excellence customarily used by health providers, such as more years of training, positive motivation of the physician toward patients and peer supervision of physicians (for a review of these data see Lebow 1983a). Interesting findings have been found recently in the work done by Sheppard (1993) that correlates levels of patients' satisfaction to the nature of the intervention and the quality of some skills used by practitioners in extended intervention in a community mental health centre. Considerable differences have been identified between satisfied and dissatisfied clients in the service received and their perception of the service; satisfaction is clearly related to the use of interpersonal skills such as communication, empathy, listening, openness and genuineness. Another aspect of professionals' mistrust of patients is that they tend to believe that the patient is responsible for whatever problems have arisen in the treatment; it may frequently happen, for example, that they believe that the patient's complaint arises from "transference distortions" rather than from real problems in the treatment relationship. It is often further assumed that such transference problems would inevitably recur with subsequent therapists. This belief has been disproved in a paper by Andrews et al. (1986), which has demonstrated that most requests for a change in therapists in an outpatient psychotherapy service result from patient-therapist mismatch and the majority of patients who change therapists remain in treatment with the new therapist and report being satisfied with the change.

With Sheppard (1993) we think that "... while it would be foolish to dismiss the themes which underlie these reservations about satisfaction, which emphasize both social context and background assumptions, it is also important to be aware of their limits. It is, first of all, useful to examine factors 'internal' to interviews and interventions, as well as the social context of the client's involvement in the first place. It is also helpful to ... unravel the meaning for clients of intervention. In addition, by emphasizing differences between clients' and workers' views, we may underestimate the potential for common ground and shared meanings between participants. Finally, the concept of satisfaction may itself be rather aggrandized. It may be helpful to assign it a more humble, but correspondingly more powerful, role indicating a general sense in which the clients, overall, felt positive or negative about interventions."

Measuring satisfaction with services may enlighten results obtained when measuring other types of variables (such as psychopathology, social functioning, quality of life, burden of relatives, etc.), but satisfaction should be considered a *complement* of rather than a *substitute* for the information provided by research utilizing these variables and of professional judgement. Moreover, one should be clear that increasing a service recipient's satisfaction is not necessarily the main goal of a service and psychiatrists should not feel, as they often do, threatened by the assessment of clients' satisfaction or obliged to fulfil all patients requests in order to be judged positively.

It is obvious that there may be times when fulfilling clients' requests may prove too difficult or too costly, or may not be clinically indicated. *Short-term dissatisfaction* in some cases can be legitimately considered a side effect of a therapeutic intervention that changes the patient's perspective (such as, for example, putting into practice a shift from institutional to community care or pursuing a change in the relationship of the patient with significant others): apart from the risk of early dropout from treatment, dissatisfaction itself may not be a worrying event here. A certain relevance should, instead, be given to consumers' dissatisfaction in the long-term. *Long-term dissatisfaction,* in fact, may indicate that the planned change did not contribute to a real improvement in the consumers' life: in this case, optimality of such intervention should be seriously reconsidered. It may also indicate that consumers do not have enough personal resources to appreciate the advantages of that intervention: in this case, if not a change in the therapeutic strategy, at least an improvement in communication between consumers and professionals is necessary.

Short-term dissatisfaction can easily become satisfaction in the long run if professionals perceive it correctly, communicate their perception to the consumer and discuss with him/her problems that are occurring. Moreover, it should be stressed that different perspectives do not necessarily result in dissatisfaction. In fact, when consumers feel that their viewpoint has been taken into account and an acceptable therapeutic management plan has been worked out through a process of mutual negotiation, they may still feel satisfied even if their initial requests are not fully met.

In conclusion, though being an important variable to be measured in service evaluation, it should be clearly stressed that consumers' satisfaction is only *one* evaluative perspective and that it is resonable to consider satisfaction a *necessary,* but not a *sufficient,* component in the assessment of quality and effectiveness of care.

A major review of existing literature in this field up to the early 1980s has been published (Attkisson and Pascoe 1983). In that monograph, work done in the field until 1982 has been comprehensively reviewed (Pascoe 1983; Lebow 1983a, b; Lehman and Zastowny 1983). In the years following, a few other attempts were made (Kalman 1983; Zastowny and Lehman 1988; Corrigan 1990; Ricketts 1992) that, however, lacked comprehensiveness. The aims of the present paper are: (1) to update the Attkisson and Pascoe monograph by considering work done in the field of satisfaction with mental health services in the last decade; (2) to describe the main instruments currently available to measure patients' and relatives' satisfaction with mental health services; (3) to provide guidelines for the future development of instruments and their use in mental health settings.

Review Methodology

This review was based on a computerized library search of the literature (Medlars, National Library, Bethesda, USA) published in the period 1982–1993 and made by using the following strategy: the key words *Patient satisfaction/Client satisfaction* were crossed with the key words *Mental Health Services/Community-based Mental Health Services/Community Psychiatry.* Moreover, all issues of *Psychological Abstracts* published from January 1982 to December 1993 were systematically consulted and papers classified under the key word *Satisfaction* and referring to work done in mental health services were selected. References found are reported in Table 1 and classified into three categories: (1) empirical studies; (2) editorials / commentaries / letters; (3) reviews/chapters. Main empirical studies were then analysed in detail: reported in Table 2 are the characteristics of the instruments used, and in Table 3, some characteristics of the study design and of the results.

The term 'consumer satisfaction' has been used to describe a broad range of research. According to Lebow (1983a), studies based on both a broad and a narrow definition of satisfaction are available in the literature. Studies based on a *broad definition* of satisfaction are, for example, those that use measures of self-perception of improvement, records of complaints or praise for treatment, suggestions for improving treatment and inquiries into what is found helpful and unhelpful in treatment. Studies based on a *narrow definition* of satisfaction are ". . . all enquiries into the extent to which services gratify the client's wants, wishes, or desires for treatment. Included here are inquiries into both the felt adequacy of treatment and of surrounding milieu; specific aspects may include reactions to the quality of care, to its helpfulness, its cost and continuity, the availability and accessibility of the practitioner, and the reaction to supporting services" (Lebow 1983a). Lebow has basically reviewed studies published that fall within this narrow definition. Here, we will give secondary attention to papers based on a broad definition of satisfaction and will mainly consider the latter kind of studies. With a few exceptions, major emphasis will be given to the papers in which the authors explicitly mention their intent to study "satisfaction with mental health services".

A considerable effort was made to locate all relevant published studies; however, the disparate locations in which this work appears, coupled with the inconsistent labelling of these studies, were not easy problems to overcome and the author cannot fully guarantee the comprehensiveness of the review with respect to all material published in the period. Another limit of this review is that, with few exceptions, it doesn't consider unpublished reports or work in progress.

Theory and Definition

A number of investigators have criticized satisfaction research as having little theory guiding the variables chosen for study or the hypotheses being tested. Locker and Dunt (1978), in particular, state that ". . . it is rare to find the concept of patient satisfaction defined and there has been little clarification of what the term means either to researchers who employ it or respondents who respond to it." The little attention directed towards developing a well-defined sociopsychological theory of satisfaction limits the scientific knowledge in this field; it must, however, be emphasized that the concept of satisfaction is itself difficult to conceptualize. Ware et al. (1983) suggest that ". . . the term 'satisfaction' is defined differently by individuals as a result of varying backgrounds and experiences". Thus, *subjectivity* causes problems in formulating a clear and generalizable definition of satisfaction; on the other hand, assessing subjective variables seems to be a unique opportunity in service evaluation to take account of and examine the perspective of consumers. Moreover, clinicians should never forget that finding the best treatment for the *individual* patient (a person with his/her own opinions, needs and desires) is the ultimate goal of a good quality care.

Expectancy approaches are the major conceptual models used. According to these models, individuals seek help for a variety of reasons and their judgements may have to do not only with the nature of the intervention received but also with the process

Table 1. References quoted in the period 1982–1993 under key words 'patient satisfaction/consumer satisfaction and mental health services/community mental health services/community psychiatry' in Medlars and Psychological Abstracts

	1982–1983	1984–1985	1986–1987
Empirical studies	Bene-Kociemba et al. (1982)[1] P	Bugge et al. (1985)[1] P	Andrews et al. (1986) P, S
	Damkot et al. (1983)[1] P	Greenley et al. (1985)[1] P	Azim and Joyce (1986)[1] P
	Dyck and Azim (1983)[1] P	Hersch and Lathan (1985) P	Bennett and Feldstein (1986)[1] P
	Distefano et al. (1983)[1] P	Hoult et al. (1984) P	Bennun (1986) R
	Holden and Lewine (1982) R	Lemoine and Carney (1984) P	Bulow et al. (1987)[1] P, R, S
	Hoult et al. (1983) P	Lorefice and Borus (1984) P, S	Depp et al. (1986) P
	Lindholm (1983) P	MacPheeters (1984) P	Long and Bourne (1987) P
	Lorefice et al. (1982)[1] P, S	Roberts et al. (1984)[1] P	McGuire et al. (1986)[1] P
	Mangen and Griffith (1982)[1] P	Rothman (1984)[1] P	Sishta et al. (1986)[1] P
	Mangen et al. (1983) P		Urquhart et al. (1986)[1] P
	Slavinsky and Krauss (1983) P		
	Wood (1982) P		
Editorials/ commentaries/ letters	Breyer and Malafonte (1983)		Vousden (1986)
	Conway (1983)		
	Kiesler (1983)[1]		
	Lebow (1982)		
	Lewine (1982)[1]		
Reviews/ chapters	el-Guebaly et al. (1983)	Greenley (1984)	
	Kalman (1983)[1]	Molde and Diers (1985)	
	Lebow (1983a, b)		
	Ley (1982)[1]		

P, patients' satisfaction measured; R, relatives' satisfaction measured; S, staff's satisfaction measured.
[1]   Satisfaction is main topic.

→

Table 1 continued

of becoming clients. Expectancy approaches consider satisfaction both a cognitive and an emotional perspective (Linder-Peltz 1982a) determined by a comparison between the subject's experience and the subject's expectations (Linder-Pelz 1982b). That expectations are somehow correlated with satisfaction is supported also by everyday clinical experience with patients and relatives: it isn't rare to find that a subject whom a doctor considers uncooperative is, for example, looking for something in the consultation process that is quite different from that being provided. This dissonance of expectations may determine dissatisfaction, dissatisfaction may cause reactive behaviours such as uncooperativeness. How dissonance of expectations between consumers and professionals may be managed is discussed in the Introduction to this chapter.

The three basic expectancy models that have been formulated are the contrast model, the assimilation model and the assimilation-contrast model. According to the *contrast model*, the consumer magnifies discrepancies between expectations and performance; performance that is somewhat higher than expectations will be

Table 1. continued

	1988–1989	1990–1991	1992–1993
Empirical studies	Conte et al. (1989)[1] P Greenfield and Attkisson (1989)[1] P Grella and Grusky (1989)[1] R Hansson (1989)[1] P Krulee and Hales (1988) P Lesage and Pollini (1989)[1] R MacDonald et al. (1988)[1] P Morgan (1989)[1] R Perkins et al. (1989) P Solomon et al. (1988) R Wright et al. (1989) P	Andrews et al. (1990) P Carscaddon et al. (1990)[1] P Elbeck and Fecteau (1990)[1] P Elzinga and Barlow (1991)[1] P Grosser and Vine (1991) R Harkness and Hensley (1991) P MacDonald et al. (1990)[1] P, R, S Smylie et al. (1991) P, S Tessler et al. (1991) R	Allen et al. (1993) P Burns et al. (1993) P Corrigan and Jakus (1993)[1] P Dean et al. (1993) P Eisen and Grob (1992)[1] P Ferguson et al. (1992) P Hanson and Rapp (1992) R Huxley and Warner (1992) P Merson et al. (1992) P O'Driscoll et al. (1993) P Perreault et al. (1993)[1] P Polowczyk et al. (1993)[1] P Ruggeri and Dall' Agnola (1993)[1] P, R, S Sheppard (1993)[1] P Solomon (1992) P Thornicroft et al. (1993) P Vicente et al. (1993a,b)[1] P, R, S
Editorials/ commentaries/ letters		Bernheim (1990) Rees (1990) Romeo et al. (1990) Silva (1990)	Crowe et al. (1993)[1] Gersons et al. (1992) van Hoorn (1992)
Reviews/ chapters	Zastowny and Lehman (1988)[1]	Corrigan (1990)[1]	Attkisson and Greenfield (1994)[1] Ricketts (1992)[1]

evaluated as satisfactory, performance less than expected will be judged as unsatisfactory. According to the *assimilation model,* performance that is moderately lower than expectations will not cause dissatisfaction because perceptions of performance will be assimilated to match higher expectations. The *assimilation-contrast model* is a hybrid of the previous ones and assumes that assimilation effects occur in reaction to ambiguous attributes of the subject's experience, whereas contrast effects result when responding to less ambiguous attributes.

Most patient satisfaction studies have implicitly employed a contrast approach. However, the relationship between expectations and satisfaction, though certainly a major issue in this field, is not always straightforward. It is reasonable to hypothesize that many other factors may intervene and have a moderating effect on both expectations and satisfaction. Moreover, expectancy models should be complemented by other models in order to achieve a full understanding of satisfaction. Work to clarify these theoretical aspects is needed. For a review of the main theories on consumer satisfaction, see Pascoe (1983).

Table 2. Characteristics of the instruments used in the main studies on satisfaction with mental health services in the period 1982–1993

Authors of the study	Type of instrument	Variable measured	Validation	Items (n)	Aspects considered	Scale
Bene-Kociemba et al. (1982), UK	Ad hoc; interview	Patients' satisfaction with aftercare services	Interrater agreement	n.s.	Hospitalization / Types of assistance / Relationship with key professionals	Three-point Likert scale
Mangen and Griffith (1982), UK	Ad hoc; interview	Patients' satisfaction with community-based psychiatric nursing	Not reported	n.s.	Overall satisfaction	Fixed format
Damkot et al. (1983), USA	Client Satisfaction Survey; self-administration	Patients' satisfaction with community-based psychiatric services	Consensus of experts / Pilot testing / Factor analysis	16	Services scheduling / Problem resolution / Therapist cost of service / Medication / Length of service	Varying
Dyck and Azim (1983), Canada; Azim and Joyce (1986), Canada	User Satisfaction Survey (Love et al. 1979); Client Satisfaction Questionnaire (Larsen et al. 1979); self-administration	Patients' satisfaction with health services	Construct validity / Split-half reliability / Factor analysis / Various psychometric tests	6 + 8	Respect from staff members / Recognition of needs / Therapeutic skills / Kind and quality of the service	Four-point Likert scale
Sishta et al. (1986), Canada	Client Satisfaction Questionnaire-8; 3 items from Client Satisfaction Questionnaire-31 (Larsen et al. 1979); self-administration	Patients' satisfaction with health services	Construct validity / Split-half reliability / Factor analysis / Various psychometric tests	12	Overall satisfaction	Four-point Likert scale
Urquart et al. (1986), USA	Ad hoc; self-administration	Patients' satisfaction with psychiatric outpatient services	Reliability / Stability (not published)	9	Appearance / Courtesy / Treatment delivery / Overall satisfaction	Four-point Likert scale
Long and Bourne (1987), UK	Ad hoc; self-administration	Patients' satisfaction with an anxiety self-help management group course	Not reported	8	Overall satisfaction / Deal with problems / Meet needs / Length of course	Varying
Grella and Grusky (1989), USA	Family Service Satisfaction Scale; self-administration	Relatives' satisfaction with community support programmes	Internal consistency	6	Information / Assistance in finding services / Information on how to cope / Contact with other people / Understanding of problems / Participation in treatment	Four-point Likert scale

Study	Instrument; administration	Focus	Reliability/validity	No.	Dimensions	Scale
Hansonn (1989), Sweden	Ad hoc (based on Kelstrup et al. 1985 and Hansonn et al. 1988); self-administration	Patients' satisfaction with in-hospital psychiatric care	Not reported	44	Physical environment; Staff-patient relationship; Information/influence; Treatment design; Treatment programme; General satisfaction	Seven-point Likert scale
Wright et al. (1989), USA	Ad hoc; self-administration	Patients' satisfaction with community-based psychiatric services	Not reported	6	Improvement; Living situation; Contact with other people; Medication; Help from support programme; Quality of services	Five-point Likert scale
Carscaddon et al. (1990), USA	Ad hoc; self-administration	Patients' satisfaction with psychotherapy in community-based psychiatric services	Split-half reliability	16	Therapist; Therapy; Overall satisfaction	Likert scale
McDonald et al. (1988), UK; Elzinga and Barlow (1991), Australia	Interview	Patients' satisfaction with psychiatric hospitals	Interrater reliability; Test-retest reliability; Cluster analysis	40	Restrictiveness; Autonomy; Lack of individualization; Unsatisfactory environment; Restriction of action; Lack of control; Homeliness of the environment	Yes/no
Huxley and Warner (1992), UK, USA	General Satisfaction Questionnaire (derived from the CSQ, Larsen et al. 1979); self-administration	Patients' satisfaction with health services	Not reported	20	General satisfaction; Access; Help given; Acceptability (reception/competence)	Four-point Likert scale; Seven-point Likert scale
Ruggeri and Dall'Agnola (1993), Italy	Verona Service Satisfaction Scale (partly derived from the SSS-30, Greenfield and Attkisson 1989); self-administration	Patients', relatives and professionals' satisfaction with community-based psychiatric services	Acceptability; Content validity; Sensitivity; Test-retest reliability; Factor analysis	82	Overall satisfaction; Professionals' skills and behaviour; Information; Access; Efficacy; Types of intervention; Relative's involvement	Five-point Likert scale
Vicente et al. (1993a, b), Chile, UK, Italy	Ad hoc; self-administration/interview	Patients', relatives' and professionals attitudes and satisfaction with mental health services	Not reported	46	Overall satisfaction; Hospital and community care; Compulsory admission	Five-point Likert scale

n.s., not specified.

Methodological Problems in Measurement

Efforts to measure satisfaction have varied widely in method, and systematic knowledge within the area has been scattered. Description of methodology is usually lacking in the vast majority of papers published to the point that one must carefully comb the text to find even partial information. The main limits of studies published are the following: (1) inadequacy of the study design or implementation, (2) inadequacy in the instrument's construction; (3) lack of attention to the psychometric properties of the instruments.

Study Design or Implementation

Major limits in the study design are the scarce representativeness of subjects interviewed, the high number of refusals and the lack of confidentiality in the study conduct.

The *representativeness* of responders with respect to the larger population of consumers is of concern in evaluating the usefulness of a patient satisfaction measure. Nguyen et al. (1983) suggest that satisfied clients are often more likely to return questionnaires than those who are not pleased. Lebow (1983a) has reported that more satisfied respondents tend to reply to the first inquiry. However, findings are not unanimous: Ware et al. (1983), for example, have found that those who are more satisfied with the quality of their care are less likely to return questionnaires.

Response rates in satisfaction studies are usually low, even though they vary slightly according to the method used. Many studies of client satisfaction done utilizing mailed questionnaires have achieved very low response rates of between 30 % and 40 %. Lebow (1983a) has reviewed 49 studies done in mental health settings, finding that mail-in surveys have the lowest average rate of return (40 %), followed by telephone surveys (43 %), interviews in the home (64 %) and a combination of these methods (82 %). Lower percentages of refusals have been found in some recent studies (see Table 3, fifth column), suggesting some improvement in systematic data collection.

Those methods that yield the highest rate of return are more costly, both in money and personnel time, and can be biased by undifferentiated high satisfaction ratings if *confidentiality* is not carefully pursued. LeVois et al. (1981) have found, for example, that oral administration of questionnaires increases the degree of positiveness of the ratings by 10 % over other methods of administration. Soelling and Newell (1983) have found that lack of anonymity determines scores on the average notably higher. Polowczyk et al. (1993) have demonstrated that surveys conducted by patients elicit lower satisfaction than surveys conducted by staff members. Conversely, Greenfield (1983) has found that optional identification, not of the respondent but of the practitioner, does not reduce the response rate or change mean satisfaction scores.

Construction of Instruments

Major limits found in the construction of available instruments include the *low range of choices* in the response (often reduced to the dichotomy satisfied/dissatisfied) and taking into consideration only general aspects of consumers' interaction with a service. The former limit has been considered to greatly contribute to the lack of sensitivity of instruments in measuring dissatisfaction, the latter contributes to the lack of content validity of the majority of available instruments (see the paragraph on psychometric properties).

Most studies on satisfaction in mental health settings published before 1982 used measures that were composed of either a few broad questions about satisfaction or unstandardized, single-item subscales that tapped reactions to one or two dimensions (Pascoe 1983; Lebow 1983a, b; Westbrook and Oliver 1981), and this notwithstanding findings available in the literature on satisfaction in other medical settings supported the idea that satisfaction is a *multidimensional* concept. Ware et al. (1978) reviewed 111 theoretical and empirical articles on health services published prior to 1976 in order to determine the nature of the concept of satisfaction and to identify its major dimensions. On the basis of the content of these studies, they identified "... eight distinguishable dimensions which constitute the major sources of satisfaction and dissatisfaction with care: art of care, technical quality of care, accessibility/convenience, finances, physical environment, availability, continuity and efficacy/outcomes of care". Ware later (1981) reduced his original eight major dimensions of patient satisfaction to five: quality of care, accessibility/convenience, finances, physical environment and availability.

Between 1982 and 1993 a tendency to use multidimensional instruments became clearly dominant in mental health settings also. But, as shown in Table 2, sixth column, there is a marked heterogeneity of aspects considered in the various instruments. This reflects the confusion that still exists on the dimensions that constitute the domain of satisfaction. A trend for an increase in the number of items can be found in more recent works (see Table 2, fifth column) in an attempt to assess the various dimensions more precisely. Still further studies that would clarify the dimensionality of satisfaction in mental health settings are needed. Another problem should be faced. Ware's approach indicates those aspects of care that have been inquired about most frequently by researchers; increasing the number of dimensions in a questionnaire and the number of items is considered a progress in the instrument's construction; but this work does not really address the issue of which dimensions constitute the domain of satisfaction from the point of view of consumers. For further discussion on this issue see below.

Psychometric Properties

Although the importance of demonstrating that a test instrument exhibits good psychometric properties is widely recognized, psychometric analysis has too often been neglected in the field of client satisfaction. In the last few years the need for research that develops and refines measures of client satisfaction and establishes their psychometric properties has been considered a priority in service evaluation by a growing number of authors (Steinwachs et al. 1992). In spite of this, in the mental health field very few validated instruments for the measurement of satisfaction are currently available. The acceptability, sensitivity, validity, and reliability of the instruments used are rarely, if ever, reported.

Table 3. Characteristics of the main studies on satisfaction with mental health services published in the period 1982–1993

Authors	Diagnosis of patients/affected relatives	Services/treatments assessed	Number of patients/relatives	Refusals (%)	Main results
Bene-Kociemba et al. (1982), UK	Schizophrenia (60%) Alcoholism (14%)	After-care service	22	39	Higher satisfaction with aftercare than hospitalization Satisfaction positively correlated with continuity of care and quality of relationship with key worker
Mangen and Griffiths (1982), UK	Neurosis	Community-based psychiatric service	71	15	Higher satisfaction with psychiatric nurses than psychiatrists
Dyck and Azim (1983), Canada	Mainly neurosis and adjustment disorders	Psychiatric walk-in clinic	323	n.s.	Lower satisfaction with group psychotherapy than individual psychotherapy or clinical assessment
Damkot et al. (1983), USA	n.s.	Community-based psychiatric service	>600	42.3	Various considerations on the methodology of satisfaction measurement Various considerations on local services
Azim and Joyce (1986), Canada	Mainly neurosis and adjustment disorders	Group psychotherapy in a psychiatric walk-in clinic	85 (time 0) 41 (f.u.)	−9.4 (time 0) −7.3 (f.u.)	Improvement at f.u. of satisfaction with group psychotherapy if modifications are made according to criticisms recorded at time o
Sishta et al. (1986), Canada	Psychosis (46%) Neurosis (28%)	Inpatient facility	87	53	Various considerations on the methodology of satisfaction measurement High overall satisfaction with the inpatient facility ("better facility"?) Satisfaction not correlated with demographic characteristics or consultant
Long and Bourne (1987), UK	– Anxiety and agoraphobia	Anxiety self-help management group course	106	0	High satisfaction with self-help groups
McDonald et al. (1988), UK	– Schizophrenic psychosis (49%) – Residual schizophrenia (19%) – Organic psychosis (11%) – Manic-depressive psychoses (8%) – Anxiety state (8%)	Long-stay ward	104	27	High satisfaction with life in hospital, although levels of satisfaction varied significantly among wards Factors causing greatest dissatisfaction related to failure to be treated as individuals and to feelings of isolation and apathy
Grella and Grusky (1989), USA	Relatives of patients affected by Schizophrenia (75%) Bipolar depression (25%)	Community support programme for relatives	56	27	Low relatives' satisfaction with relationship with professionals Satisfaction positively correlated with good relationship with professionals

Hansson (1989), Sweden	Psychosis (65%) Non-psychosis (35%)	In-hospital psychiatric care	173	56.5	Higher satisfaction with staff-patient relationship, treatment programmes, physical environment Lower satisfaction with patient information, influence on management and design of treatments Satisfaction positively correlated with quality of treatment process, global improvement, being male and being older Satisfaction negatively correlated with compulsory admissions
Wright et al. (1989), USA	Schizophrenia (75%) Major depression (25%)	Community care	93	56	Higher satisfaction with life and support programme in the community than in the hospital
Carscaddon et al. (1990), USA	Anxiety Depression	Rural community based psychiatric service	−88 (time 0) −17 (3-month f.u.)	15.4	Satisfaction negatively correlated with number of symptoms and distress Satisfaction positively correlated with symptom amelioration at f.u.
Elzinga and Barlow (1991), Australia	Chronic psychiatric in-patients Psychogeriatric patients	Psychiatric hospital	112	43	Satisfaction more correlated with autonomy of the patient and a greater say in the running than with physical surroundings
Huxley and Warner (1992), UK, USA	Psychotic patients	Case management	68	9.3	Satisfaction with acceptability negatively correlated with brokerage Satisfaction with accessibility positively correlated with monitoring Satisfaction negatively correlated with number of contacts (intrusiveness?)
Ruggeri and Dall'Agnola (1993), Italy	Schizophrenia (36%) Affective psychosis (16%) Depressive neurosis (17%) Personality disorder (13%)	Community care	75 patients 76 relatives		Various considerations on the methodology of satisfaction measurement Higher patients' and relatives' satisfaction in the dimensions "Overall – Satisfaction", "Professionals Skills and Behaviour", "Access", "Efficacy" Lower patients' and relatives' satisfaction in the dimensions "Information", "Types of Intervention", "Relative's Involvement"
Vicente et al. (1993), Chile, UK, Italy	All but mental handicap, dementia, acute psychotic states	Mental health services in three countries	172 (UK) 105 (Chile) 55 (Italy)	n.s.	Patients in UK interested in improvement of institutional facilities Patients in Italy supportive of community care Patients in Chile satisfied with institutional care

n.s., not specified; f.u., follow-up.

Acceptability

In public psychiatric settings problems in acceptability of instruments to clients can easily arise due to the poor education of many subjects, the possible limitations in subjects' understanding and patients' symptoms such as suspiciousness and passivity. This a fundamental but mostly unexplored methodological issue. While, in fact, these limitations have greatly contributed in determining uncertainty about the possibility of measuring satisfaction, their effects on instruments' psychometric properties have almost never been substantiated by empirical findings.

Sensitivity

Concern exists about the sensitivity of available instruments in detecting dissatisfaction. In fact, it is often said that most studies on satisfaction with health care and mental health services find that the majority of respondents are satisfied (approximately 75 %). This has been regarded as a phenomenon occurring regardless of the method used, population sampled or object of rating. Thus, satisfaction has not been considered to be a discriminant variable, and the lack of variability has been seen as a problem in correlating satisfaction with other variables; all of this taken together has been considered to severely limit the usefulness of the information that studies on satisfaction provide.

However, such a problem in the measurement of satisfaction is not universal and reports of measures' lack of variability are greatly exaggerated, and are much more frequently due to methodological problems in the study design or in the construction of specific instruments than to intrinsic characteristics of the underlying construct being measured. For example, Lebow (1982, 1983a, b) has found that, in those studies that propose a range of choice wider than the dichotomy satisfied/dissatisfied, only 49 % of clients rate themselves as highly satisfied. We have already mentioned that studies where confidentiality and anonymity are guaranteed provide more differentiated satisfaction ratings. Moreover, high dissatisfaction ratings have been reported in the few studies that consider relatives' satisfaction (Grella and Grusky 1989; Morgan 1989). This finding seems correlated to another problem existing in the literature on satisfaction: the scarce attention given to the representativeness of the subjects. Among the other factors, high dissatisfaction among relatives seems to be due to the fact that often opinions of relatives involved in family associations, probably more prone to criticisms toward services than the average relative, have been selectively elicited. This area needs further research.

Content Validity

Differences in the views of patients and professionals on service delivery have been reported (Sorensen et al. 1979; Dowds and Fontana 1977; Mayer and Rosenblatt 1974; Ruggeri and Dall'Agnola 1993); if the user's perspective is not included, then there is a risk that service evaluation may be distorted within the narrow perception of the provider. Still, instruments on client satisfaction rely heavily on standards generated by professionals, and the content validity of instruments measuring satisfaction according to the views of the clients has seldom been studied.

A major problem in measuring this psychometric property has been the difficulty in assessing consumers' true feelings. A few efforts have been made to overcome this limitation. Some of them were made by using unstructured interviews assessing the domain of satisfaction according to the patients' views. Eisen and Grob (1978), for example, asked discharged psychiatric patients to generate a list of pleasing and unsatisfying aspects of their experience of the inpatient setting. Elbeck and Fecteau (1990) promoted focus-group discussions where psychiatric inpatients were asked to generate a pool of attributes describing an ideal acute care unit; this method resulted in a 50-item questionnaire, which was then factor analysed and resulted in two main factors: "behavioural autonomy" and "supportive care". Perreault et al. (1993) combined structured and unstructured measures in order to identify service dimensions associated with satisfaction from the patients' viewpoints in an outpatient psychiatric service. They have found that service dimensions most frequently evoked by patients are physical environment and atmosphere, personnel qualities, and intervention characteristics. Ruggeri and Dall'Agnola (1993) and Ruggeri et al. (1994) have assessed the importance of various aspects of care in a community-based psychiatric service in patients, relatives and professionals by combining an unstructured interview with a questionnaire, the *Verona Expectations for Care Scale*. They have demonstrated that both unstructured and structured methods are necessary to fully survey the domain of satisfaction and have shown that a key characteristic of content validity is the instrument's multidimensionality, with major contributions from dimensions regarding the skills and behaviour of professionals and types of intervention provided. In addition, patients' and relatives' views, though differing to some extent, have been found globally similar, while professionals' views markedly differ from those of the other two groups.

A common finding of studies on content validity is that cross-setting and setting-specific aspects both contribute to content validity. Omission of combining cross-setting and setting-specific aspects is a major limitation of most existing instruments; this issue, however, needs further clarification. Various evidences suggest that dimensions may be constituted by both cross-setting and setting-specific aspects. Various studies emphasize the importance of the relationship between patient and professional in both health and mental health settings (Conte et al. 1989; Bene-Kociemba et al. 1982; Jones and Zuppell 1982; Bugge et al. 1985; Lorefice and Borus 1984; Ruggeri and Dall'Agnola 1993): this seems to be mainly a cross-setting dimension. Other work indicates that enquiring about satisfaction with the types of intervention provided and other setting-specific programme aspects (a rarely assessed dimension) enhances greatly the instrument validity (Elbeck and Fecteau 1990; Rees 1990; Perreault et al. 1993; Ruggeri and Dall'Agnola 1993; Ruggeri et al. 1994): this seems to be mainly a setting-specific dimension.

Reliability

Ware et al. (1983) have reported that reliability estimates are rarely published for studies on satisfaction with medical care, and even more rarely do estimates of test-retest reliability appear in the literature. In their review, they found that only in 11 of 81 empirical studies were reliability coefficients reported, often limited to the internal consistency. Similarly, Lebow's review (1983a) noted that reliability was seldom assessed in studies done in mental health services before 1982. More efforts have been made since 1982 by studying internal consistency (Urquart et al. 1986; Carscaddon et al. 1990; Attkisson and Greenfield 1994) and test-retest reliability (Elzinga and Barlow 1991; Ruggeri and Dall'Agnola 1993). The two last studies, one done with patients in an inpatient setting, the other one done with patients and relatives in a community-based setting, have reported a test-retest percentage agreement of around 70%. This indicates that, contrary to the common belief, satisfaction is an acceptably stable concept for mental health service consumers.

Main Studies in Mental Health Services

As shown by the number of references reported in Table 1, there has been sustained interest in the last decade for the measurement of satisfaction. As Lebow suggests (1983a), empiricial studies on satisfaction with psychiatric services can be divided into four general categories: (1) poorly controlled studies conducted generally in community mental health facilities in naturalistic settings with a crude methodology; (2) better-controlled studies, usually conducted in counselling settings but involving atypical brief treatments and often assessing satisfaction after only a few sessions; (3) well-controlled evaluations of the efficacy of psychotherapy and psychopharmacology in which consumer satisfaction is employed as a tangential measure; (4) well-controlled studies aimed at assessing satisfaction in typical mental health treatments and treatment settings.

Studies belonging to category 1 are often unpublished, or published in local journals; for the time being they remain the more numerous category; they are underrepresented in this review due to the selection criteria that guided our work. A smaller number of studies in the literature belong to category 4; however, the trend is toward an increase, and, as shown in Tables 1 and 3, an expansion of this kind of study can be detected when comparing studies made at the beginning of the 1980s with studies done at the beginning of the 1990s. Especially noteworthy is the attempt by some groups to compare *satisfaction with different settings*. In the work done by McDonald et al. (1988) and by Elzinga and Barlow (1991), satisfaction with British and Australian inpatient psychiatric settings has been compared. In the work by Vicente et al. (1993a), satisfaction ratings obtained in Italian, English and Chilean mental health centers have been compared. Work done and in progress with the Verona Service Satisfaction Scale (Ruggeri and Dall'Agnola 1993) will provide a comparison of satisfaction with community-based psychiatric services in Italy, the United Kingdom, Canada, Spain, Greece, Denmark and Holland.

Very few studies have compared *views of different subjects*, but the trend for such a design is clearly emerging in the 1990s. As Table 1 shows, from 1982 to 1989 only three papers considered two perspectives (Lorefice et al. 1982; Andrews et al. 1986; Bulow et al. 1987); from 1990 to 1993, four studies have considered more than one perspective, with increasing complexity in the study design (McDonald et al. 1990; Smylie et al. 1991; Ruggeri and Dall'Agnola 1993; Vicente et al. 1993). The work done by McDonald et al. (1990) is an interesting attempt to evaluate a mental health service by considering different perspectives; its main limit is the instrument used, consisting of an ad hoc, semistructured interview whose results seem unlikely to be replicable. Similarly, the work by Vicente et al., though having an interesting study design, used an ad hoc, unvalidated instrument. The work by Ruggeri and Dall'Agnola has tried to overcome these limitations by using both a comprehensive study design and validated instruments. Even though it is believed that relatives can have contrasting opinions and different priorities than patients, few studies have examined the satisfaction of patients' relatives as well as of patients (Dowds and Fontana 1977; Prager and Tonaka 1980); most of them have been done recently (Morgan 1989; Grella and Grusky 1989; Lesage and Pollini 1989; McDonald et al. 1990; Ruggeri and Dall'Agnola 1993; Vicente et al. 1993). Conflicting results have been found. A high degree of dissatisfaction among relatives with mental health services, and especially with community-based psychiatric services, is frequently but not always reported. In some instances, relatives appear satisfied; Ruggeri and Dall'Agnola, for example, have shown that relatives, notwithstanding a certain differentiation in the ratings obtained in the various dimensions, are highly satisfied with the service provided by the South-Verona community-based psychiatric service. In some cases, the representativeness of the relatives interviewed, as opposed to the larger group of relatives attending a specific service, may partly explain those conflicting results. However, what variables influence satisfaction or dissatisfaction among relatives is a question of utmost relevance to studies on satisfaction that should be better clarified in the future. Emotional resources and aftercare services, requests for information and greater participation in care appear of particular concern for the family members.

Available Instruments

The major problem in the field of satisfaction research is the inadequacy of the instruments used in the vast majority of studies. As already mentioned, researchers conducting studies on satisfaction have tended to develop their own instruments; therefore, there are very few widely used instruments with the vast majority of ad hoc instruments developed for use only in the original study. Often instruments have been developed on the basis of an unclear concept of satisfaction; others are based on a broad definition of satisfaction, having the aim to measure, for example, attitudes towards services, expectations and usefulness of a service (see, for example, Lorefice et al. 1982; Lorefice and Borus 1984; Bennett and Feldstein 1986; Thornicroft et al. 1993). We will not consider that kind of instrument here.

With few exceptions, the distinction between instruments for research or clinical use is not made by the developers and the state of the art in this field doesn't allow a clear distinction at present. However, it should be stressed that this will probably not be a major issue even with further methodological development. Instruments for measuring satisfaction should, in fact, be simple and possibly self-administered in order to be highly acceptable to clients; potentially, the number of items seems to be the main differentiating characteristic (higher in research settings, lower in clinical settings).

Some scales have been developed in the 1970s and 1980s for assessing psychiatric outpatient treatment by Love et al. (1979), Slater et al. (1981) and Deiker et al. (1981), a scale has been developed by Strupp et al. (1964) for assessing psychotherapy. Several excellent scales are also available that assess satisfaction with medical care (Doyle and Ware 1977; Hulka et al. 1970; Ware and Snyder 1976) and that could easily be adapted to assess mental health treatment. It should be said that, in reality, the former instruments have rarely been used in the last decade and the latter ones have rarely been adapted to psychiatric settings. Undoubtedly, the most sustained effort in this field has been done by Attkisson and his colleagues at the University of California, San Francisco. They first developed the *Client Satisfaction Questionnaire* (CSQ; Attkisson and Zwick 1982; Larsen et al. 1979; LeVois et al. 1981; Nguyen et al. 1983) in a 31-item form. This form was then shortened to an 18-item version and an 8-item version. The latter version has a high degree of internal consistency and correlates highly with the longer instrument. All CSQ version assess a general satisfaction factor, use a 4-point Likert scale, have been developed through careful validation, are practically the only instruments for measuring patients' satisfaction that have had widespread use in many types of health and mental health service settings (Sishta et al. 1986; Dyck and Azim 1983; Azim and Joyce 1986; Greenfield 1983; Huxley and Warner 1992) and have been translated into other languages, notably Spanish, Dutch and French (de Brey 1983; Roberts et al. 1984; Sabourin et al. 1987).

However, the monodimensionality of the CSQ constitutes a severe limit to its sensitivity and content validity. Based on experience with the CSQ, Greenfield and Attkisson (1989) have recently developed another instrument, the *Service Satisfaction Scale* (SSS-30), specifically designed as a multidimensional scale that, on a 5-point Likert scale (terrible/delighted) adapted from life satisfaction research (Andrews and Withney 1976), assesses several components of satisfaction with health outpatient services (Practitioner Manner and Skill, Perceived Outcome, Office Procedures and Access). For a detailed description of research on the CSQ and the SSS-30, their scoring, administration, validation and service-type norms, see Attkisson and Greenfield (1994).

The SSS-30 can be considered an excellent instrument for cross-setting studies or studies in general practice but, though being a substantial improvement on previous questionnaires, may not assess some domains of specific importance in a variety of mental health setting-specific studies. The *Verona Service Satisfaction Scale* (VSSS), developed in Italy by the author of this review within the frame of the quantitative and qualitative evaluation of the South-Verona community-based psychiatric service (Tansella 1991), is an attempt to combine cross-setting and setting-specific items to enhance content validity in measuring satisfaction with community-based psychiatric services. The VSSS covers seven dimensions (Overall Satisfaction, Professionals Skills and Behaviours, Information, Access, Efficacy, Types of Intervention, Relative's Involvement) and consists of 82 items to be rated on a 5-point Likert scale slightly modified with respect to the one used in the SSS-30 (terrible/excellent). Of these items, 36 have been adapted from the SSS-30 and two derivative scales (the SSS-38 and the Family Satisfaction Scale; Greenfield and Attkisson 1989; Attkisson and Greenfield 1994; Ruggeri and Greenfield, 1995); they cover aspects considered to be relevant across a broad array of both medical and psychiatric settings. Forty-six items were newly developed and added: the new items involve aspects considered to be relevant specifically in psychiatric settings, particularly in community-based psychiatric services, such as, for example, satisfaction with service's efficacy on social skills and satisfaction with various interventions provided (i.e. psychotherapy, rehabilitation etc). Acceptability, sensitivity, content validity and test-retest reliability of the VSSS have been studied in patients and relatives in an Italian community based psychiatric service (Ruggeri et al. 1994) and proved to be good. To our knowledge, the findings presented in this validation study constitute the first complete study available in the literature on the psychometric properties of the measurement of satisfaction in a community-based psychiatric setting. Based on results from the validation study and factor analysis, shorter forms of the VSSS more suitable for routine clinical use have been developed (Ruggeri et al., 1996) and cross-cultural work on the psychometric properties of the VSSS in other countries is in progress. To date, the VSSS has been translated into English, French, Spanish, Dutch and Greek; VSSS testing in these countries is in progress.

Among the studies published between 1982 and 1993 and mentioned in Tables 2 and 3, seven took place in a community-based psychiatric service (see Table 3, third column). In one case the aim of the instrument used was to assess only psychotherapy (Carscaddon et al. 1990), in another case the instrument used was a cross-setting instrument lacking in specificity for the setting (Huxley and Warner 1992); five ad hoc instruments (Bene-Kociemba et al. 1982; Lorefice et al. 1982; Mangen and Griffith 1982; Damkot et al. 1983; Wright et al. 1989) were designed to assess integrated interventions in community-based psychiatric services (see Table 2, third column). As shown in Table 2, fourth column, only in one case (Damkot et al. 1983) was some attention given to psychometric properties of the instrument and to comprehensiveness of the domain studied. Damkot et al. describe carefully the development, implementation and findings of the *Client Satisfaction Survey*. This instrument, though not fully satisfactory from the point of view of the face and content validity and developed on the basis of concepts that appear to a certain extent out of date, is easily administered and constitutes one of the very few methodologically acceptable instruments that has been used (locally) on a regular basis. Some attentions to methodological problems has been deserved in the work by Urquhart et al. (1986), still the instrument developed suffers from various methodological drawbacks. Among the instruments developed for measuring satisfaction in a community-based psychiatric service the VSSS seems to be the instrument of choice; more information on the performance of the VSSS in other community-based settings, presently under study, will be necessary to confirm the properties of this instrument.

As shown in Table 2, fourth column, two main instruments have been developed for measuring satisfaction in inpatient settings. The *Patient Opinion Survey,* developed by McDonald et al. (1988) and used later by Elzinga and Barlow (1991), has some validation and shows a good face validity; its main limit appears to be the dichotomous rating scale used, reducing sensitivity. The instrument proposed by Hansson et al. (1985) and Hansson (1989) shows good face validity, but validation is not reported. Further work is needed in this area.

Few instruments have been developed to assess relatives' satisfaction with psychiatric services, most research in this field having been conducted by analysing relatives' spontaneous reports. Among the few instruments developed, the VSSS, version for relatives, seems to be the only comprehensive and validated instrument for assessing relatives' satisfaction with community-based psychiatric services: The development of shorter versions for easier use in routine clinical work is in progress. The *Family Service Satisfaction Scale* developed by Grella and Grusky (1989), though being of some interest, appears very limited from the point of view of the content validity and has not been fully validated. An interesting instrument is the *Family Ser-*

vice Satisfaction, a 27-item scale derived from the SSS-30 for assessing relatives' satisfaction with residential facilities for severely ill patients (Greenfield and Attkisson 1989, unpublished report). Work in this area is clearly needed.

Conclusions and Future Perspectives

Compared to the state of the art in satisfaction research described in 1983 by Attkisson and Pascoe, the present review indicates steady progress and sensible improvement introduced during the last decade. Data available indicate that most of the reservations on the meaning and measurability of client satisfaction do not have a scientific basis. The capability of clients to judge service delivery has been demonstrated by various findings, and the value of measuring satisfaction (point 1 in the Introduction) should not be questioned any more. Some methodological questions have been clarified by recent studies, such as the stability of opinions expressed by consumers' (point 5 in the Introduction) and the fact that enquiring about consumers' satisfaction doesn't necessarily attenuate criticism if a correct methodology is applied (point 4 in the Introduction). The fact that satisfaction may be co-determined by clients' background and expectations (point 6 in the Introduction) has been demonstrated to be the case in some instances but, rather than being a reason for not considering satisfaction, seems instead to provide a theoretical justification for more penetrating analyses of the concept of satisfaction and its determinants. This review reveals more awareness today of the complexities of the theoretical definition and methodological problems affecting the measurement of satisfaction. A few attempts to develop instruments that can measure satisfaction correctly both in patients and relatives have been made. As Zastowny and Leeman (1988) have said "... The study of satisfaction with mental health services is just now entering a new era that promises a more integrate development similar to the progress seen earlier in medical care."

To make further progress more research on specific concerns in now indicated. Continued research should better define the measurement of satisfaction and clarify its theoretical and substantive meaning. Other work to clarify the correlation between satisfaction and other outcome and quality of care variables is urgently needed (point 2 in the Introduction). Whether satisfaction measurement is biased by other factors, such as, for example, knowing little of the alternatives available (point 3 in the Introduction), should be better ascertained. Moreover, today, as in 1983, considerable effort is needed in developing and spreading the use of validated instruments and discouraging the use of ad hoc measures. A problem still partially to be solved is the content validity of the measurement of clients' satisfaction with specific types of psychiatric services. Work should be done in order to more clearly define the dimensions that contribute to the domain of satisfaction according to differing perspectives, such as those of patients, relatives and professionals. Instruments should provide the basis for conducting a *multiaxial evaluation* of satisfaction so as to simultaneously consider the views of all these subjects. This seems to be a fundamental requisite in settings, such as in community-based psychiatric services where these subjects interact continuously.

The practise of developing ad hoc instruments should be replaced by the use of well-validated instruments that combine cross-setting and setting-specific items.

The same instruments, possibly selected among those indicated in this review that have already undergone some validation, should be preferred and used in different countries, in various settings and in subjects with various characteristics who have received various kinds of interventions. *Comparability* between studies should be pursued more vigorously. Results obtained on a large scale should then be reviewed again. Limits and advantages of the various instruments in the settings studied should then become clearer and this will allow both refinement of existing instruments or development of new instruments. In 1988, Zastowny and Lehman stated "... It may be said that the study of satisfaction with mental health services is still in its infancy, while the study of satisfaction with medical care has probably entered its early childhood". By undertaking this kind of collaborative research, we can reasonably expect mental health consumer satisfaction research to quickly grow to childhood too.

Acknowledgements. This work was carried out at the Servizio di Psicologia Medica, Universita' di Verona (WHO Collaborating Centre for Research and Training in Mental Health), Italy, directed by Professor M. Tansella and was supported by a Grant from the Minsitero dell'Universita' e della Ricerca Scientifica e Tecnologica (MURST, Roma), Fondi 60 %. I am grateful to Professor Tansella for his generous and continuous support, for his most valuable advice and for having revised the manuscript. I thank also Dr. Thomas Greenfield (Department of Psychiatry, University of California, San Francisco and California Pacific Medical Center Research Institute) for helpful advice and revision of the manuscript.

References

Allen H, Baigent B, Kent A, Bolton J (1993) Rehabilitation and staffing levels in a 'new look' hospital hostel. Psychol Med 23: 203–211

Andrews FM, Withey SB (1976) Social indicators of wellbeing: American perceptions of life quality. Plenum Press, New York

Andrews S, Leavy A, DeChillo N, Frances A (1986) Patient – therapist mismatch: we would rather switch than fight. Hosp Community Psychiatry 37: 918–922

Andrews G, Teesson M, Stewart G, Hoult J (1990) Follow-up of community placement of the chronic mentally ill in New South Wales. Hosp Cummunity Psychiatry 41: 184–188

Attkisson CC, Greenfield TK (1994) The Client Satisfaction Questionnaire-8 and the Service Satisfaction Questionnaire-30. In: Maruish M (ed) Psychological testing: treatment planning and outcome assessment. Lawrence Erlbaum Associates, San Francisco, pp 402–420

Attkisson CC, Pascoe GC (eds) (1983) Patient satisfaction in health and mental health services. Eval Program Plann 6. Special Issue. Pergamon Press, New York

Attkisson CC, Zwick R (1982) The Client Satisfaction Questionnaire: psychometric properties and correlation with service utilization and psychotherapy outcome. Eval Program Plann 5: 233–237

Azim HFA, Joyce AS (1986) The impact of data-based program modifications on the satisfaction of outpatients in group psychotherapy. Can J Psychiatry 31: 119–122

Bene-Kociemba A, Cotton PG, Fortgang RC (1982) Assessing patient satisfaction with state hospital and aftercare services. Am J Psychiatry 139: 660–662

Bennett MJ, Feldstein ML (1986) Correlates of patients satisfaction with mental health services in a health maintenance organization. Am J Prev Med 2: 155–162

Bennun I (1986) Evaluating family therapy: a comparison of the Milan and problem solving approaches. J Fam Ther 8: 225–242

Bernheim KF (1990) Promoting family involvement in community residences for chronic mentally ill persons. Hosp Community Psychiatry 41: 668–670

Brandon D (1981) Voices of experience: consumer perspectives of psychiatric treatment. MIND, London

de Brey H (1983) A cross-national validation of the client satisfaction questionnaire: the Dutch experience. Eval Program Plann 6: 395–400

Breyer P, Malafonte D (1983) Promoting community involvement in deinstitutionalization planning: the experience in one community. Hosp Community Psychiatry 33: 655–657

Bugge I, Hendel DD, Moen R (1985) Client evaluations of therapeutic process and outcomes in a university mental health center. Coll Health 33: 141–146

Bulow S, Sweeney JA, Shear MK, Friedman R (1987) Family satisfaction with psychiatric evaluations. Health Soc Work 12: 290–295

Burns T, Beadsmoore A, Bhat AS, Oliver A, Mathers C (1993) A controlled trial of home-based acute psychiatric services. I. Clinical and social outcome. Br J Psychiatry 163: 49–54

Carscaddon DM, George M, Wells G (1990) Rural community mental health consumer satisfaction and psychiatric symptoms. Community Ment Health J 26: 309–318

Conte HR, Plutchik R, Buckley P, Spence DW, Karasu TB (1989) Outpatients view their psychiatric treatment. Hosp Community Psychiatry 40: 641–643

Conway A (1983) Psychiatric management: change in the 1980s. Hosp Community Psychiatry 33: 310–311

Corrigan PW (1990) Consumer satisfaction with institutional and community care. Community Ment Health J 26: 151–165

Corrigan PW, Jakus MR (1993) The Patient Satisfaction Interview for partial hospitalization programs. Psychol Rep 72, 2: 387–390

Crowe M, Strathdee G, Sair A, Caan W (1993) Patients' satisfaction with psychiatric care. BMJ 307: 130

Damkot DK, Pandiani JA, Gordon LR (1983) Development, implementation, and findings of a continuing client satisfaction survey. Community Ment Health J 19: 265–278

Dean C, Philipps J, Gadd EM, Joseph M, England S (1993) Comparison of community based service with hospital based service for people with acute, severe psychiatric illness. BMJ 307: 473–476

Deiker T, Osborn SM, Distefano MR, Pryer NW (1981) Consumer accreditation: development of a quality assurance patient evaluation scale. Hosp Community Psychiatry 32: 565–567

Depp FC, Dawkins JE, Selzer N, Briggs C et al (1986) Subsidized housing for the mentally ill. Soc Work Res Abstr 22: 3–7

Distefano M, Pryer M, Baker B (1983) Factor structure of a clients' satisfaction scale with psychiatric inpatients. Psychol Rep 53: 1155–1159

Donabedian A (1966) Evaluating the quality of medical care. Mildbank Memorial Fund Q 44: 166–203

Dowds B, Fontana A (1977) Patients' and therapists' expectations and evaluations of hospital treatment. Compr Psychiatry 18: 295–300

Doyle B, Ware J (1977) Physician conduct and other factors that affect consumer satisfaction with medical care. J Med Educ 52: 793–801

Dyck RJ, Azim HF (1983) Patient satisfaction in a psychiatric walk-in clinic. Can J Psychiatry 28: 30–33

Eisen SV, Grob MC (1978) Assessing consumer satisfaction from letters to the hospital. Hosp Community Psychiatry 30: 344–346

Eisen SV, Grob MC (1992) Patient outcome after transfer within a psychiatric hospital. Hosp Community Psychiatry 43: 803–806

Elbeck M, Fecteau G (1990) Improving the validity of measures of patient satisfaction with psychiatric care and treatment. Hosp Community Psychiatry 9: 998–1001

El-Guebaly N, Toews J, Leckie A, Harper D (1983) On evaluating patient satisfaction: methodological issues. Can J Psychiatry 28: 24–29

Elzinga RH, Barlow J (1991) Patient satisfaction among the residential population of a psychiatric hospital. Int J Soc Psychiatry 37: 24–34

Ferguson B, Cooper S, Brothwell J, Markantonakis A, Tyrer P (1992) Clinical evaluation of a new community psychiatric service based on general practice psychiatric clinics. Br J Psychiatry 160: 493:497

Gersons B, vanDeGraaf W, Rijkschroeff R, Schramejer F (1992) The mental health care transformation process: the Amsterdam experience. Int J Soc Psychiatry 38: 50–58

Greenfield TK (1983) The role of client satisfaction in evaluating university counseling services. Eval Program Plann 6: 315–327

Greenfield TK, Attkisson CC (1989) Steps toward a multifactorial satisfaction scale for primary care and mental health services. Eval Program Plann 12: 271–278

Greenley JR (1984) Social factors, mental illness, and psychiatric care: recent advances from a sociological perspective. Hosp Community Psychiatry 35: 813–820

Greenley JR, Schulz R, Nam SH, Peterson RW (1985) Patient satisfaction with psychiatric inpatient care: issues in measurement and application. Res Community Ment Health 5: 303–319

Grella CE, Grusky O (1989) Families of the seriously mentally ill and their satisfaction with services. Hosp Community Psychiatry 40: 831–835

Grosser RC, Vine P (1991) Families as advocates for the mentally ill: a survey of characteristics and service needs. Am J Orthopsychiatry 61: 282–290

Hansson JG, Rapp CA (1992) Families' perceptions of community mental health programs for their relatives with a severe mental illness. Community Ment Health J 28: 181–195

Hansson L, Berglund M, Ohman R, Lihencrantz C, Andersson G (1985) Patient attitudes in short term psychiatric care. Relations to social and psychiatric background, clinical symptoms and treatment model. Acta Psychiatr Scand 72: 193–201

Hansson L (1989) Patient satisfaction with in-hospital psychiatric care. Eur Arch Psychiatry Neurol Sci 239: 93–100

Harkness D, Hensley H (1991) Changing the focus of social work supervision: effects on client satisfaction and generalized contentment. Soc Work 36: 506–512

Hersh JB, Lathan C (1985) The mental health walk-in clinic: the University of Massachusetts experience. J Am Coll Health 34: 15–27

Holden DF, Lewine RRJ (1982) How families evaluate mental health professionals, resources, and effect of illness. Schizophr Bull 8: 626–634

van Hoorn E (1992) Changes? What changes? The views of the European patients' movement. Int J Soc Psychiatry 38: 30–35

Hoult J, Reynolds I, Charbonneau-Powis M et al (1983) Psychiatric hospital versus community treatment: the results of a randomized trial. Aust N Z J Psychiatry 17: 160–167

Hoult J, Rosen A, Reynolds I (1984) Community orientated treatment compared to psychiatric hospital orientated treatment. Soc Sci Med 18: 1005–1010

Hulka B, Zyzansky L, Cassel J, Thompson S (1970) Scale for the measurement of attitudes toward physicians and primary health care. Med Care 8: 429–430

Huxley P, Warner R (1992) Case management, quality of life, and satisfaction with services of long-term psychiatric patients. Hosp Community Psychiatry 43: 799–803

Kalman T (1983) An overview of patient satisfaction with psychiatric treatment. Hosp Community Psychiatry 34: 48–54

Kiesler C (1983) Social psychological issues in studying consumer satisfaction with behavior therapy. Behav Ther 14: 226–236

Krulee DA, Hales RE (1988) Compliance with psychiatric referrals from a general hospital psychiatry outpatient clinic. Gen Hosp Psychiatry 10: 339–345

Jones EE, Zuppell CL (1982) Impact of client and therapist gender on psychotherapy, process, and outcomes. J Consult Clin Psychol 50: 259–272

Larsen D, Attkisson CC, Hargreaves W, Nguyen T (1979) Assessment of client/patient satisfaction: development of a general scale. Eval Program Plann 2: 197–207

Lebow JL (1982) Consumer satisfaction with mental health treatment. Psychol Bull 91: 244–259

Lebow JL (1983a) Client satisfaction with mental health treatment: methodological considerations in assessment. Eval Rev 7: 729–752

Lebow JL (1983b) Similarities and differences between mental health and health care evaluation studies assessing consumer satisfaction. Eval Program Plann 6: 237–245

Lehman AF, Zastowny TR (1983) Patient satisfaction with mental health services: a metanalysis to establish norms. Eval Program Plann 6: 265–274

Lemoine RL, Carney A (1984) The Louisiana mental health client-outcome evaluation project: an initial progress report. Community Ment Health J 20: 90–100

Lesage A, Pollini D (1989) A new schedule to assess relatives satisfaction with psychiatric services: preliminary results on a sample of relatives living with a mentally retarded young adult. New Trends Exp Clin Psychiatry 3: 151–159

Le Vois M, Nguyen TD, Atkisson CC (1981) Artifact in client satisfaction assessment: experience in community health settings. Eval Program Plann 4: 139–150

Lewine RR (1982) A dialogue among patients' relatives and professionals. Overview and reflections. Schizophr Bull 8: 652–654

Ley P (1982) Satisfaction, compliance and communication. Br J Clin Psychol 21: 241–254

Like R, Zyzanski J (1987) Patient satisfaction with the clinical encounter: social psychological determinants. Soc Sci Med 24: 351–357

Linder-Pelz S (1982a) Toward a theory of patient satisfaction. Soc Sci Med 16: 577–582

Linder-Pelz S (1982b) Social psychological determinants of patient satisfaction: a test of five hypotheses. Soc Sci Med 16: 583–589

Lindholm H (1983) Sectorized psychiatry. A methodological study of the effects of reorganization on patients treated at a mental hospital. Acta Psychiatr Scand 304: 1–127

Locker D, Dunt D (1978) Theoretical and methodological issues in sociological studies of consumer satisfaction with medical care. Soc Sci Med 12: 283–292

Long CG, Bourne V (1987) Linking professional and self-help resources for anxiety management: a community project. J R Coll Gen Pract 37: 199–201

Lorefice LS, Borus JF (1984) Consumer evaluation of a community mental health service, II: perceptions of clinical care. Am J Psychiatry 141: 1449–1452

Lorefive LS, Borus JF, Keefe C (1982) Consumer evaluation of a community mental health service, I: care delivery patterns. Am J Psychiatry 139: 1331–1334

Love RE, Caid CD, Davis A (1979) The User Satisfaction Survey: consumer evaluation of an inner city community mental health center. Eval Health Profession 2: 42–54

McDonald L, Sibbald B, Hoare C (1988) Measuring patient satisfaction with life in a long-stay psychiatric hospital. Int J Soc Psychiatry 34: 292–304

McDonald L, Ochera J, Leibowitz JA, McLean EK (1990) Community mental health services from the user's perspective: an evaluation of the Doddington Edward Wilson (DEW) mental health service. Int J Soc Psychiatry 36: 183–193

McPheeters HL (1984) Statewide mental health outcome evaluation: a perspective of two southern states. Community Ment Health J 20: 44–55

Mangen SP, Griffith JH (1982) Patient satisfaction with community psychiatric nursing: a prospective controlled study. J Adv Nurs 7: 477–482

Mangen SP, Paykel ES, Griffith JH, Burchell A, Mancini P (1983) Cost-effectiveness of community psychiatric nurse or out-patient psychiatrist care of neurotic patients. Psychol Med 13: 407–416

Mayer J, Rosenblatt A (1974) Clash in perspective between mental patients and staff. Am J Orthopsychiatry 44: 432–441

McGuire J, Borowy T, Kolin I (1986) Attitudes towards mental health professionals in a hospital-based community mental health center. Community Ment Health J 22: 39–48

Merson S, Tyrer P, Onyett S, Lack S, Birkett P et al (1992) Early intervention in psychiatric emergencies: a controlled clinical trial. Lancet 339: 1311–1314

Molde S, Diers D (1985) Nurse practitioner research: selected literature review and research agenda. Nurs Res 34: 362–367

Morgan SL (1989) Families' experiences in psychiatric emergencies. Hosp Community Psychiatry 40: 1265–1269

Nguyen TD, Attkisson CC, Stegner BL (1983) Assessment of patient satisfaction: development and refinement of a service evaluation questionnaire. Eval Program Plann 6: 299–314

O'Driscoll C, Wills W, Leff J, Margolius O (1993) The TAPS project. 10. The long-stay population of Friern and Claybury hospitals. The baseline survey. Br J Psychiatry 162: 30–35

Pascoe GC (1983) Patient satisfaction in primary health care: a literature review and analysis. Eval Program Plann 6: 185–210

Perkins RE, King SA, Hollyman JA (1989) Resettlement of old long-stay psychiatric patients: the use of the private sector. Br J Psychiatry 155: 233–238

Perreault M, Leichner P, Sabourin S, Gendreau P (1993) Patient satisfaction with outpatient psychiatric services: qualitative and quantitative assessments. Eval Program Plann 16: 109–118

Polowczyk D, Brutus M, Orvieto A, Vidal J, Cipriani D (1993) Comparison of patient and staff surveys of consumer satisfaction. Hosp Community Psychiatry 44: 589–591

Prager E, Tonaka H (1980) Self-assessment: the client' perspective. Soc Work 25: 32–34

Rees C (1990) Family satisfaction. Hosp Community Psychiatry 41: 201–202

Ricketts T (1992) Consumer satisfaction surveys in mental health. Br J Nurs 1: 523–527

Roberts R, Attkisson C, Mendias RM (1984) Assessing the Client Satisfaction Questionnaire in English and Spanish. Hispanic J Behav Sci 6: 385–396

Romeo TD, Mauch D, Morrison E (1990) A catalyst for change. The art of strategic mental health planning in Rhode Island. Am Psych 11: 1253–1256

Rothman GH (1984) Needs of female patients in a veterans' psychiatric hospital. Soc Work 29: 380–385

Ruggeri M, Dall'Agnola R (1993) The development and use of the Verona Expectations for Care Scale (VECS) and the Verona Service Satisfaction Scale (VSSS) for measuring expectations and satisfaction with community-based psychiatric services in patients, relatives and professionals. Psychol Med 23: 511–523

Ruggeri M, Dall'Agnola R, Agostini C, Bisoffi G (1994) Acceptability, sensitivity and content validity of VECS and VSSS in measuring expectations and satisfaction in psychiatric patients and their relatives. Soc Psychiatry Psychiatr Epidemiol 29: 265–276

Ruggeri M, Greenfield T (1995) The Italian version of the Service Satisfaction Scale (SSS-30) adapted for community-based psychiatric services: development, factor analysis and application. Evaluation and Program Planning 18: 191–202

Ruggeri M, Dall'Agnola R, Greenfield T, Bisoffi G (1996) Factor analysis of the Verona Service Satisfaction Scale-82 and development of reduced versions. International Journal of Methods in Psychiatric Research 6: 23–38

Sabourin S, Gendreau P, Frenette L (1987) Le neveau de satisfaction des cas d'abandon dans un service universitaire de psychologie. Can J Behav Sci 19: 314–323

Sheppard M (1993) Client satisfaction, extended intervention and interpersonal skills in community mental health. J Adv Nurs 18: 246–259

Silva EL (1990) Collaboration between providers and client-consumers in public mental health programs. New Dir Ment Health Serv 46: 57–63

Sishta SK, Rinco S, Sullivan JCF (1986) Clients' satisfaction survey in a psychiatric inpatient population attached to a general hospital. Can J Psychiatry 31: 123–128

Slater V, Linn MW, Harris R (1981) Outpatient evaluation of mental health care. South Med J 74: 1217–1219

Slavinsky AT, Krauss JB (1983) Two approaches to the management of long-term psychiatric outpatients in the community. Nurs Res 31: 284–9

Smylie JA, Calvert BL, Gerber GJ (1991) Program evaluation as a measure of a new approach to community psychiatric care. Quality Assurance Health Care 3: 247–255

Soelling ME, Newell TG (1983) Effects of anonymity and experimenter demand on client satisfaction with mental health services. Eval Program Plann 6: 329–333

Solomon P (1992) The closing of a state hospital: what is the quality of patients' lives one year post-release? Psychiatr Q 63: 279–296

Solomon P, Beck S, Gordon B (1988) Family member's perspectives on psychiatric hospitalization and discharge. Community Ment Health J 24: 108–117

Sorensen J, Kantor L, Margolis R, Galano J (1979) The extent, nature and utility of evaluating consumer satisfaction in community mental health centers. Am J Community Psychol 7: 329–337

Steinwachs DM, Cullum H, Dorwart RA, Flynn L et al (1992) Service systems research. Schizophr Bull 18: 627–668

Strupp HH, Wallach ML, Wogan M (1964) The psychotherapy experience in retrospect: a questionnaire survey of former patients and their therapists. Psychol Monogr 78: 11–18

Tansella M (ed) (1991) Community-based psychiatry: long term patterns of care in South-Verona. Psychological Medicine Monograph Supplement 19, Cambridge University Press, Cambridge

Tessler RC, Gamache GM, Fisher GA (1991) Patterns of contact of patients' families with mental health professionals and attitudes toward professionals. Hosp Community Psychiatry 42: 929–935

Thornicroft G, Gooch C, O'Driscoll C, Reda S (1993) The TAPS project. 9. The realiability of the Patient Attitude Questionnaire. Br J Psychiatry 162: 25–29

Urquhart B, Bulow B, Sweeney J, Shear K, Frances A (1986) Increased specificity in measuring satisfaction. Psychiatr Q 58: 128–134

Vicente B, Vielma M, Jenner AF, Mezzina R, Lliapas (1993a) Users' satisfaction with mental health services. Int J Soc Psychiatry 39: 121–130

Vicente B, Vielma M, Jenner AF, Mezzina R, Lliapas (1993b) Attitudes of professional mental health workers to psychiatry. Int J Soc Psychiatry 39: 131–141

Vousden M (1986) MIND conference: removing labels. Nurs Times 82: 48: 18–19

Ware JE (1981) How to survey patient satisfaction. Drug Intell Clin Pharm 15: 892–899

Ware JE, Davies AR (1983) Behavioural consequences of consumer dissatisfaction with medical care. Eval Program Plann 6: 291–298

Ware JE, Snyder MK (1976) Dimensions of patients' attitudes regarding doctors and medical care services. Med Care 13: 669–683

Ware JE, Davies-Avery A, Stewart AL (1978) The measurement and meaning of patient satisfaction: a review of the recent literature. Health Med Care Serv Rev 1: 1–15

Ware JE, Snyder MK, Wright WR, Davies AR (1983) Defining and measuring patient satisfaction with medical care. Eval Program Plann 6: 247–263

Westbrook RA, Oliver RL (1981) Developing better measures of consumer satisfaction: some preliminary results. In: Munroe KB (ed) Advances in consumer research (vol. 8). Association for consumer research, Ann Arbor, pp 150–168

Wood WD (1982) Do fees help heal? J Clin Psychol 38: 669–673

Wright RG, Heiman JR, Shupe J, Olvera G (1989) Defining and measuring stabilization of patients during 4 years of intensive community support. Am J Psychiatry 146: 1293–1298

Zastowny TR, Lehman AF (1988) Patient satisfaction with mental health services. Quality Revision Bull 14, 9: 284–289

CHAPTER 5

Instruments Measuring Family or Caregiver Burden in Severe Mental Illness

AART H. SCHENE, RICHARD C. TESSLER and GAIL M. GAMACHE

Abstract

The consequences of psychiatric disorders for family members, usually called family or caregiver burden, have been studied during the last 4 decades. During this period a variety of instruments have been developed to measure the impact of mental illness on family members, but not all instruments have been described systematically in the published literature. The authors review 21 instruments that have been used or developed during the last 10 years, including several that have not previously been reported. The protocols are described in terms of their method and comprehensiveness, precursors and theoretical foundations, and types of psychometric information available. The instruments are assessed for potential use as research tools, and also for application in routine clinical practice.

Introduction

Until the middle of this century, neither society nor psychiatry as the principal responsible discipline could offer people with severe mental illness much more than hospital care for periods ranging from months to years. The recognition of the detrimental effects of hospitalization and developments in psychopharmaceutical, psychotherapeutic and social treatments gave impetus to deinstitutionalization and opened doors to new approaches now associated with community psychiatry and community care.

Over the past 4 decades this movement away from hospital care has resulted in a great interest in the community adjustment of psychiatric patients (Weissman 1975, 1981). Treating the patient in the least restrictive environment and consumer empowerment have made social functioning and social performance important concepts, not only for patients, practitioners and researchers, but certainly also for family members and close relatives of patients (Fisher et al. 1990). Confronted with caregiving tasks taken away from them since the start of institutionalism in the early nineteenth century, family members have had to learn to cope again with the dysfunctional behavior inherent in most of the severe mental illnesses.

A. H. Schene
Academisch Ziekenhuis bij de Universiteit van Amsterdam, Academisch Medisch Centrum, Meibergdreef 9, 1105 AZ Amsterdam Zuidoost, The Netherlands

R. C. Tessler and G. M. Gamache
Social and Demographic Research Institute, Machmer, University of Massachusetts, Box 34830, Amherst, MA 01003-4830, USA

The adverse consequences of psychiatric disorders for relatives, known as family or caregiver burden, have been studied since the early 1950s for different reasons: at first, to determine the feasibility of discharging patients into the community; later, to refine the concept of caregiving, its content and its underlying structure; most recently, to measure burden as an outcome variable in program evaluations and controlled clinical trials (Schene et al. 1994). Although a number of instruments or scales have been developed to measure caregiver burden, there is still no standard instrument generally accepted within the scientific community. The application of burden measures in routine clinical settings, i.e., to screen for burden, to identify individual family members at risk, and to monitor changes in burden over time, is in its infancy.

The present article seeks to extend two earlier reviews of family burden instruments (Platt 1985; Schene 1990) by focusing on instruments in recent use, by using a broad net for identifying relevant instruments, and by discussing the suitability of these instruments for both routine clinical and research use. The protocols are described in terms of their method and comprehensiveness, precursors and theoretical foundations, and types of psychometric information available. The following instruments were not included in the review because to our knowledge they have not been used in the last 10 years, or because they have been superceded by other instruments that have built upon them and that are included in the current review: Grad and Sainsbury (1963, 1968), Pasamanick (1967), Hoenig and Hamilton (1966a,b), Spitzer et al. (1971), Test and Stein (1980), and Creer et al. (1982).

Family or Caregiver Burden

Caregiving refers to the relationship between two adult individuals who are typically related through kinship. One, the caregiver, assumes an unpaid and unanticipated responsibility for another, the care recipient, whose mental health problems are disabling and long-term in nature, with no curative treatment available. The care recipient is unable to fulfill the reciprocal obligations associated with normative adult relationships and the mental health problems are serious enough to require substantial amounts of care. What makes it burdensome is the addition of the caregiving role to the already existing family role (Gubman et al. 1987; Tessler et al. 1989; Gallop et al. 1991).

Although the concept is referred to as "family" burden, most studies have sampled primary "caregivers". Caregiver burden has a narrower perspective than family burden, which includes the consequences for family members other than the main caregiver, such as the interpersonal relations within the family, the consequences for children of patients, and the social network of the whole family.

Method

There are two reasons to contact researchers personally about their work in progress when the goal is to provide an up-to-date overview of instrument development in a specific area. First, there is a lag between the use of an instrument and the publication of results based upon it in scientific journals. This is a particular problem for researchers in countries where English is not the first language, and where language problems may further delay or inhibit publication. A second reason is that scientific journals are not eager to publish papers about instrument development, leaving researchers ignorant of important developments in instrumentation.

To address these issues we turned to family burden researchers to identify instruments available in English. We used our own personal knowledge of researchers in the field, identified others from the literature on family burden, and searched the database of the European Network for Mental Health Service Evaluation (ENMESH). This resulted in an original list of 96 names. A letter describing the purpose of this review article asked researchers if they were adapters or developers of family burden instrumentation, and also to name other persons who might be working in the area of family burden. This snow-ball sampling method resulted in 32 more names.

In order to build a database from which to systematically evaluate the instruments, the authors developed an 80-item Family Burden Researchers Questionnaire. Questionnaires were sent to 52 of the original 128 researchers that the authors believed had developed or adapted measures that could be shared with other researchers. When possible the original author was contacted. When the senior author was not available, a second author or an active current user was contacted and asked to complete the questionnaire. One additional questionnaire was filled in using published information (Morosini et al. 1991). Reminders were sent to all those receiving the questionnaire who did not respond within 4 weeks. Researchers were *not* sent a questionnaire if they failed to respond to the first letter, if they replied that they were not developers or adapters, or if they were using an instrument developed by someone already represented in the sample. Instruments developed primarily for use with caregivers other than those of the severely mentally ill (e.g., geriatric patients) were also excluded.

The final count of completed questionnaires received was 28. Of these, seven were eliminated: three were dropped because they were in too early a phase of development, two because they had not been used in the last 10 years, and two because they used already existing instruments without adaptation. Thus, the final sample consisted of 21 family burden instruments.

Results

Table 1 shows the names of the 21 instruments, as well as their developers and the year of the main reference(s) However, the instruments are listed according to the year in which they were first printed and/or included in a published report (see Table 4 for these years). The difference between the year the instrument was introduced and the year of the main reference exists because of the lag between instrument development and publication in scientific journals. Three instruments have not yet resulted in published reports. To the best of our knowledge this list represents the state of the art of burden measures that are currently in use or in advanced stages of development. For brevity of presentation, the numbers shown in Table 1 are used to identify specific instruments throughout the text and in the other tables.

Conceptual Issues and Content

Researchers were asked to describe the theoretical foundations underlying their measures and to check from a list of 20 the dimensions included in their instruments. All researchers considered burden to be a multidimensional concept (see Table 2). Some researchers considered patient symptoms and behaviors to be the origin of burden. Dysfunctional behavior results in disruption of household routine and in caregiving tasks for close relatives. Others suggested that caregiving may result in role strain because it is added to the culturally defined roles that define relationships between family members. Some researchers also referred to the stress research literature. They considered patients' dysfunctioning and its different consequences as chronic stressors with which family members must learn to cope. Standard neoclassical economic theory was the basis for a specialized instrument (no. 20).

Table 1. Family or caregiver burden instruments and main references

No.	Instrument	References
1.	Social Behaviour Assessment Schedule	Platt et al. (1980); Platt et al. (1983)
2.	Burden on Family Interview Schedule	Pai and Kapur (1981, 1982, 1983)
3.	Subjective Burden Scale	Potasznik and Nelson (1984)
4.	Family Distress Scale for Depression	Jacob et al. (1987)
5.	Scale for Assessment of Family Distress	Gopinath and Chaturvedi (1986, 1992)
6.	Family Burden Scale	Madianos et al. (1987); Madianos and Madianou (1992)
7.	Family Distress Scale	Birchwood and Smith (1992)
8.	Thresholds Parental Burden Scale	Cook and Pickett (1987)
9.	Family Members Perceptions of Enforced Psychiatric Institutionalization	Axelsson-Ostman (no references)
10.	Texas Inventory of Grief-Mental Illness Version	Miller et al. (1990)
11.	Family Burden Questionnaire	Fadden (1984); Fadden et al. (1987a, b)
12.	Significant Other Scale	Herz et al. (1991)
13.	Questionnaire for Family Problems	Morosini et al. (1991)
14.	Involvement Evaluation Questionnaire	Schene (1990); Schene and Van Wijn-gaarden (1992, 1993)
15.	Family Burden Interview Schedule	Tessler et al. (1992)
16.	Family Caregiving of Persons with Mental Illness Survey	Biegel et al. (1994)
17.	Family Burden and Services Questionnaire	Greenberg et al. (1993)
18.	Burden Assessment Scale	Reinhard et al. (1994)
19.	The Norwegian Family Impact Questionnaire	Sorensen (no references)
20.	Family Economic Burden Interview	Clark and Drake (1994)
21.	Impact of Mental Illness on Family/Household Members	Vine (no references)

A major theoretical distinction made by almost all researchers was that between objective and subjective burden. However, definitions of objective and subjective burden are implicit rather than explicit and operationalizations differ. The following approaches can be distinguished. Platt (no. 1) considers symptoms and dysfunctioning as objective and assesses the informant's distress (subjective burden) in relation to each particular problem or difficulty associated with the patient's illness. Gopinath (no. 5) and Tessler (no. 15) also use this approach. However, the latter also includes measures of subjective burden such as anger, depression, and embarrassment that are separate from measures of objective caregiving. Schene (no. 14) argues that burden should be measured objectively, i.e., how often do relatives have to perform caregiving tasks. Like Tessler, he measures distress, tension, and worrying, but not directly related to patient behavior. Pai (no. 2) measures subjective burden by one question: "How much would you say you have suffered owing to the patient's illness?" Reinhard and Horwitz (no. 18) consider subjective burden to be affective di-

Table 2. Dimensions assessed by family or caregiver burden instruments

Dimension									Instruments												
	1	2	3	4	5	6	7	8	9	10	11	12	13	14	15	16	17	18	19	20	21
Effect on:																					
Family interaction		+	+	+	+	+	+	+			+	+	+	+	+	+		+	+		+
Family routine		+	+	+	+	+	+	+	+		+	+	+	+	+	+	+	+	+	+	+
Leisure	+	+	+	+		+	+	+	+		+	+	+	+	+	+	+	+	+		+
Work/employment	+			+	+	+		+			+	+	+		+	+	+	+	+	+	+
Mental health	+	+	+	+	+	+		+	+	+	+	+	+			+			+		+
Physical health	+	+			+		+	+				+	+			+			+		+
Use of psychotropics						+						+	+								
Social network	+	+		+	+	+	+	+			+	+	+	+		+	+	+	+		+
Others outside household	+			+	+	+	+				+	+	+	+		+		+	+		
Children	+		+		+	+	+	+			+		+	+		+		+	+		+
Financial consequences	+	+		+	+	+	+				+	+	+	+	+	+	+	+	+	+	+
Helping the patient with ADL			+	+	+	+	+	+			+		+	+		+		+	+	+	+
Supervising the patient				+	+	+	+				+	+	+	+	+	+			+	+	+
Encouraging the patient						+	+	+					+	+		+		+	+	+	+
Distress	+	+	+	+	+		+	+	+	+	+	+	+	+	+	+	+		+		+
Stigma		+			+	+	+	+			+	+	+			+	+	+	+		+
Worrying	+	+	+	+	+	+	+	+	+		+	+	+	+	+	+	+	+	+		+
Shame		+			+	+	+				+		+	+		+	+		+	+	+
Guilt		+			+	+	+						+			+	+	+	+	+	+
Global burden		+	+		+	+	+	+				+	+		+	+		+		+	+
Total no. of dimensions	10	11	10	7	12	16	17	18	14	2	15	14	15	16	14	16	11	12	19	6	18

ADL, activities of daily living.

mensions subjectively felt such as shame, stigma, guilt, resentment, grief, and worry. The instruments developed by Axelsson-Ostman (no. 9) and Potaszik and Nelson (no. 3) only measure subjective burden.

Table 2 shows that some dimensions are included in almost all instruments. Worrying and the effect of patient's disorder on family routine are most frequently included ($n = 19$). Effects on leisure ($n = 18$), distress ($n = 18$), and financial consequences ($n = 17$) are also typical. Among the least frequently measured dimensions are use of psychotropics ($n = 3$), having to encourage the patient ($n = 9$), effects on the physical health of the caregiver ($n = 10$), and caregivers' feelings of guilt ($n = 10$) and shame ($n = 10$).

In the category "other" more than half of the researchers mention additional burden dimensions including: cognitive preoccupation (no. 8), feelings of loss and grief (no. 10), positive aspects of caregiving and knowledge about the illness (no. 11), problems with patients using alcohol or drugs, feeling threatened (no. 14), having to change personal plans for the future, and being upset about the change in the patient from his or her former self (no. 18).

The average number of dimensions is 13. These may be represented by a single item or by a fully developed scale. A measure of global burden is included in 62 % of the instruments. These may include a single general item, summary scales or cumulative indexes constructed from items, or interviewer assessments.

Another way to examine the structure underlying the burden concept is to use results from factor analyses (see Table 4). These results show some empirical basis for the dimensions of worrying, effect on family routine/interaction (tension, familial discord, disruption), care and control (supervision, urging, ongoing responsibility), behavioral problems, economic hardship, preoccupation (also emotional overinvolvement), distress, and stigma.

Specialized Instruments

Some instruments have been developed for specific purposes. Those of Jacob (no. 4) and Fadden (no. 11) have been designed in particular for family members of patients with depression. Cook's instrument (no. 8) has been developed for parents residing with chronically mentally ill offspring. Coverage includes parental feelings of connection to the ill child, preoccupation, and feelings of ongoing responsibility, among others. Axelsson-Ostman's instrument (no. 9) has a special aim, namely to interview relatives within a psychodynamic frame of reference about their experience in relation to enforced psychiatric institutionalization. Miller (no. 10) has adapted an instrument used to measure both initial and present symptoms of grief. In his view, families of the severely mentally ill undergo a syndrome of grief and mourning akin to that experienced by individuals suffering other forms of real or psychic loss. Finally, Clark (no. 20) has developed an instrument especially to measure economic burden. Costs are defined as direct dollar expenditures, time expended, and opportunities forgone.

Precursors and Influences

Table 3 summarizes the influence of older existing instruments on the development of new ones. The vast majority of burden instruments in current use are adapted or influenced at least in part by the work of earlier researchers. The instruments of Grad and Sainsbury (1963), Platt et al. (1980), Creer et al. (1982), Pasamanick et al. (1967), and Tessler et al. (1987) appear to have had the most influence. While some instruments were influenced by one or two precursors, others acknowledge multiple influences. The instruments developed by Schene (no. 14), Greenberg (no. 17), Reinhard (no. 18), and Vine (no. 19) give credit to a variety of sources.

How did researchers collect their items if not by using already existing instruments? Gopinath (no. 5) held open interviews with a number of relatives and chose the most frequent and important distressing behaviors. Cook (no. 8) used the work of Hatfield (1978, 1981), Hatfield and Lefley (1987) and Falloon et al. (1984). Axelsson-Ostman (no. 9) developed her items from clinical experience and Miller

Table 3. Instruments based on or influenced by other (earlier) instruments

Based on/influenced by	1	2	3	4	5	6	7	8	9	10	11	12	13	14	15	16	17	18	19	20	21
Freeman and Simmons (1958)																+	+			+	
Grad and Sainsbury (1963)	+	+	+										+			+	+			+	
Hoenig and Hamilton (1966a, b)	+												+								
Pasamanick et al. (1967)				+		+							+		+					+	
Spitzer et al. (1971)												+					+				
Test and Stein (1978)				+												+	+				
Platt et al. (1980)											+		+	+		+	+			+	
Pai and Kapur (1982)					+								+								
Thompson and Doll (1982)				+												+	+		+		
Creer et al. (1982)											+		+	+		+			+		
Fadden et al. (1987a, b)												+	+								
Coyne et al. (1987)													+							+	
Jacob et al. (1987)													+								
Tessler et al. (1987)													+			+	+		+	+	

(no. 10), as noted above, modified an already existing griefinstrument. Sorensen (no. 19) organized meetings with patients, relatives, and staff to aid in developing his instrument, and Morosini (no. 13) used the expressed emotion literature.

Structure and Psychometrics

Table 4 contains an overview of the instruments, country of origin, and most important psychometric characteristics. Twelve instruments are from the United States, 3 from the United Kingdom, 2 from India, and 1 each from Greece, Italy, Norway, Sweden, and the Netherlands. Nine instruments are self-administered questionnaires, of which three can also be used as personal interviews, three also as mail questionnaires, and one also as a telephone interview. Fourteen instruments can be used as personal interviews of which 9 can only be used as such, 2 can also be used as a telephone interview, and 3 also as self-administered questionnaires. One instrument can only be used as a telephone interview.

The 15 instruments using an interview format all require an interviewing background. Ten also require that the interviewers have a special background. Seven require knowledge of severe mental illness, and seven require a clinical background. For eight of the instruments the interviewers require special training, for four instruments a training guide is currently available (others are being developed), and for six instruments interviewer judgments or ratings are required.

The number of questions ranges from 19 to 300, with a mean of 73 (this does not include no. 21, the longest instrument, which did not provide an item count). One-third of the instruments have less than 30 questions. Most of the briefer instruments

Table 4. Psychometric characteristics of family or caregiver burden instruments

Instrument (year of publication)	Authors (country)	Number of questions / Completion time / Time frame / Type of instrument	Information available on					Subscale scores	Summary score	Factor analyses
			CV	IC	IR	TRR	SFC			
1. Social Behaviour Assessment Schedule (1980)	Platt, Weyman, Hirsch, Hewett (United Kingdom)	186 / 90 min / 4 weeks / SPI	0	0	+	+	0	+	0	0
2. Burden on Family Interview Schedule (1981)	Pai, Kapur (India)	28 / 25 min / No time frame / SSPI	+	+	+	0	+	+	+	0
3. Subjective Burden Scale (1983)	Potasznik, Nelson (USA)	20 / 20 min / No time frame / SAQ	+	+	n.a.	+	0	0	+	0
4. Family Distress Scale for Depression (1983)	Jacob, Frank, Kupfer, Carpenter (USA)	25 / 10 min / several weeks / SSPI	0	0	0	0	0	0	+	0
5. Scale for Assessment of Family Distress (1986)	Gopinath, Chaturvedi (India)	26 / 20 min / 4 weeks / SAQ, SSPI	+	+	+	+	0	+	+	six factors (data not yet reported)
6. Family Burden Scale (1987)	Madianos, Economou (Greece)	34 / 30 min / ? / SPI	0	0	+	+	0	+	+	0
7. Family Distress Scale (1987)	Birchwood, Smith (United Kingdom)	46 / 10 min / 4 weeks / SAQ	0	+	n.a.	+	+	+	+	0

Instrument	Authors (Country)	n / Time / Timeframe / Methods								Dimensions
8. Thresholds Parental Burden Scale (1988)	Cook, Pickett (USA)	29, 10 min, Current time, SAQ, SPI, SSPI	+	+	+	+	+	+	+	Feelings of connection, preoccupation, ongoing responsibility, behavioral problems, familial discord, worries
9. Family Members Perceptions of Enforced Psychiatric Institutionalization (1989)	Axelsson-Ostman (Sweden)	128, 60 min, Past month, SSPI	0	0	+	+	0	0	+	0
10. Texas Inventory of Grief-Mental Illness Version (1990)	Miller, Dworkin, Ward, Barone (USA)	24, 10 min, Current time, SAQ	+	0	n.a.	0	0	+	0	0
11. Family Burden Questionnaire (1990)	Fadden, Bebbington, Kuipers (United Kingdom)	95, 90 min, Not specified, SSPI	0	0	0	+	0	0	0	0
12. Significant Other Scale (1991)	Herz, Glazer, Mostert (USA)	50, 15 min, Last month, SPI	0	0	+	0	0	+	+	0
13. Questionnaire for Family Problems (1991)	Morosini, Rancone, Veltro Palombo, Casacchia (Italy)	72, 45 min, 4 weeks, SAQ, MQ	+	+	+	+	0	+	+	Objective and subjective burden, critical attitudes, emotional involvement, economic hardship
14. Involvement Evaluation Questionnaire (1992)	Schene, Van Wijngaarden (The Netherlands)	77, 30 min, 4 weeks, SAQ, MQ	+	+	n.a.	0	+	+	+	Tension, worrying, supervision, urging

Table 4. (Continued)

Instrument (year of publication)	Authors (country)	Number of questions Completion time Time frame Type of instrument	Information available on					Subscale scores	Summary score	Factor analyses
			CV	IC	IR	TRR	SFC			
15. Family Burden Interview Schedule (1992)	Tessler, Fisher Gamache (USA)	100 60 min 4 weeks TIS, SPI	+	+	0	0	+	+	+	Care, control, disruption
16. Family Caregiving of Persons with Mental Illness Survey (1992)	Biegel, Milligan (USA)	437 70 min No time frame SPI	+	+	0	0	0	+	+	Overall burden, family disruption, client dependency, stigma, strain
17. Family Burden and Services Questionnaire (1992)	Greenberg, Greenley, Benedict (USA)	300 90 min 4 weeks TIS	+	+	0	0	0	+	0	Subjective burden, worry, patient harming self, patient harming others, stigma, positive/negative feelings about involvement
18. Burden Assessment Scale (1992)	Reinhard, Horwitz (USA)	19 5 min 6 months SAQ, TIS, SPI	+	+	0	0	+	+	+	Disrupted activities, personal distress, time perspective, guilt, basic social functioning
19. The Norwegian Family Impact Questionnaire (1993/94)	Sorensen (Norway)	30 15 min Current time SAQ, MQ	0	0	n.a.	0	0	0	0	0

20. Family Economic Burden Interview (1993/94)	Clark, Drake (USA)	70	30 min	2 and 4 weeks	TIS, SPI	0	0	0	0	+	0	Different factors analyzed for each module
21. Impact of Mental Illness on Family/ Household Members (1993/94)	Vine, Stueve Streuning (USA)	437	120 min	4 weeks	SPI	+	+	0	0	+	0	

SAQ, self-administered questionnaire; MQ, mail questionnaire; TIS, telephone interview [structured]; TISS, telephone interview [semi-structured]; SPI, structured personal interview; SSPI, semi-structured personal interview; CV, construct validity; IC, internal consistency; IR, interrater reliability; TRR, test-retest reliability; SFC, sensitivity to change; n.a., not applicable; 0, not available.

contain caregiving burden questions only. The instruments with more than 70 questions also incorporate other nonburden items, e. g., asking about the patient, the family, the caregiver, social support, use of mental health services, opinions about mental health services, coping, and patients' contributions to the household.

Of the nine self-administered questionnaires, more than half have less than 30 questions and take 5–45 min to complete (the average is 18 min). The self-administered questionnaires of Morosini (no. 13) and Schene (no. 14) take the most time because they also gather information about the patient, the family, the household, contact with the patient, etc. Of the personal and telephone interviews, six have over 100 questions and take between 1 and 2 h to complete. Nine interviews take 30 min or less, with a mean of 37 questions.

For the majority of instruments the time frame is the past 4 weeks or 30 days, and for one it is 6 months. Approximately one-fourth use no time frame. For two others it is the "current time." In longitudinal studies, the time frames may vary from baseline to follow-up.

Table 4 also shows whether information is available about construct validity, internal consistency, interrater reliability (if applicable), test-retest reliability, and sensitivity to change. Slightly more than half of the researchers have information on construct validity and internal consistency. Of the six instruments that require interviewer ratings, four have information about interrater reliability. Of the 21 instruments, 7 have information about test-retest reliability and 5 have information about sensitivity to change. Ten instruments produce subscale scores, as well as a summary score, six only produce subscale scores, three only produce summary scores, and two produce neither. For eight instruments, subscale scores are probably associated with factor analyses.

Types of Studies, Diagnoses, and Kinship

Table 5 summarizes the type of studies that have been conducted until now using the instruments under review. A total of 17 instruments have been used in descriptive studies. Eight have been used in program evaluation, eight in randomized clinical trials, and four in both.

Regarding the type of patient populations in relation to which burden was measured, researchers' descriptions in the questionnaires were used. Most have studied family members of severely mentally ill patients. Neurotic patients have only been studied by two researchers. Another two only studied relatives of patients with affective disorders. Parents have been most often studied ($n = 13$), followed by siblings ($n = 11$), indicating a tendency to focus on the family of origin. Significant others, partners, and offspring have been studied less often.

Individual Instruments

In the following section, a summary description of each instrument will be given. Instruments are divided into two categories: suitable for research use only and suitable for both research and clinical use, according to the authors of the instruments. All 21 instruments are considered suitable for research use, while 13 are also considered suitable for clinical use.

Table 5. Conducted studies for each instrument: patient populations, caregivers, type of study, and suitability for research and clinical use

	Instruments																				
	1	2	3	4	5	6	7	8	9	10	11	12	13	14	15	16	17	18	19	20	21
Patient populations studied																					
Schizophrenia	+	+		+	+	+			+		+			+							
Psychosis	+													+							
Affective disorders		+		+	+				+	+				+							
Chronic patients	+	+																+			
Neurotic patients		+												+							
Severely mentally ill			+					+	+			+	+			+	+		+		
Generic									+				+	+						+	
Caregivers studied																					
Parents	+	+	+			+	+	+				+	+	+	+	+	+		+		
Siblings	+	+				+		+				+	+	+	+	+	+		+		
Partners								+		+		+	+	+	+	+			+		
Offspring		+						+				+	+	+		+			+		
Close relative					+						+	+	+	+			+			+	+
Most significant other				+	+		+														
Type of study																					
Exploratory/descriptive	+		+	+	+	+	+	+	+	+	+	+		+	+	+	+	+	+	+	+
Epidemiological																					+
Program evaluation	+	+		+	+	+									+		+	+			
Randomized clinical trial	+	+					+				+	+		+	+				+		
Others		+						+													
Instrument suitable for																					
Research use	+	+	+	+	+	+	+	+	+	+	+	+	+	+	+	+	+	+	+	+	+
Clinical use		+		+	+	+		+	+	+			+	+	+		+		+		+

Scales Suitable for Research Use Only

Social Behaviour Assessment Schedule (no. 1)

This interview, developed in the United Kingdom, is still widely used (we found at least six groups using this instrument), although the author himself is not active in the field any longer (personal communication to the senior author of the current review). This instrument is administered by trained interviewers, for whom a training guide is available, and information on interrater reliability is available. The instrument is comprehensive, and measures social behavior, as well as burden. For routine clinical use this interview might be too lengthy.

Subjective Burden Scale (no. 3)

This self-administered questionnaire is short and has good psychometric properties. It was designed to measure subjective burden in conjunction with Test and Stein's objective burden scale. It served as the basis for an article on stress and social support (Potaszik and Nelson 1984), but to our knowledge has not been adopted yet by other research groups.

Family Distress Scale (no. 7)

This self-administered questionnaire, developed in the United Kingdom, is an expanded version of Pasamanick's scale. It measures in particular subjective burden (Smith et al. 1993), and was designed for use with first-degree relatives of schizophrenic patients. It takes 10 min to complete and covers a large number of burden dimensions. The psychometric properties are well established.

Family Burden Questionnaire (no. 11)

This 95-item interview, developed in the United Kingdom, is one of two that concentrate especially on family members of patients with depression. It has been used effectively in descriptive studies. Psychometrics are not well established, but are currently under study and will be available soon. According to the author, the interview would probably be perceived as too long for routine clinical work.

Family Burden Interview Schedule (no. 15)

This 100-item structured personal interview was developed in the United States. It takes about 60 min to administer in person and can also be used as a briefer telephone interview as has been done in two follow-up assessments (Tessler and Gamache 1994). Interviewers do not need special background, and a manual is available describing the modular structure of the instrument. Some psychometric information is also available.

Family Burden and Services Questionnaire (no. 17)

This telephone interview was developed in the United States. Interviewers do not need special background, but have to be trained. It contains approximately 300 questions, of which some 57 are about burden. The other items measure attributions as to the cause of the illness, coping, opinions about mental health services, patient behavior, and client contributions to the family. The entire instrument takes 90 min to administer, of which about 45 min are devoted to burden. Factor analysis has resulted in a 6-factor structure, and information is available pertaining to reliability and validity.

The Norwegian Family Impact Questionnaire (no. 19)

This questionnaire was developed in Norway. It contains 79 questions of which 27 are about the type of treatment the family member thinks the patient needs and satisfaction with patient services. It was developed for long-term patients in the community and is now in field trials. Psychometrics are not yet known. The author states that it may also be suitable for clinical use.

Family Economic Burden Interview (no. 20)

This personal and/or telephone interview was developed in the United States. It contains 70 questions, and is the only instrument that is devoted mainly to economic burden. It has been used for relatives of people with severe mental disorder who also suffer from substance abuse. Its primary focus is on objective burden. This is a recently developed instrument, and psychometric information has not yet been reported.

Scales Suitable for Both Clinical and Research Use

Burden on Family Interview Schedule (no. 2)

This interview, developed in India, takes 25 min to administer, its psychometric properties are well established, and information about sensitivity to change is available. Interviewer ratings and special training are required. Developed in the early 1980s, this instrument has since then been used by a number of other researchers (e. g., Raj et al. 1991; Chakrabarti et al. 1992).

Family Distress Scale for Depression (no. 4)

This interview is based on Pasamanick's instrument, but has been greatly modified to assess the distress associated with depressive symptoms and behavior. It takes 10 min to complete. Its brevity and ease of administration are advantages for use in routine clinical practice. However, its comprehensiveness of coverage falls in the low end, and the psychometric properties are not well established.

Scale for Assessment of Family Distress (no. 5)

This self-administered questionnaire, a second Indian contribution to burden measurement, takes 20 min to complete. The scale focuses on the distress that psychotic symptoms and behavior produce in family members, rather than on the measurement of caregiving per se. It can also be used as an interview, for which interviewers require clinical background, but not special training. This scale has been used mainly in association with psychiatric patients, but a variant scale is available for patients with substance abuse disorders. Extensive psychometric analyses have been done. The scale, available in English, may soon be translated into Kanarese and Tamil.

Family Burden Scale (no. 6)

This instrument, developed in Greece, is a structured personal interview requiring 30 min to administer. It is designed for use with first-degree relatives of schizophrenic patients. Interviewers require clinical background but no special training. Some psychometric information is currently available, and the authors report that the scale is undergoing standardization. The authors also developed The Family Atmosphere Scale, which is a supplementary instrument (Madianos and Economou 1994).

Thresholds Parental Burden Scale (no. 8)

This 29-item self-administered questionnaire, developed in the United States, was designed to be used for parents of offspring with severe mental illness. Recently it has been used in analyses of the relationship of parental burden to race, age, residence, and stage in the life course. The psychometric properties are well established and will soon be available in the published literature (Cook et al. 1994; Pickett and Cook 1994; Pickett et al. 1994). The scale has also been administered to the parents of a sample of nondisabled, same-aged offspring.

Family Members Perceptions of Enforced Psychiatric Institutionalization (no. 9)

This personal interview, developed in Sweden, includes eight dimensions of burden, as well as measures of family attitudes toward mental health care in a general hospital. The instrument takes 60 min to administer, of which the burden items take about 40 min. The interview has been administered to parents, spouses, siblings, and adult children of both committed and voluntarily admitted psychiatric patients. Although information on interrater reliability is available, no other psychometric data are reported by the author.

Texas Inventory of Grief – Mental Illness Version (no. 10)

This 24-item self-administered questionnaire can be completed in 10 min. It concentrates on grief reactions of family members of persons with severe mental disorder. Although this is one of the least comprehensive burden instruments, it provides the most extensive measures of grief available. Separate subscale scores are produced for initial and present feelings about the relative's loss of mental health. Psychometric information is available pertaining to internal consistency and construct validity.

Significant Other Scale (no. 12)

This personal interview with family members whose relative is a patient with schizophrenia takes 15 min to administer. It is comprehensive and designed to generate separate scores for subjective and objective burden. The instrument has been used in a randomized trial, comparing intermittent and maintenance medication. Psychometric information is only available pertaining to interrater reliability.

Questionnaire for Family Problems (no. 13)

Developed in Italy for use in routine clinical practice, this comprehensive self-administered questionnaire takes 25–45 min to complete. It has been administered to a variety of relatives of recently admitted psychiatric patients at two points in time. Its psychometric properties are well established. Factor analysis has identified four factors (see Table 4).

Involvement Evaluation Questionnaire (no. 14)

This instrument was developed in the Netherlands initially to study the family impact of day hospitalization versus inpatient hospitalization (Schene 1987). It was subsequently revised to survey a large organization of relatives of patients with psychotic disorders. This 77-item instrument takes about 30 min to administer, and may be used as a self-administered or mail questionnaire. Psychometric properties are well established. Factor analysis has identified four factors (see Table 4). It also includes a distress scale and a separate section about children.

Family Caregiving of Persons with Mental Illness Survey (no. 16)

This structured personal interview was developed in the United States. It includes 53 burden items contained within a broader instrument that also measures client and caregiver demographic characteristics, client illness characteristics and behavioral problems, social network and social support, and health status. The burden items take 10 min to administer, while the larger instrument requires 70 min. It has been administered to a heterogeneous population of relatives of persons with mental illness. Extensive psychometric information is available, including results from factor analysis (see Table 4).

Burden Assessment Scale (no. 18)

This instrument, developed in the United States, can be administered as a personal interview and as a self-administered questionnaire. The 19 questions can be answered in 5 min. A 6-month time frame is recommended, which contrasts with the 4 weeks used in most other instruments. The instrument is appropriate for use with a variety of family members of the severely mentally ill, including, but not limited to, the primary caregiver. Psychometric information is available. Factor analysis has identified five factors (see Table 4).

Impact of Mental Illness on Family/Household Members (no. 21)

This is a structured personal interview that was developed in the United States. It is part of a family burden study funded explicitly for scale development. The instrument is organized as a series of 16 modules but only some deal directly with family burden. The senior author suggests that some modules are suitable for use in routine clinical settings. Psychometrics are not yet established but will be available in the future.

Discussion

Family or caregiver burden research has a history that begins after the second world war. During the last decade, however, the field has undergone rapid growth. Some years ago the first author was able to identify 12 burden instruments (Schene 1990). The current review identifies 21 instruments, not including 6 older instruments that are included in the last review. The emergence of 15 new family burden instruments indicates the growing importance accorded to burden within the mental health field. This scientific tradition continues in the United States and to some lesser extent in the United Kingdom. Not only were the "classic" scales developed in those two countries, but also most of the recent ones. However, we were able to identify five instruments from other European countries and two from India.

Researchers thus have 21 scales from which to make a selection. Since the authors of this review are each identified with their own burden instruments, we do not feel it is appropriate to recommend one instrument over another. In any case, the final choice of an instrument depends on a variety of considerations including the purpose(s) for which the study is being conducted. Depending on the research aims, the following should be considered as guidelines in making a selection.

If the purpose is to conduct a theoretical study linking burden with other constructs, then the following instruments may be relevant: nos. 1, 9, 11, 15, 16, 17, 19, and 21. If the purpose is to study the family burden associated with caring for a person with depression, then the following instruments should be considered: nos. 1, 4,

11, and 14. For those whose research interest is in studying relatives of persons with schizophrenia, the following instruments are appropriate: nos. 1, 5, 6, 7, 10, 12, and 14. For more general use with heterogeneous patient populations, researchers may find the following instruments useful: nos. 1, 2, 5, 9, 10, 14, 15, 16, 17, 18, and 21. For specialized studies when the focus is economic burden, no. 20 should be consulted. For studying grief reactions, no. 10 is appropriate. For measuring change in longitudinal studies, the following instruments should be considered as they have previously been used for this purpose: nos. 2, 7, 14, 15, 17, 20, and 21.

The section on individual instruments and Table 4 may also be useful in helping researchers to select an instrument that meets other specific requirements, such as time to administer, interviewer background, and method of administering. For example, if one knows in advance that a brief self-administered questionnaire is to be used, then this narrows down considerably the range of options. However, we recommend that researchers do not make final choices based on this review alone, but contact the authors of the instruments directly and obtain copies of their instruments before making a final choice. A list of addresses is available from the first author of this article upon request.

Morisini and his colleagues suggest that "family evaluation should not be performed only at specific requests for help, but offered routinely to families at the first contact with the patient." (Morisini et al. 1991). If we take this as a modus operandi, then the following criteria may be applied in choosing an instrument for clinical use: brevity and ease of administration, comprehensiveness of coverage, appropriateness for different types of patients and family members, and adequate psychometric properties. While a number of the instruments reviewed appear to meet these criteria rather well, and thus have potential use in routine clinical settings, it should be noted that the measurement of burden in routine clinical practice is relatively new. No authors have reported clinical norms or cutoff points that can be used to detect individual family members at risk from burden or to serve as a basis for clinical intervention for the family member.

Conclusions

Researchers more or less agree about the dimensions that comprise the family burden concept. There is less agreement with regard to definition of burden and how best to measure objective and subjective burden. These disagreements influence how specific dimensions are operationalized. Some burden researchers use single items denoting different aspect of burden as part of a summary scale, while others have turned to a modular approach with multi-item scales devoted to separate dimensions.

It is promising to see that some theoretical models describing the structure of burden or caregiving have recently been presented or published (Biegel et al. 1991; Schene 1990; Tessler et al. 1989, 1991). This is significant because the measurement of burden hinges largely on how it is conceptualized. Further research is needed to elaborate these models so that the theory and measurement of family burden are better integrated. The relationship between the characteristics of patient and caregiver, caregiving tasks, and the role of social and professional support needs further empirical and theoretical work.

In conclusion, although it is encouraging to see that the field is growing, this can end in a situation comparable to that of social support or social functioning research where there are too many instruments, and none that is really accepted as a standard measure. We believe that some standardization is needed and, therefore, recommend that burden researchers join and develop a few standard instruments with acceptable psychometric properties for both research and routine clinical use.

References

Biegel DE, Sales E, Schulz R (1991) Family caregiving in chronic illness. Sage Publications, London

Biegel DE, Milligan SE, Putman PL, Song L (1994) Predictors of burden among lower socioeconomic status caregivers of persons with chronic mental illness. In: Kahana E, Biegel D, Wykle M (eds) Family caregiving across the lifespan. Family caregiver applications series, vol 4. Sage Publications, Newbury Park CA, (in press)

Birchwood M, Smith J (1992) Specific and non-specific effects of educational intervention for families living with schizophrenia. Br J Psychiatry 160: 645–652

Chakrabarti S, Kulhara P, Verma SK (1992) Extent and determinants of burden among families of patients with affective disorders. Acta Psychiatr Scand 86: 247–252

Clark RE, Drake RE (1994) Expenditures of time and money by families of people with severe mental illness and substance use disorders. Community Ment Health J (in press)

Cook JA, Pickett SA (1987) Feelings of burden and criticalness among parents residing with chronically mentally ill offspring. J Appl Soc Sci 12: 79–107

Cook JA, Lefley HP, Pickett S, Cohler BJ (1994) Parental aging and family burden in major mental illness. Am J Orthopsychiatry (in press)

Coyne JC, Kessler RC, Tal M, Turnbull J, Wortman CB, Greden JF (1987) Living with a depressed person. J Consult Clin Psychol 55: 347–352

Creer C, Sturt E, Wykes T (1982) The role of relatives. In: Wing JK (ed) Long term community care experience in a London borough. Psychol Med [Monogr Suppl] 2: 29–39

Fadden GB (1984) The relatives of patients with depressive disorders: a typology of burden and strategies of coping. M. Phil Thesis, Institute of Psychiatry, University of London

Fadden G, Bebbington P, Kuipers L (1987a) The burden of care: the impact of functional psychiatric illness on the patient's family. Br J Psychiatry 150: 285–292

Fadden G, Bebbington P, Kuipers L (1987b) Caring and its burdens. A study of the spouses of depressed patients. Br J Psychiatry 151: 660–667

Falloon IRH, Boyd JL, McGill CW (1984) Family care of schizophrenia. Guilford Press, New York

Fisher GA, Benson PR, Tessler RC (1990) Family response to mental illness: developments since deinstitutionalization. Res Community Ment Health 6: 203–236

Freeman HE, Simmons OG (1958) Mental patients in the community. Family settings and performance level. American Sociological Review 22: 147–154

Gallop R, McKeever P, Mohide EA, Wells D (1991) Family care and chronic illness: the caregiving experience. A review of the literature. Faculty of Nursing, Toronto

Gopinath PS, Chaturvedi SK (1986) Measurement of distressful psychotic symptoms perceived by the family: preliminary findings. Indian J Psychiatry 28: 343–345

Gopinath PS, Chaturvedi SK (1992) Distressing behaviour of schizophrenics at home. Acta Psychiatr Scand 86: 185–188

Grad J, Sainsbury P (1963) Mental illness and the family. Lancet I 8: 544–547

Grad J, Sainsbury P (1968) The effects that patients have on their families in a community care and a control psychiatric service. Br J Psychiatry 114: 265–278

Greenberg JS, Greenley JR, McKee D, Brown R, Griffin-Francell C (1993) Mothers caring for an adult child with schizophrenia: the effects of subjective burden on maternal health. Fam Relations 42: 205–211

Gubman GD, Tessler RC (1987) The impact of mental illness on families. J Fam Issues 8: 226–245

Gubman GD, Tessler RC, Willis G (1987) Living with the mentally ill: factors affecting household complaints. Schizophr Bull 13: 727–736

Hatfield A (1978) Psychological costs of schizophrenia to the family. Soc Work 23: 355–359

Hatfield AB (1981) Coping effectiveness in families of the mentally ill: an exploratory study. J Psychiatr Treat Eval 3: 11–19

Hatfield AB, Lefley HP (1987) Families of the mentally ill. Coping and adaptation. Cassell, London

Herz MI, Glazer W, Mostert M (1991) Intermittent vs maintenance medication in schizophrenia. Arch Gen Psychiatry 48: 333–339

Hoenig J, Hamilton MW (1966 a) The schizophrenic patient in the community and the effect on the household. Int J Soc Psychiatry 26: 165–176

Hoenig J, Hamilton MW (1966 b) The burden on the household in an extramural psychiatric service. In: Freeman HL, Farndale WAJ (eds) New aspects of the mental health services. Pergamon Press, Oxford, pp 612–635

Jacob M, Frank E, Kupfer DJ, Carpenter LL (1987) Recurrent depression: an assessment of family burden and family attitudes. J Clin Psychiatry 48: 395–400

Madianos MG, Economou M (1994) Schizophrenia and family rituals: measuring family rituals among schizophrenics and normals. Eur Psychiatry (in press)

Madianos M, Madianou D (1992) The effects of long-term community care on relapse and adjustment of persons with chronic schizophrenia. Int J Ment Health 21: 37–49

Madianos M, Gournas G, Tomaras V, Kapsali A, Stefanis C (1987) Family atmosphere on the course of chronic schizophrenia treated in a community mental health center; a prospective-longitudinal study. In: Stefanis C, Rabavilas A (eds) Schizophrenia: recent biosocial developments. Human Sciences Press, New York, pp 246–256

Miller F, Dworkin J, Ward M, Barone D (1990) A preliminary study of unresolved grief in families of seriously mentally ill patients. Hosp Community Psychiatry 41: 1321–1325

Morosini P, Roncone R, Veltro F, Palomba U, Casacchia M (1991) Routine assessment tool in psychiatry: a case of questionnaire of family attitudes and burden. Ital J Psychiatry Behav Sci 1: 95–101

Pai S, Kapur RL (1981) The burden on the family of a psychiatric patient; development of an interview schedule. Br J Psychiatry 138: 332–335

Pai S, Kapur RL (1982) Impact of treatment intervention on the relationship between dimensions of clinical psychopathology, social dysfunction and burden on the family. Psychol Med 12: 651–658

Pai S, Kapur RL (1983) Evaluation of home care treatment for schizophrenic patients. Acta Psychiatr Scand 67: 80–88

Pasamanick B, Scarpitti FR, Dinitz S (1967) Schizophrenics in the community; an experimental study in the prevention of hospitalization. Appleton-Century-Crofts, New York

Pickett SA, Cook JA (1994) Caregiving burden experienced by parents of offspring with severe mental illness: the impact of off-timedness. J Appl Soc Sci (in press)

Pickett SA, Vraniak DA, Cook JA (1994) Strength in adversity: blacks bear burden better than whites. Professional psychology; research and practice, vol 24, issue 4. (in press)

Platt S (1985) Measuring the burden of psychiatric illness on the family: an evaluation of some rating scales. Psychol Med 15: 383–393

Platt S, Weyman A, Hirsch S, Hewett S (1980) The Social Behaviour Assessment Schedule (SBAS); rationale, contents, scoring and reliability of a new interview schedule. Soc Psychiatry 15: 43–55

Platt S, Weyman A, Hirsch S (1983) Social Behaviour Assessment Schedule (SBAS, 3rd edn). NFER-Nelson, Windsor, Berkshire

Potasnik H, Nelson G (1984) Stress and social support. The burden experienced by the family of a mentally ill person. Am J Community Psychol 12: 589–607

Raj L, Kulhara P, Avasthi A (1991) Social burden of positive and negative schizophrenia. Int J Soc Psychiatry 37: 242–250

Reinhard S, Gubman G, Horwitz A, Minsky S (1994) Burden assessment scale for families of the seriously mentally ill. Eval Program Plann (in press)

Schene AH (1987) The burden on the family scale. Department of Ambulatory and Social Psychiatry, University of Utrecht, Utrecht

Schene AH (1990) Objective and subjective dimensions of family burden. Toward an integrative framework for research. Soc Psychiatry Psychiatr Epidemiol 25: 289–297

Schene AH, van Wijngaarden B (1992) The Involvement Evaluation Questionnaire. Department of Psychiatry, University of Amsterdam, Amsterdam

Schene AH, van Wijngaarden B (1993) Familieleden van mensen met een psychotische stoornis; een onderzoek onder Ypsilonleden. (Family members of people with a psychotic disorder; a study among members of Ypsilon). Department of Psychiatry, University of Amsterdam, Amsterdam

Schene AH, Tessler RC, Gamache GM (1994) Caregiving in severe mental illness; conceptualization and measurement. In: Knudsen HC, Thornicroft G (eds) Mental health service evaluation. Cambridge University Press, Cambridge, (in press)

Spitzer RL, Giboon M, Endicott J (1971) Family Evaluation Form. New York State Department of Mental Hygiene, New York

Smith J, Birchwood M, Cochrane R, George S (1993) The needs of high and low expressed emotion families: a normative approach. Soc Psychiatry Psychiatr Epidemiol 28: 11–16

Tessler RT, Gamache G (1994) Continuity of care, residence, and family burden in Ohio. Milbank Q (in press)

Tessler RC, Killian LM, Gubman GD (1987) Stages in family response to mental illness: an ideal type. Psychosoc Rehabil J 10: 3–16

Tessler R, Fisher G, Gamache G (1989) A role strain approach to the measurement of family burden: the properties and utilities of a new scale. Paper presented at the Annual Meetings of the Eastern Sociological Society, Baltimore

Tessler R, Fisher G, Gamache G (1991) Conceptualizing and measuring the burden of caregiving on families of the severely mentally ill. Social and Demographic Research Institute, University of Massachusetts, Amherst

Tessler RC, Fisher GA, Gamache GM (1992) The Family Burden Interview Schedule; Manual. Social and Demographic Research Institute, University of Massachusetts, Amherst

Test MA, Stein LI (1978) Alternatives to mental hospital treatment. Plenum Press, New York

Test MA, Stein LI (1980) Alternative to mental hospital treatment: III social cost. Arch Gen Psychiatry 37: 409–412

Thompson EH, Doll W (1982) The burden of families coping with the mentally ill; an invisible crisis. Fam Relations 31: 379–388

Weissman MM (1975) The assessment of social adjustment. A review of techniques. Arch Gen Psychiatry 32: 357–365

Weissman MM (1981) The assessment of social adjustment. An update. Arch Gen Psychiatry 38: 1250–1258

Measures of Quality of Life Among Persons with Severe and Persistent Mental Disorders

ANTHONY F. LEHMAN

Abstract

In order to provide clinicians, researchers, program evaluators, and administrators with current information on the assessment of humanistic outcomes of services for persons with severe and persistent mental illnesses (SPMI), the literature on measuring quality of life (QOL) for these persons is summarized. The literature on QOL assessment procedures up to the end of October 1992 for persons with SPMI is reviewed, covering QOL measures that at a minimum assess subjective well-being. Measures are summarized according to purpose, content, psychometric properties, patient subgroups with whom used, and key references. Ten QOL measures are summarized and reflect considerable variability on the parameters examined. Comprehensive, reliable, and valid measures of QOL are available although further development of QOL assessment methodologies is needed. More importantly, we must strive for a better understanding of how to interpret and use QOL outcome information.

Introduction

The broad impact that severe and persistent mental illnesses have on persons' lives and the resulting complexity of the needs generated by such illnesses pose a particular challenge in the assessment of the outcomes of services for these persons [1, 2]. Relevant outcome domains include psychiatric symptoms, functional status, access to resources and opportunities, subjective well-being, family burden, and community safety. Because of this broad array of relevant outcomes and because of a prevailing concern that outcome assessments should include the patient's perspective, there has been increased attention paid over the past decade to the development of measures of patient "quality of life". This report summarizes these measures of humanistic outcomes or quality of life (QOL) that have been developed specifically for persons with severe and persistent mental illnesses.

Before describing the measures that are reviewed, it is important to acknowledge those that are not. "Humanistic" is a broad term and conceptually could cover all outcome measures, including measures of clinical symptoms and functional status. Indeed, a recent review in *Medical Care* (vol. 28, no. 12, 1990) of QOL measures for general medical conditions includes many such measures. However, many of these measures are reviewed elsewhere in this issue or have been reviewed previously [3–

Department of Psychiatry, University of Maryland, Center for Mental Health Services Research, 645 West Redwood Street, Baltimore, MD 21201, USA

5]. Therefore, they are not included in this review. Also excluded are measures of such concepts as "family burden" and client satisfaction with services, because these are considered not to be patient outcomes per se.

Rather, the measures reviewed here are those that emphasize the patient's QOL, that is, measures covering patients' perspectives on what they have, how they are doing, and how they feel about their life circumstances. At a minimum, QOL covers persons' sense of well-bring; often it also includes how they are doing (functional status) and what they have (access to resources and opportunities). The measures selected for this review were identified in the literature on QOL up to the end of October 1992. In order to be selected a measure had to at least assess the domain of subjective well-being; as will be seen, most of these measures also cover the broad areas of functioning and resources.

In the first section, each measure is described. The subsequent section includes summary tables describing the measures, their contents, psychometric properties, the populations with whom they have been used, and an instrument-specific bibliography. The final section discusses needs for future measure development and the potential utility of QOL assessments for planning and evaluating services.

Description of the measures

(In order of chronological development; Tables 1–3)

Standardized Social Schedule

The Standardized Social Schedule (SSS; Clare and Cairns, 1978) was developed in London to assess the nature and extent of social maladjustment and dysfunction in patients attending their family doctors' surgery. This semistructured interview is administered to the patient (and key informant, if available) by a trained interviewer, and item ratings are completed by both interviewer judgment and respondent self-report. The interview consists of 48 items and its administration requires approximately 45 min. A manual to guide administration is available.

The SSS covers six major life areas: Housing; Occupation/social role; Economic situation; Leisure/social activities; Family and domestic relationships; Marital situation. For each area the interview asks about (a) material conditions (what the person has), (b) social management (what the persons does), and (c) satisfaction (how the person feels about it).

The individual items can be combined in a variety of ways to produce summary scales, and individual items can also be used separately. Summary scales are computed as the number of items within a designated set of items that are scored as either "marked or severe difficulties" or "dissatisfaction". Summary scales include Overall, Material conditions, Social management, and Satisfaction. Individual items include: Extent of leisure activities; Housing conditions; Occupational stability; Family income; Household care; Housekeeping; Quality of relations with workmates, neighbors and family; Marital relationship quality; Extent of social activities; Satisfaction with housing, work, income, leisure, social relationships, family relationships, parental role, and marriage; Residential stability; Opportunities for leisure and social activities; Interaction with neighbors and relatives.

Table 1. Description and psychometric properties of humanistic outcome measures

Measure	Type	Length (min)	Reliability	Validity	Manual
Standardized Social Schedule	Semistructured interview (IR/SR)	45	+	+	Y
Community Adjustment Form	Semistructured interview (SR)	45	NA	NA	N
Quality of Life Checklist	Semistructured interview/ checklist (IR)	60	NA	NA	N
Satisfaction with Life Domains Scale	Structured interview (SR)	10	NA	+ / –	N
Oregon Quality of Life Scale	Structured interview (SR)	45	+	+	Y
Lehman Quality of Life Interview	Structured interview (SR)	45	+	+	Y
Quality of Life Scale	Semistructured interview (IR)	45	+	NA	N
Client Quality of Life Interview	Structured interview (SR)	30	NA	–	N
Well-Being Project Client Interview	Structured interview/ques- tionnaire (SR)	?	NA	NA	N
Lancashire Quality of Life Profile	Structured interview (SR)	55	+	+	Y

IR, interviewer-rated; SR, self report; Y, yes; N, no; NA, not available

Interrater K_w on items range from 0.55 to 0.94 (median = 0.76) and interrater agreement ranges from 64% to 100% (median = 82%). The factor structure is *not* stable across study populations, however. The interview differentiated as predicted across three populations studied. The three patient populations included: (a) 48 non-psychiatric patients referred by their doctors because of "adverse" social circumstances, (b) 221 patients with "chronic neurotic illnesses", and (c) 104 women with premenstrual complaints. Of the 373 patients included, 79% were women, 41% were 45 years of age or less, and ethnicity was not specified. Data are presented mainly as frequencies of persons scoring in the maladaptive range on various items across populations.

Community Adjustment Form

The semistructured self-report interview, Community Adjustment Form (CAF; Stein and Test, 1980) was developed to assess life satisfaction and other QOL outcomes in a randomized study of an experimental system of community-based care for the severely mentally ill versus standard care in Dane County, Wisconsin. It consists of 140 items and takes approximately 45 min to complete.

The areas assessed include: Leisure activities; Quality of living situation; Employment history and status; Income sources and amounts; Free lodging and/or meals;

Table 2. Content areas covered by the humanistic outcome measures

Measure	Subjective wellbeing	Resources and opportunities	Functional status	Other
Standardized Social Schedule	Overall satisfaction; Satisfaction with housing, work, income, leisure, social relations, family relations, parental role, marriage	Overall material conditions; Housing conditions; Family income; Residential stability; Opportunities for leisure and social activities	Overall social management; Extent of leisure activities; Household care; Housekeeping; Quality of relations with workmates, neighbors, and family; Marital relationship quality; Extent of social activities; Interaction with neighborhood and relatives	
Community Adjustment Form	Life satisfaction scale	Quality of living situation; Income sources and amounts; Free lodging and/or meals; Medical care; Agency utilization	Leisure activities; Employment history and status; Contact with friends; Family contact; Legal problems	
Quality of Life Checklist	Psychological dependency; Inner experience	Housing standard; Medical care; Religion; Vocational rehabilitation; Economic dependency	Leisure activities; Work; Relationships	Knowledge and education
Satisfaction with Life Domains Scale	Overall satisfaction; Satisfaction with housing, neighborhood, food, clothing, health, people, lived with, friends, family, relationships with other people, work/day programming, spare time, fun, services and facilities in the area, economic situation, place lived in now			
Oregon Quality of Life Questionnaire	Psychological distress; Psychological well-being; Tolerance of stress	Total basic need satisfaction; Social support	Independence; Interpersonal interactions; Spouse role; Work at home; Employability; Work on the job; Meaningful use of time	Negative consequences of alcohol use and drug use

Measure				
Lehman Quality of Life Interview	Global life satisfaction; Satisfaction with living situation, daily activities, family relations, social relations, finances, work, safety, health, (religion, neighborhood)	Residential stability; Hopelessness; Quality of living circumstances; Monthly spending money; Adequacy of financial supports; Victim of crimes	Leisure activities; Frequency of family contacts; Frequency of social contacts; Current employment status; Nights in jail	
Quality of Life Scale	Intrapsychic foundations; Sense of purpose; Motivation; Curiosity; Anhedonia; Empathy; Emotional interaction; Work satisfaction	Possession of commonplace objects	Interpersonal relations; Instrumental role; Occupational role; Work functioning; Work level; Interpersonal relations; Aimless inactivity	
Client Quality of Life Interview	Peace of mind	Essentials of life; Job training and education; Privacy; Social supports	Daily activities and recreation; Social time; Selfreliance	
Well-being Project Client Interview	Well-being quotient			
Lancashire Quality of Life Profile	General wellbeing; Satisfaction with work, leisure, religion, finances, living situation, family relations, social relations, health	Living circumstances (independence, comfort, influence); Safety	Leisure activities; Employment status; Family relations; Social contacts; Health status; Religious activity	Self-concept

Contact with friends; Family contact; Legal problems; Life satisfaction (21 items); Self-esteem (Rosenberg scale); Medical care; agency utilization. No psychometric properties are reported.

The original patient sample studied included 130 patients seeking admission to a state hospital. Over half were men (55%), and their mean age was 31 years. Half carried a diagnosis of schizophrenia. They were treated both in the state hospital and in a community-based assertive community treatment program. The results of the original Wisconsin study have been replicated in Australia using the same measures [8].

Quality of Life

The Quality of Life Checklist (QLC; Malm et al., 1981) checklist was developed to provide information about which aspects of QOL are particularly important to patients and clinician raters to assist in therapeutic planning. This 93-item rating scale is completed by a trained interviewer after a 1-h semistructured interview. Scoring for all areas assessed is dichotomized as "satisfactory" or "unsatisfactory". The areas assessed include: Leisure activities; Work; Vocational rehabilitation; Economic dependency; Social relationships; Knowledge and education; Psychological dependency; Inner experience; Housing standard; Medical care (psychiatric and general); Religion.

No psychometric properties are reported. Data analyses report simple frequencies of *"satisfactory"* vs *"unsatisfactory"* by items. The patients studied included 40 persons with chronic schizophrenia in a Swedish outpatient clinic. They ranged in age from 18 to 50 years, and 68% were men.

Satisfaction with Life Domains Scale

The Satisfaction with Life Domains Scale (SLDS; Baker and Intagliata 1982) was developed to evaluate the impact of the Community Support Program in New York State on the quality of life of chronically mentally ill patients. It is a self-report scale administered by a trained interviewer; it consists of 15 items and takes approximately 10 min to administer. Its individual items cover: Satisfaction with housing, neighborhood, food to eat, clothing, health, people lived with, friends, family, relations with other people, work/day programming, spare time, fun, services and facilities in area, economic situation, and place lived in now compared with state hospital. These can be summed into a total life satisfaction score.

The total life satisfaction score correlates at $r = 0.64$ with the Bradburn Affect Balance Scale and at $r = 0.29$ with the Global Assessment Scale. No other psychometric data are provided. The frequencies and means on these items can be compared with item scores in a national QOL survey of the general population [11].

The patients studied included 118 chronically mentally ill outpatients aged 18–86 years in two community support programs. They had a mean age of 53.3 years, 61% were women, and 84% lived in supervised residential settings. Diagnoses included schizophrenia (56%), affective disorders (14%), substance use disorders (5%), and organic mental syndromes (3%).

Table 3. Populations studied with humanistic outcome measures

Measure	Women	Men	Caucasian group	Minority groups	Age (years)	Types of patients	Nonmental comparison
Standardized Social Schedule	Y	Y	NA	NA	18–65 +	Outpt, CMI	Y
Community Adjustment Form	Y	Y	NA	NA	31 (mean)	Inpt/outpt CMI, schiz	N
Quality of Life Checklist	Y	Y	NA	NA	18–50	Outpt, schiz	N
Satisfaction with Life Domains Scale	Y	Y	NA	NA	53 (mean)	CMI, schiz, outpt	Y
Oregon Quality of Life	Y	Y	Y	?	34 (mean)	Outpt, CMI	Y
Lehman Quality of Life	Y	Y	Y	Y	18–65	Inpt/outpt CMI	Y
Quality of Life Scale	Y	Y	Y	Y	29 (mean)	Outpt, schiz	N
Client Quality of Life Interview	Y	Y	Y	Y	41.5 (mean)	Outpt, CMI	N
Well-Being Project Client Interview	Y	Y	Y	Y	35 (median)	Outpt/inpt CMI	N
Lancashire Quality of Life Profile	Y	Y	Y	NA	NA	Outpt, CMI	N

inpt, inpatient; outpt, outpatient; schiz, schizophrenic; CMI, chronic mental illness; N, no; Y, yes; NA, not available.

Oregon Quality of Life Questionnaire

The Oregon Quality of Life Questionnaire (OQLQ; Bigelow et al., 1982, 1991) was originally developed based upon the Denver Community Mental Health Scale and has undergone a series of developments since 1981. The original purpose of the OQLQ was to assess QOL outcomes among clients served by community mental health programs, especially those developed under the NIMH Community Support Program (CSP) initiative. Originally published in 1982, the OQLQ has recently been updated by its developer with more recent psychometric data, alternative versions, and further program applications.

The OQLO exists in two versions: a structured self-report interview (263 items) and a semistructured interviewer-rated interview (146 items). Both are administered by a trained (not necessarily clinical) interviewer. The theory underlying the OQLQ states that QOL derives from the social contract between an individual and society. Individuals' *needs* are met to the extent that persons fulfill the *demands* placed upon them by society. Most of the items use fixed, ordinal response categories, and the interview takes approximately 45 min to administer.

The OQLQ yields 14 scale scores: Psychological distress; Psychological well-being; Tolerance of stress; Total basic need satisfaction; Independence; Interpersonal interactions; Spouse role; Social support; Work at home; Employability; Work on the job; Meaningful use of time; Negative consequences of alcohol use; Negative consequences of drug use.

The psychometric properties of the OQLQ have been evaluated extensively. Cronbach's alpha for the 14 scales on the self-report interview versions ranges from 0.05 to 0.98, with a median of 0.84. Eight of the scales have excellent reliability (alpha > 0.8), two have intermediate reliability (alpha between 0.8 and 0.4), and four have poor reliability (< 0.4). Test-retest reliabilities (interval not specified) range from 0.37 to 0.64 with a median of 0.50. The interrater reliability for the interviewer-rated version has been assessed in a small sample study ($n = 6$) and has produced interrater agreement levels between 58% and 100% on the interviewer judgments. More than half of the items showed greater than 90% agreement, and Cronbach alpha ranged from 0.32 to over 0.80 (more than half over 0.80).

The predictive validity of the OQLQ has been evaluated by comparing; (a) clients in different types of community mental health programs (CSP, drug, alcohol, and general psychiatric clinics), (b) general community respondents from economically distressed and nondistressed communities, and (c) changes in community mental health clients over time. Results of these analyses support the overall predictive validity of the OQLQ.

The OQLQ has been applied to outpatients of mental health programs, as well as to samples of the general population. The outpatient samples included patients at intake to community mental health programs in Oregon (including chronically mentally ill patients, drug abusers, alcoholics, and general psychiatric patients). Their mean age was 33.8 years (range 18–85) and included 60% men and 96% "non-Hispanics". The community sample had 43% men, with a mean age of 36.8, and was 92% non-Hispanic.

Lehman Quality of Life Interview

The overall purpose of the Lehman Quality of Life Interview (QOLI; 1982, 1988 [1]) is to assess the life circumstances of persons with severe mental illnesses both in terms of what they actually do and experience ("objective" QOL) and their feelings about these experiences ("subjective" QOL). The interview provides a broad-based assessment of the recent and current life experiences of the respondent in a wide variety of life areas of potential interest, including living situation, family relations, social relations, leisure activities, finances, safety and legal problems, work and school, and health (as well as religion and neighborhood in some versions).

The QOLI is a structured self-report interview administered by trained lay interviewers. It consists of 143 items and takes approximately 45 min to administer. It has undergone a variety of revisions over the past 10 years, primarily to improve its psychometric properties and to shorten it. The core version contains a global measure of Life satisfaction, as well as measures of objective and subjective QOL in eight life domains: Living situation; Daily activities and functioning; Family relations; Social relations; Finances; Work and school; Legal and safety issues; Health. The sections *on each life domain* are organized in such a way that information is first obtained about objective QOL and then about level of life satisfaction in that life area. This pairing of objective and subjective QOL indicators by domain is essential to the QOL assessment model [13].

All the life satisfaction items in the interview utilize a fixed interval scale, that was originally developed in a national survey of the quality of American life [11]. The types of objective QOL indicators utilized vary considerably across the domains. In general, they can be viewed as of two types: measures of functioning (e. g., frequency of social contacts or daily activities) and measures of access to resources and opportunities (e. g., income support or housing type). The QOL indicators include both individual items (e. g., monthly income support) and scales (e. g., frequency of social contacts).

The variables generated by the QOLI include:
A. *Objective QOL indicators.* Length of time at current residence; Residential stability; Homelessness; Quality of living circumstances; Leisure activities; Frequency of family contacts; Frequency of social contacts; Total monthly spending money; Adequacy of financial supports; Current employment status; Number of nights in jail during the past year; Victim of violent crime during past year; Victim of nonviolent crime during the past year
B. *Subjective QOL indicators.* Satisfaction with: Living situation; Leisure activities; Family relations; Social relations; Finances; Work and school; Legal and safety; Health (Religion and Neighborhood)

The psychometric properties of the QOLI have been extensively assessed. Internal consistency reliabilities range from 0.79 to 0.88 (median = 0.85) for the life satisfaction scales, and from 0.44 to 0.82 (median = 0.68) for the objective QOL scales. These reliabilities have been replicated in two separate studies of persons with severe mental illnesses. Test-retest reliabilities (1 week) have also been assessed for the QOLI: life satisfaction scales: 0.41–0.95 (median = 0.72); objective QOL scales: 0.29–0.98 (median = 0.65). Construct and predictive validity have been assessed as good by confirmatory factor analyses and multivariate predictive models. The QOLI also differentiates between patients living in hospitals and supervised community residential programs in the United States and Britain [14, 15]. Individual life satisfaction items clearly discriminate between persons with severe mental illness and the general population [1]. Further construct validation has been assessed in studies of the predictors of QOL among day treatment patients in Britain [16] and the relationship between QOL and feelings of empowerment among persons with severe mental illnesses in the United States [17]. A variety of methodologic papers have explored such other issues as the relationship between QOL and clinical symptoms [18], gender and age [19], and housing type [20, 21].

The QOLI has been used almost exclusively with persons with severe mental disorders. The samples in published studies have included approximately equal numbers of men and women, about 75% of whom are Caucasian, ranging in age from 18–65 years. The predominant diagnosis in these studies has been schizophrenia, ranging from 57% to 76% of patients. General pupulation norms for individual life satisfaction items are available [11].

Quality of Life Scale

The Quality of Life Scale (QLS; Heinrichs et al., 1984) was developed to assess the deficit syndrome in patients with schizophrenia. It is a semistructured interview rated by trained clinicians. Its 21 items are rated on fixed interval scales based upon the interviewer's judgment of the patient's functioning in each of the 21 areas. The interview takes approximately 45 min.

The 21 items of the QLS cover: Commonplace activities; Occupational role; Work functioning; Work level; Possession of commonplace objects; Interpersonal relations (household, friends, acquaintances, social activity, social network, social initiative, social withdrawal, sociosexual functioning); Sense of purpose; Motivation; Curiosity; Anhedonia; Aimless inactivity; Empathy; Emotional interaction; Work satisfaction. These items reduce to four scales: Intrapsychic foundations, Interpersonal relations, Instrumental role, and Total score.

The interrater reliabilities on conjointly conducted interviews range from 0.84 to 0.97 on summary scales. Individual item intraclass correlations range from 0.5 to 0.9. Confirmatory factor analysis has been conducted. This scale is widely used in the evaluation of psychopharmacologic treatments for schizophrenia, predominantly in outpatients (e.g., see [23]).

Client Quality of Life Interview

The Client Quality of Life Interview (CQLI; 1986) was developed as part of a battery of instruments to assess outcomes among persons with severe mental disorders who were served by the NIMH CSP. These instruments include the Uniform Client Data Instrument (UCDI), the UCDI-Short Form, the CSP Participant Follow-up Form, and the CQLI. The contents of these instruments overlap to a considerable degree. All but the CQLI are completed by case managers or other professionals serving the clients, and generally focus on functioning, services, and clinical outcomes. Only the CQLI asks clients directly about the quality of their lives and, therefore, only it is reviewed here. The conceptual model underlying the CQLI assumes that certain life essentials are necessary precursors to a quality life. One major purpose of the CSP was to provide these essentials and thus to enhance QOL.

The CQLI is a structured self-report interview administered by a trained lay interviewer. It consists of 46 items rated by the respondent, as well as 19 interviewer ratings. Ratings are done on fixed, ordinal scales. The content areas covered include: Essentials of life (food, clothing, shelter, health and hygiene, money, and safety); Job training and education; Daily activities and recreation; Privacy; Social supports; Social time; Self-reliance; Peace of mind. In each area questions generally cover both the quantity or resources or activity, as well as the respondents' subjective feelings about these resources and activities. Many of the item sets lend themselves readily to composite scales, although the development or scoring of these scales is not available for the CQLI. Some of the scales parallel the UCDI, for which scale computation guidelines, as well as psychometric properties are available.

No formal psychometric analyses of the CQLI are available. Correlations of CQLI items rated by the clients with comparable items from the UCDI rated by the case manager were quite low. The CQLI ratings remained stable over a 14-month follow-up period. The subsample in the CSP study who completed the CQLI were 109 severely mentally ill clients from six exemplary CSP programs. They included 51% men: 82% Caucasian, 11% black, 6% Hispanic, and 1% other; and the mean age was 41.5 years. No diagnoses were indicated, but all were severely mentally ill.

California Well-Being Project Client Interview

The California Well-Being Project was a 3-year initiative funded by the California Department of Mental Health to develop a better understanding of the health and well-being concerns of persons who have been treated for mental illness, the so-called psychiatrically labeled. The most individual aspect of this initiative is that it was designed and conducted entirely by mental health care consumers. The project consisted of three components: (1) research and analysis of well-being factors for individuals assessed through a structured survey of consumers, family members, and professionals; (2) production of educational materials based upon this survey; (3) dissemination of these educational materials to consumers, family members, and mental health providers.

Three versions of the survey questionnaire on well-being (California Well-Being Project Client Interview; CWBPCI; 1989 [25]) were developed for consumers (151 items), family members (76 items), and mental health professionals (77 items). The time required for administration is not indicated. The questionnaires consist predominantly of Likert-scaled questions, but with some open-ended questions interspersed. The questionnaires are designed to be administered either in face-to-face interviews (conducted by trained consumers), self-administered by mail, or group self-administration with an interviewer available to answer questions. The instrument is thus designed for flexibility in administration to provide the multiple perspectives of consumers, family members, and professionals.

In the California survey the CWBPCI was administered to 331 persons who were psychiatrically labeled and living in various settings, including psychiatric hospitals (nonstate), skilled nursing facilities, board-and-care homes, satellite houses, single occupancy hotels, community residential treatment centers, drop-in centers, client self-help groups, organizations serving people identified as "homeless mentally ill", and the streets. The final sample consisted of 61 randomly selected members of the California Network of Mental Health Consumers (surveyed by mail), 249 volunteer respondents from various facilities in California (face-to-face interviews, not randomly selected), and 21 randomly selected Project Return clients. The sample comprised 52% men, 67.5% Caucasian, 14.7% black, and 4.6% Hispanic. They were predominantly young with 41% below the age of 35 years and 75% below the age of 45 years; the authors describe them as predominantly chronically mentally ill, but no further clinical details are given.

No information is provided on the instrument's psychometric properties, and, for the most part, data from individual items are reported as frequencies (or percentages) in a narrative section that discusses the many concerns of the respondents. Topics covered in this narrative include: Adequate resources; Age; Alternatives to psychiatric hospitalization; Aspirations; Benefit agencies; Board and care residents; Boredom; Causes of psychological and emotional problems; Children; Client/consumer; Conservatorship; Control of emotional problems; Creativity; Stereotype of dangerousness; Discrimination; Electroconvulsive therapy; Empowerment; Ethnic/cultural group; Family relationships; Freedom; Friends; Gender; General population; Hallucinations and/or voices; Happiness; Health; Homelessness; Hospitalization; Income; Informed consent; Internalized stigma; Involuntary treatment/hospitalization; Labeling; Loneliness/isolation; Mass media; Meaningful work and achievement/activity; Medications; Misdiagnosis; Neighborhood resistance; "Normal" people; Patients' rights; Personhood; Poverty; Privacy; Pro-choice; Professional/client relationship; Public policy; Quality of life; Seclusion and restraint; Self-esteem; Self-help; Sexual life; Side-effects; Social life; Spiritual life; Stigma; Stress; Tolerance; Stereotype of unpredictability; Validation; Vocational rehabilitation; Warmth and intimacy; Well-being; Young adult chronic mentally ill.

A key measure derived from the interview is the Well-Being Quotient. This measure is derived from two questions providing information about the relative importance assigned to various factors that may affect well-being and whether the respondent currently lacks these factors. The questions read: (1) "Below is a list of things that some people have said are essential for their well-being. Please mark all of those things that you believe are *essential* for your well-being." (2) "Of the things that people have mentioned that are essential for well-being, which of the following, if any, do you lack in your everyday life?" The response factors include happiness, health, adequate income, meaningful work or achievement, comfort, satisfying social life, satisfying spiritual life, adequate resources, good food and a decent place to live, satisfying sexual life, creativity, basic human freedoms, warmth and intimacy, safety, and other. Besides simply rank-ordering these factors according to the percentages of respondents who identify each factor in each of the questions, four well-being profiles are computed: (1) for each factor, the proportion of respondents who indicate that they lack a well-being factor that they consider essential; (2) the proportion of respondents who do not lack a factor they consider essential; (3) the proportion of clients who consider a factor essential regardless of whether they have it; (4) the proportion of respondents who lack a given factor regardless of its essentialness.

The most noteworthy aspect of this instrument is that it was entirely consumer generated. The fact that it is consumer generated enhances its face validity even though no formal psychometric analyses were conducted. The researchers consider this instrument to be still in a developmental stage.

Lancashire Quality of Life Profile

The Lancashire Quality of Life Profile (LQOLP; 1991 [26]) was developed in the United Kingdom during the late 1980s by Oliver et al. in response to a mandate by the British government that all community care programs serving persons with severe mental disorders assess the impact of their services on patients' QOL. The LQOLP is based upon the Lehman QOLI, but is modified to reflect cultural variations and the broader survey intent of the government mandate for service-based evaluation of QOL. The theory underlying the LQOLP is essentially the same as that described for the Lehman QOLI.

The LQOLP is a structured self-report patient interview designed for administration by clinical staff in community settings. It consists of 100 items and requires approximately 1 h to administer. It assesses objective QOL and life satisfaction in nine life domains: Work/education; Leisure/participation; Religion; Finances; Living situation; Legal and safety; Family relations; Social relations; Health. In addition, it includes a measure of General well-being and self-concept. Objective QOL information is collected by means of categorical or continuous measures depending upon the content area. Life satisfaction ratings are on a seven-point Likert scale.

Psychometric properties of the life satisfaction have been evaluated in a series of pilot studies [26]. Test-retest reliabilities for life satisfaction scores range from 0.49 to 0.78, depending upon the patient sample. Internal consistency reliabilities (Cronbach's alpha) of these scales range from 0.84 to 0.86. Content, construct, and criterion validities were also assessed using a variety of techniques and judged to be adequate.

The LQOLP has been used with chronically mentally ill patients in a variety of community care settings in the United Kingdom and in Colorado. Details of sample characteristics are not available. A briefer version of the LQOLP is currently being piloted in 12 European countries and is being considered by the World Health Organization in conjunction with their broader studies of QOL.

Discussion

Selecting a QOL Measure

Given that none of these QOL measures has been widely used or accepted as a standard, the choice of a measure must rest with the investigator's particular purpose and needs. The most comprehensive and best characterized scales from a psychometric standpoint are the Oregon Quality of Life Questionnaire, the Lehman Quality of Life Interview, and the Lancaster Quality of Life Profile. All three cover similar domains of QOL functioning, are based upon comprehensive QOL models, and have acceptable psychometric properties. They have been used with typical samples of severely mentally ill patients in the United States, which means that high percentages of psychotic patients are involved. These instruments take approximately 45 min to administer.

The remaining instruments have had much more limited usage and/or are less comprehensive. The Satisfaction with Life Domains Scale is a reasonably well-characterized and brief measure of life satisfaction that has been used with severely mentally ill populations. Since it only measures life satisfaction, measures of QOL functioning and resources would have to be added to provide a comprehensive QOL assessment. The Quality of Life Checklist was developed specifically for use in a clinic setting and seems particularly adapted to help clinicians assess the various areas of QOL functioning. However, it has no known psychometric properties and apparently has only been used in one small study. The Standardized Social Schedule has only been used with chronic neurotic patients in Britain. It has adequate reliability properties, but its factor structure is not stable. The Community Adjustment Form has demonstrated sensitivity to changes over time among patients assigned to alternative community treatment programs, but lacks adequate psychometric analysis. The Quality of Life Scale is a relatively comprehensive and well-characterized instrument, and thus, is similar to the first three discussed. However, it was developed for the more focal purpose of assessing the deficit functional symptoms of schizophrenia and requires administration by a trained clinician. As such it does not fit readily into the mainstream of QOL assessment and must be viewed as more disease-specific than the others. The Well-Being Project Client Interview has not undergone any psychometric evaluation and has been used in only one study, but it has the important distinction of being the only instrument developed primarily by service consumers. Finally, the Client Quality of Life Interview has been used as a companion to the Uniform Client Data Instrument in the major evaluation of the NIMH CSP. Its major shortcoming is that it also has not been characterized adequately from a psychometric perspective.

For some of the measures described above, there are published norms for different samples of patients, thus allowing some comparisons of new patient samples with these samples. For the life satisfaction measures in the Lehman Quality of Life Interview and Satisfaction with Life Domains Scale, there are also national normative data, because these measures draw heavily upon prior work assessing general QOL in the United States [11].

Beyond these instrument-specific comments, some general comments and caveats are warranted for the investigator or program evaluator seeking a QOL measure for the severely mentally ill, whether one of those described above or some other. First, a major concern with using normative QOL measures in this population is that floor effects are frequently encountered, especially in role-functioning domains (e.g., spouse, parent, employment roles). Therefore, special attention must be paid to instrument sensitivity. Such floor effects are typically not a problem in the domains of life satisfaction and resources. Second, significant numbers of these patients have problems with task perseverance and comprehension. Therefore, pencil-and-paper questionnaires are ill-advised. Note that nearly all of the instruments discussed here are interviews. Finally, psychopathology affects patients' ratings of their QOL. In the only study of this phenomenon, anxiety and depression had significant effects on patients' perceived life satisfaction [18]. Therefore, QOL assessments of these patients should be accompanied by a concomitant assessment of psychopathologic symptoms to reduce the confounding effects of psychiatric syndromes on QOL assessments.

Interpreting QOL Information

Because of the newness of this field in psychiatric research, it is not possible to make specific recommendations about the interpretation of QOL data. Conceptually, QOL is generally seen as related to, but distinct from, such clinical syndromes as depression and anxiety. Perhaps the most important point about interpretation that can be made at present is the need to distinguish psychological QOL, e.g. life satisfaction or morale, from clinical symptomatology, particularly depression. We know that measures of subjective QOL are clearly affected by clinical symptomatology [13]. However, at least conceptually, subjective QOL equivalents are viewed as distinct from clinical syndromes. This distinction has particular relevance with regard to implications for interventions. That is, one might attempt to effect various changes in a patient's environment to improve housing, financial, or work dissatisfaction, whereas one might prescribe a clinical intervention, such as an antidepressant, to alleviate symptoms of depression. Certainly we can foresee the development of an interactive model between QOL and clinical symptomatology, but at the very least we can say that for adequate interpretation of QOL data from psychiatrically impaired populations both QOL and clinical syndromes need to be assessed.

A common dilemma encountered in the assessment of QOL among persons with severe and persistent mental illnesses (SPMI) is that at times they may perceive the quality of their lives differently than social norms would predict. Such findings of counterintuitive QOL results are frequently met with concerns about the reliability or validity of the QOL data. While such basic psychometric concerns may be reasonable, the fact is that the psychometric properties of the better QOL measures for the SPMI are comparable to those in the general population. Rather than reflecting measurement limitations, such intuitively inconsistent QOL findings may offer valuable information for clinical interventions and service planning.

Counterintuitive QOL results may reflect idiosyncratic views and values of persons afflicted by SPMI and should affect the clinician's approach to service planning. Patients are unlikely to be motivated to change circumstances with which they are content even if the clinician and family feel otherwise. Conversely, failure to address an area of life with which a patient is dissatisfied, even though the clinician and family view the patient's circumstances as satisfactory, can adversely affect the treatment alliance with the patient. Such disagreements about QOL may signal the need for a period of negotiation regarding treatment and service goals.

Counterintuitive QOL findings also may represent patients' accomodation to adversity. Patients who have lived with social isolation, unemployment, poverty, or adverse living circumstances for extended periods of time may report relative positive life satisfaction. Their satisfaction reflects an accommodation to adversity and does not necessarily mean that they would not desire an improvement in life circumstances if the hope and opportunity for such changes were offered. Conversely, interventions that promote positive change, e.g., vocational rehabilitation or a novel antipsychotic medication (e.g., clozapine), may produce transient decreases in life satisfaction because of patients' renewed awareness of how their lives could be better. Such possibilities form the basis for caution and more thoughtful consideration about how we expect interventions to affect QOL.

Research Needs

In order to advance QOL assessment for severely mentally ill persons to the point that more scientifically and clinically meaningful applications can be achieved, work is needed in several areas. First, we need a clearer definition of what QOL is and what it is not. The existing literature is characterized by conceptually clear but disparate models of QOL, as well as overly broad and vague definitions of the phrase "quality of life". Definitions include life satisfaction, illness-related "deficit states", very comprehensive multidimensional models of well-being, and ill-defined, though appealing, humanistic notions. Second, with the adoption of a common definition, there needs to be some agreement about how to measure QOL. This will allow us to begin to accumulate comparable data across studies and populations. Third, we need to compare QOL data from psychiatrically impaired populations with those from other nonpsychiatric groups, particularly the physically disabled, the general population, and other economically disadvantaged groups, to establish some normative perspective. Fourth, we need a better understanding about how QOL varies naturally over time in psychiatric populations, the predictive validity of QOL measures for subsequent illness course and outcome, and the sensitivity of QOL measures for detecting treatment effects among these patients, who may at best experience very modest improvements. Finally, there is a need for basic conceptual work to develop better models for integrating QOL data into a general model of outcome for persons with severe mental illnesses.

Acknowledgement. Preparation of this paper was supported by a contract from the National Institute of Mental Health, Rockville, MD, USA.

Bibliography

(Arranged according to instruments in chronological order, asterisks indicating key references to individual measures)

Standardized Social Schedule

*   Clare AW, Cairns VE (1978) Design, development and use of a standardized interview to assess social maladjustment and dysfunction in community samples. Psychol Med 8: 589–604

Community Adjustment Form

*   Stein LI, Test MA (1980) Alternative to mental hospital treatment. I. conceptual model, treatment program and clinical evaluation. Arch Gen Psychiatry 37: 392–397
Hoult J, Reynolds J (1984) Schizophrenia: a comparative trial of community oriented and hospitals oriented psychiatric care. Acta Psychiatr Scand 69: 359–372

Quality of Life Checklist

*   Malm U, May PRA, Dencker SJ (1981) Evaluation of the quality of life of the schizophrenic outpatient: a checklist. Schizophr Bull 7: 477–487

Satisfaction with Life Domains Scale

*   Baker F, Intagliata J (1982) Quality of life in the evaluation of community support systems. Eval Program Plann 5: 69–79
Johnson PJ (1991) Emphasis on quality of life of people with severe mental illness in community-based care in Sweden. Psychosoc Rehabil J 14: 23–37

Oregon Quality of Life Scale

Bigelow DA, Brodsky G, Steward L, Olson M (1982) The concept and measurement of quality of life as a dependent variable in evaluation of mental health services. In: Stahler GJ, Tash WR (eds) Innovative approaches to mental health evaluation. Academic Press, New York, pp 345–366
Bigelow DA, Gareau MJ, Young DJ (1990) A quality of life interview. Psychosoc Rehabil J 14: 94–98
*   Bigelow DA, McFarland BH, Olson MM (1991) Quality of life of community mental health program clients: validating a measure. Community Ment Health J 27: 43–55
Bigelow DA, McFarland BH, Gareau MJ, Young DJ (1991) Implementation and effectiveness of a bed reduction project. Community Ment Health J 27: 125–133
Bigelow DA, Young DJ (1991) Effectiveness of a case management program. Community Ment Health J 27: 115–123

Lehman Quality of Life Interview

Lehman AF, Ward NC, Linn LS (1982) Chronic mental patients: the quality of life issue. Am J Psychiatry 10: 1271–1276

Lehman AF (1983) The effects of psychiatric symptoms on quality of life assessments among the chronic mentally ill. Eval Program Plann 6: 143–151

Lehman AF (1983) The well-being of chronic mental patients: assessing their quality of life. Arch Gen Psychiatry 40: 369–373

Lehman AF, Possidente S, Hawker F (1986) The quality of life of chronic mental patients in a state hospital and community residences. Hosp Community Psychiatry 37: 901–907

Franklin JL, Solovitz B, Mason M, Clemons JR, Miller GE (1987) An evaluation of case management. Am J Psychiatry 77: 674–678

* Lehman AF (1988) A quality of life interview for the chronically mentally ill. Eval Program Plann 11: 51–62

Simpson CJ, Hyde CE, Faragher EB (1989) The chronically mentally ill in community facilities: a study of quality of life. Br J Psychiatry 154: 77–82

Levitt AJ, Hogan TP, Bucosky CM (1990) Quality of life in chronically mentally ill patients in day treatment. Psychol Med 20: 703–710

Lehman AF, Slaughter JC, Myers CP (1991) The quality of life of chronically mentally ill persons in alternative residential settings. Psychiatr Q 62: 35–49

Slaughter JC, Lehmann AF (1991) Quality of life of sverely mentally ill adults in residential care facilities. Adult Residential Care J 5: 97–111

Lehman AF, Slaughter JC, Myers CP (1992) Quality of life of the chronically mentally ill: gender and decade of life effects. Eval Program Plann 15: 7–12

Sullivan GS, Wells KB, Leake B (1992) Clinical factors associated with better quality of life in a seriously mentally ill population. Hosp Community Psychiatry 43: 794–798

Huxley P, Warner R (1992) Case management, quality of life, and satisfaction with services of long-term psychiatric patients. Hosp Community Psychiatry 43: 799–802

Rosenfeld S, Neese-Todd S (1993) Elements of a psychosocial clubhouse programm associated with a satisfying quality of life. Hosp Comm Psychiatry 44: 76–78

Rosenfield S (1992) Factors contributing to the subjective quality of life of the chronically mentally ill. J Health Soc Behav 33: 299–315

Quality of Life Scale

* Heinrichs DW, Hanlon TE, Carpenter WT (1984) The quality of life scale: an instrument for rating the schizophrenic deficit syndrome. Schizophr Bull 10: 388–398

Meltzer HY, Burnett S, Bastani B, Ramirez LF (1990) Effects of six months of clozapine treatment on the quality of life of chronic schizophrenic patients. Hosp Community Psychiatry 41: 892–897

Client Quality of Life Interview

Goldstrom ID, Manderscheid RW (1986) The chronically mentally ill: a descriptive analysis from the Uniform Client data Instrument. Community Support Serv J 2: 4–9

* Mulkern V, Agosta JM, Ashbaugh JW, Bradley VJ, Spence RA, Allein S, Nurczynski P, Houlihan J (1986) Community Support Program Client Follow-up Study. Report to NIMH Rockville, Maryland, USA

Well-Being Project Client Interview

* Campbell J, Schraiber R, Temkin T, ten Tuscher T (1989) The Well-Being Project: mental health clients speak for themselves. Report to the California Department of Mental Health

Lancashire Quality of Life Profile

* Oliver JPJ (1991–92) The social care directive: development of a quality of life profile for use in community services for the mentally ill. Soc Work Soc Sci Rev 3: 5–45

Oliver JPJ, Mohamad H (1992) The quality of life of the chronically mentally ill: a comparison of public, private, and voluntary residential provisions. Br J Soc Work 22: 391–404

References

1. Lehman AF, Ward NC, Linn LS (1982) Chronic mental patients: the quality of life issue. Am J Psychiatry 10: 1271–1276
2. Schulberg HC, Bromet E (1981) Strategies for evaluating the outcome of community services for the chronically mentally ill. Am J Psychiatry 138: 930–935
3. Weissman MM (1975) The assessment of social adjustment: a review of techniques. Arch Gen Psychiatry 11: 51–62
4. Ciarlo JA, Brown TR, Edwards DW, Kiresuk TJ, Newman FL (1986) Assessing mental health treatment outcome measurement techniques. (NIMH series FN no 9; DHHS pub no [ADM] 86-1301) Superintendent of Documents, Washington, DC
5. Kane RA, Kane RL, Arnold S (1985) Measuring social functioning in mental health studies: concepts and instruments (NIMH Series DN no 5, DHHS publ no [ADM] 85-1384) Superintendent of Documents, Washington, DC
6. Clare AW, Cairns VE (1978) Design, development and use of a standardized interview to assess social maladjustment and dysfunction in community samples. Psychol Med 8: 589–604
7. Stein LI, Test MA (1980) Alternative to mental hospital treatment. I. conceptual model, treatment program and clinical evaluation. Arch Gen Psychiatry 37: 392–397
8. Hoult J, Reynolds J (1984) Schizophrenia: a comparative trial of community oriented and hospital oriented psychiatric care. Acta Psychiatr Scand 69: 359–372
9. Malm U, May PRA, Dencker SJ (1981) Evaluation of the quality of life of the schizophrenic outpatient: a checklist. Schizophr Bull 7: 477–487
10. Baker F, Intagliata J (1982) Quality of life in the evaluation of community support systems. Eval Program Plann 5: 69–79
11. Andrews FM, Withey SB (1976) Social indicators of well-being. Plenum Press, New York
12. Bigelow DA, Brodsky G, Steward L, Olson M (1982) The concept and measurement of quality of life as a dependent variable in evaluation of mental health services. In: Stahler GJ, Tash WR (eds) Innovative approaches to mental health evaluation. Academic Press, New York, pp 345–366
13. Lehman AF (1983) The well-being of chronic mental patients: assessing their quality of life. Arch Gen Psychiatry 40: 369–373
14. Lehman AF, Possidente S, Hawker F (1986) The quality of life of chronic mental patients in a state hospital and community residences. Hosp Community 37: 901–907
15. Simpson CJ, Hyde CE, Faragher EB (1989) The chronically mentally ill in community facilities: a study of quality of life. Br J Psychiatry 154: 77–82
16. Levitt AJ, Hogan TP, Bucosky CM (1990) Quality of life in chronically mentally ill patients in day treatment. Psychol Med 20: 703–710
17. Rosenfeld S, Neese-Todd S (1993) Elements of a psychosocial clubhouse program associated with a satisfying quality of life, Hosp Comm Psychiatry 44: 76–78
18. Lehman AF (1983) The effects of psychiatric symptoms on quality of life assessments among the chronic mentally ill. Eval Program Plann 6: 143–151
19. Lehman AF, Slaughter JC, Meyers CP (1992) Quality of life of the chronically mentally ill: gender and decade of life effects. Eval Program Plann 15: 7–12
20. Slaughter JC, Lehman AF (1991) Quality of life of severely mentally ill adults in residential care facilities. Adult Residential Care J 5: 97–111
21. Lehman AF, Slaughter JC, Myers CP (1991) The quality of life of chronically mentally ill persons in alternative residential settings. Psychiatr Q 62: 35–49
22. Heinrichs DW, Hanlon TE, Carpenter WT (1984) The quality of life scale: an instrument for rating the schizophrenic deficit syndrome. Schizophr Bull 10: 388–398
23. Meltzer HY, Burnett S, Bastani B, Ramirez LF (1990) Effects of six months of clozapine treatment on the quality of life of chronic schizophrenic patients. Hosp Community Psychiatry 41: 892–897
24. Mulkern V, Agosta JM, Ashbaugh JW, Bradley VJ, Spence RA, Allein S, Nurczysnki P, Houlihan J (1986) Community Support Program Client Follow-up Study. Report to NIMH, Rockville, Maryland, USA
25. Campbell J, Schraiber R, Temkin T, Tusscher T ten (1989) The Well-Being Project: mental health clients speak for themselves. Report to the California Department of Mental Health
26. Oliver JPJ (1991–92) The social care directive: development of a quality of life profile for use in community services for the mentally ill. Soc Work Soc Sci Rev 3: 5–45

Quality of Mental Health Service Care: The Forgotten Pathway From Process to Outcome

Traolach S. Brugha and Fiona Lindsay

Abstract

The validity of the concept of outcome depends on a relationship between routine treatment and later health status. Outcome evaluations and audits are very rare in psychiatry. A substantial expansion in epidemiologically based, naturalistic, observational, process-outcome data collection in routine psychiatric practice is essential in order to identify treatment allocation biases and other reasons for unexpected outcomes. Identified causes of undertreatment should lead to locally agreed detailed clinical guidelines. Experimental evaluation should take place in routine clinical practice settings, with change in both process and outcome as the objective. Ultimately, the results of both experimental and observational outcome studies on representative service users should converge, permitting outcomes to be the ultimate arbitrator of quality.

Introduction

There should be no need to justify an article on quality in a series of papers on mental health service evaluation. What does the world of scientific evaluative research have to offer? The title of this chapter reflects two questions about medical and psychiatric care:

1. Is care being implemented according to good practice criteria?
2. Does it work?

The first of these two questions takes account of relational aspects (especially doctor patient communication), environmental aspects (for example accessibility), and the technical aspects of the process (provision of care that is most likely to lead to a better outcome; Donabedian 1989). Whether it is worth asking may depend on the answer to the second question:

Does properly implemented *care* lead to better subsequent health *status* (and functioning, satisfaction) and if not, which (combination?) of the two should we measure and rely upon: the *process* of care? or health status *subsequent* to care provision? or a *combination* of process and health status, even when they appear to be unrelated?

Department of Psychiatry, University of Leicester, Clinical Sciences Building, Leicester Royal Infirmary, PO Box 65, Leicester LE2 7LX, UK

The question of whether to monitor process or outcome is a major problem in quality assurance (Fauman 1990). The term health *status* is emphasised at this point rather than that of *outcome:* Donabedian (1992) defines outcomes as the *states* or *conditions attributable to antecedent health care.* If we accept this definition of outcome then it follows logically that we can only use this term when we are able to demonstrate that status is significantly associated with antecedent care. Within the field of psychiatry, outcomes might appear now to be at centre stage, having previously been off a stage dominated by structural measures of input and process measures (Jenkins 1990).

Medical statistics and epidemiological methods are concerned with two, related inseparable aims: estimation and uncertainty. If it seems to work, how little and how much does it work in this population? This can mean reducing complex sets of observational data to relatively simple, general statements that are an accurate representation of those data, whilst allowing for measurement error and *chance,* and in randomised studies (experiments) estimating the plausible range of the effect of a treatment by means of the *effect size* and *confidence interval* (Everitt 1989).

Review Methodology

In preparing this chapter we reviewed the literature on quality of care in medicine and psychiatry and the published literature on audit in psychiatry, which is the major area of application of this topic in service settings. A literature search was conducted by searching for articles (in PSYCHLIT and MEDLINE), textbooks, cited chapters and cross references covering historical and definitional aspects, methods of assessment and examples of their use in the field of psychiatry. A selection of relevant articles from the appropriate areas of medical statistics and epidemiology was included also.

Our first aim was to try to reach a conclusion concerning the relative benefits and feasibility of quality assessment relying on aspects of process assessment and that based on outcomes. Our second aim, also difficult to achieve, was to try to structure the evidence in the literature in a cyclical fashion as recommended in quality assurance and audit programmes: beginning with definitional issues, the establishment of quality standards, guidelines and policies; measurement and assessment issues; interpretation and appraisal as in peer group audit activities; finally, implementation strategies, including the final stage of the audit cycle and including the experimental evaluation of clinical guidelines in routine practice.

Definition and History

In 1910, Codman proposed the "end result idea" in which "every hospital should follow *every* patient it treats, long enough to determine whether or not the treatment has been successful, and then to inquire 'if not, why not?' with a view to preventing a similar failure in the future"; in essence it was equivalent to monitoring "outcomes" (Donabedian 1989). Codman suggested concurrent assessment of care and its consequences, with the occurrence of adverse outcomes being the only occasion for "process" assessment. In order to establish the relation between care and its results, observations were needed on the causes for not attaining perfection. Codman believed that the end result was the only true product of health care and the major purpose of the end result system was to bring improvements in health care (Donabedian 1989).

Quality of care is defined as the level of performance or accomplishment that characterises the health care provided (Last 1988). Structure refers to manpower, facilities, resources, numbers and qualifications of professionals, characteristics of administrative organisations and physical facilities (Tugwell 1979). Process refers to technical (investigations, physiological monitoring and treatment prescribed; diagnostic and therapeutic procedures) or interpersonal (patient education) styles (Tugwell 1979). Donabedian's (1992) definition of outcomes as the states or conditions attributable to antecedent health care is not uncontroversial. Outcome can refer to death or disability rate, disease (cure or not), effect on patient health and satisfaction (Tugwell 1979) and discomfort, social and psychological well-being.

Quality Assurance and Audit

Medical audit has been defined as "the systematic, critical analysis of the quality of medical care, including the procedures used for diagnosis and treatment, the use of resources and the resulting outcome and quality of life for the patient" (Department of Health 1989). In what way does audit relate to our basic question about the relationship between process and outcome? Audit is inclined to be insensitive to outcome, but sensitive to structure and process (Holman 1989). The government suggests that every consultant should be involved in a form of medical audit agreed between management and the profession locally, that it is now a contractual obligation. It is a condition for the training of junior staff; without it hospitals should not be accredited for higher specialist training (Department of Health 1989).

The aim of audit is to produce change but only if it extends to other health care workers and managers (Moss and Smith 1991). Quality assessment refers to the determination of the degree of quality of care and quality assurance refers to all measures used to protect, maintain and improve the quality of care (Donabedian 1992). Quality assurance implies a good quality service achieved at minimum expenditure, but in health care this means any procedure(s) improving quality of care (Jacyna 1992). Audit is about continuing improvement. Construction of an audit involved adopting a standard, defining an indicator, setting a target and defining the monitoring method (DeLacey 1992). The sequence of separate activities linked to and from the "audit cycle" loop should include stages of observation, comparison and action taking (Robinson 1991). The audit cycle must be completed if it is to be beneficial, that is to improve patient care (Hatton and Renvoize 1991; Moss and Smith 1991; McClelland 1992). Steps must be charted and measured. Identification of what improvements can be made should be followed by further assessment once improvements are instituted (Feldman 1992). The operational definitions of quality assurance all have the feedback cycle in common (McClelland 1992).

Quality Atandards and Practice Guidelines

Policy Aspects

In the United Kingdom, the Audit Commission (1992) has a statutory duty to promote economy, efficiency and effectiveness in bodies that it audits, which since 1990 has included the National Health Service (NHS). Its role is to prioritise the patient perspective, community care and joint audits, and to develop tools for direct use, quality exchange, accreditation and league tables.

Standards in Psychiatry

Standards of care will depend increasingly on regularly updated overviews and meta-analyses of evidence of the efficacy of psychiatric treatments and related interventions (Wing 1992; Depression Guideline Panel 1993). The diversity of professional providers in psychiatry has also complicated the development of standards, classifications of intervention problem groupings, and thus methods for monitoring the quality of the process of care (Wells and Brook 1988). Both national governments and agencies and the World Health Organisation have promoted standards.

The *Health Advisory Service* (HAS), The *Mental Health Act Commission Biennial Reports* (MHAC 1993), the MHAC Second Opinion system, the Mental Health Review Tribunals and the Approval Exercise of the *Royal College of Psychiatrists* are all examples of formal institutional audit (Garden et al., 1989). The introduction throughout the NHS of the *Care Programme Approach* (Royal College of Psychiatrists 1991) has been initiated through similar statutory procedures.

The Royal Australian and New Zealand College of Psychiatrists set up the "Quality Assurance in Aspects of Psychiatric Practice" project (Holman 1989), which has resulted in the development of possibly the first ever treatment recommendations for depressive disorders (Quality Assurance Project 1983). It is concerned with more than just audit; a series of treatment outlines for major conditions were developed as a basis for peer review and research. Holman (1989) has suggested that a clinical focus should be maintained in audit especially by the use of care plans and established guidelines similar to the Australian Quality Assurance Programme. More precise treatment guidelines are also being developed elsewhere (Depression Guideline Panel 1993), making use of diagnostic and treatment decision trees and algorithms. The development of more precise guidelines will facilitate quantitative audits of undertreatment leading to the prioritisation of practice altering evaluation projects (Brugha, in press).

Quality Measurement

Quality is judged by individual professionals comparing it with a standard; but it may be perceived differently by users. Donabedian (1966) consideres the sources and methods of obtaining information: sampling and selection, clinical research including the limitations of direct observation especially in general practice, measurement standards (empirical and normative), measurement scales and reliability, bias and validity.

The classic work of Donabedian is fraught with the problems of using each dimension (e. g. structure) in isolation (Turner 1989). Turner (1989) suggests other quality of care perspectives. First, patient perceptions, that is patients may judge quality more by how they are treated than by the health outcome. Second, adherence to standards, that is from industry, a multidimensional approach, but with the focus still on outcome. Monitoring quality in medical practice has come to be synonymous with the growing practice of audit.

There has been a long debate on the right way to measure the quality of care, whether to use process or outcome criteria (Ierodiakonou and Vandenbroucke 1993). These workers have argued that the ultimate judgement of quality rests on the evaluation of process (believed by the ancient (Greek) philosophers and modern theoreticians of quality assurance; Ierodiakonou and Vandenbroucke 1993). Some administrators are convinced that quality of performance should be measured according to what they assert to be outcome criteria, e. g. mortality, but there are dangers involved in ranking (Ierodiakonou and Vandenbroucke 1993). To use outcome as a quality measure, continuous evaluation of all individual patient characteristics is needed, which is a gigantic and perhaps unrealistic research effort (Ierodiakonou and Vandenbroucke 1993).

Tugwell (1979) clearly advocates process-based approaches in a quote from Cochrane: "the core of quality of medical care is the extent to which scientifically proven effective methods of treatment are properly applied to patients who can benefit from them." A strong case for a process-driven quality of care strategy has been made more recently by Micossi et al. (1993).

Evaluation of Structure and Input

The considerable emphasis on structure particularly in governmental policies, for example on deinstitutionalisation, has not been accompanied by published measures of structure. Readers may be acquainted with standard forms used in official institutional inspections and educational programme accreditation exercises (Garden et al. 1989); however, their status as measurement tools remains uncertain. The World Health Organisation (Janca and Chandrashekar 1993) has published details of six instruments designed to be used in quality assurance assessments: these consist of national assessments of mental health policy, mental health programmes, outpatient mental health facilities, and within a given setting, assessments of primary health care facilities and residential facilities for the elderly mentally ill. The former cover such matters as decentralisation, equity, community participation; the latter cover such matters as cleanliness, privacy, water and food. Both types of measure cover such matters as staffing, physical environment, interaction with families and the community. Six language versions are available or are in preparation.

Measurement of Process

Micossi et al. (1993) have argued that since an outcomes-based approach is either impracticable (randomisation is rarely feasible) and usually unreliable (due to unknown imbalances in treatment allocations) a *profiles of care* approach is preferable, being driven by the symptoms presented by patients when first seen by a physician, which determines the resources utilised and the costs incurred. Profiles of care represent blocks of symptoms and/or intermediate diagnoses that are associated with corresponding objectives and procedures. Quality control can therefore be based on the comparison between observed and expected actions.

Does psychiatry have any examples of such process-based approaches to quality assessment? Shepherd (1988) argues that the most systematic approximation to a process method of quality assessment in the field of psychiatry is the "Needs for Care Assessment" originally described by Brewin et al. (1987). This is based on an individualised assessment of clinical and social problems or deficits in functioning, linked with a schedule that prescribes appropriate actions or "forms of care" for the defined problems; progress with its use has been discussed more recently (Brewin and Wing 1993). According to this more recent report, several groups of researchers have been able to achieve an acceptable level of reliability in the use of this method, although it relies on the use of judgements both of what constitutes potentially worthwhile care and of whether realistic attempts have been made to provide it.

Process measures must be considered in the context of agreed standards of treatment, but it has been argued that there is a problem in the variety of approaches and modalities (Turner 1989). Tugwell (1979) proposes methodological criteria to assist process measurement. First, Tugwell proposes criterion validity: a statistical association is needed between process and outcome measures. His review of the literature shows few correlations in process-outcome studies. Methodological reasons have been suggested, for example sample size, inappropriate sampling and inappropriate measures. Second, he proposes clinical credibility of the process criteria with health professionals: decreased credibility would occur if items are unlikely to influence management. Third, he proposes accuracy: a measure must reflect actual clinical process. However, physician questionnaires may lead to an alteration in their usual clinical behaviour. Fourth, he proposes comprehensiveness: items must include all important aspects of the process of care. For example, patient education is often omitted. Fifth, he proposes sensitivity to differences between practices and sensitivity to improvements or deteriorations over time. Sixth, he proposes amenability to index construction: the results should enable statistical analysis. Seventh, he proposes feasibility and cost: measurement must be simple and acceptable. This could be achieved in a number of different ways, for example the use of record review, direct observation and the use of physician and patient questionnaires.

Williamson (1971) has developed a strategy for *process and outcome assessment.* The strategy is based on factors likely to have the greatest probability of effecting significant improvement in health status of a target population. The four elements of the strategy are diagnostic, therapeutic, process and outcomes. The study involves the development of outcome criteria; to determine whether process study is required, a comparison is made with the outcomes achieved. As a result of the process study, the direction and priorities for action to improve outcomes should be established. The strategy can be seen to enhance educational effectiveness.

Brook (1977) has questioned the validity of process criteria; only "technical" not "humanitarian" aspects of care were being measured. Brook (1977) cited a study that reported no relation between a process and an outcome assessment of quality of care and so invalidated process audit. He suggests that one should focus on very simple process criteria. Alternatively, efforts to bypass measuring process of care and concentrate on outcome could be considered, possibly by using short-term "proximate" outcomes (Brook 1977).

Outcome Assessment

Donabedian (1992) believes that outcomes are the paramount criteria of good quality; that is that they remain the ultimate validators of effectiveness and quality of medical care (Fessel and VanBrunt 1972). Donabedian (1992) has drawn up a classification of outcomes of health care and has discussed the uses of outcomes in quality assessment.

For example, outcomes only permit inference (not direct assessment) about process (and structure); with the role of intercurrent factors, outcomes may be misleading indicators. Outcomes are "integrative" also, that is they are of value but need process analysis.

Outcome Indicators

An indicator is a measurable variable related to facilities, treatment or outcome of care (Fauman 1990). The identification of indicators and the definition of clinical criteria is a specialised task and extra training is needed. Measurements of process and structure are only acceptable as quality indicators if they predict (outcome) functional status or patient survival (Tugwell 1979).

Jenkins (1990) has proposed a system of outcome indicators for mental health care needed for monitoring and evaluation by clinicians, District Health Authorities (DHAs) and Directors of Public Health (DPH). Jenkins (1990) considers the indicators of input, process and outcome for schizophrenia, affective psychosis, neurosis, dementia, child psychiatry, forensic psychiatry, mental handicap, disability and mortality. She regards process indicators for all illness types simply as "activity on (input indicators)". Jenkins (1990) concludes that it is more useful to measure inputs and outcomes and only use process measures when necessary to investigate shortfalls in achieving objectives.

Outcome scales are presently under development as part of the Health of the Nation target-setting strategy (Royal College of Psychiatrists Research Unit 1993, in preparation). Although these scales cover health and social functioning in the form of current status measures, their use nationally will allow variations in the distribution of health service resources to be compared with non-matching prevalence and severity rates of mental health problems in districts and regions. Their widespread introduction and storage in databases may make it possible to conduct sophisticated statistical analyses of process and outcome.

Outcome measures in psychiatry are complicated and simple quality of life measures are not available (Roy 1991). Gath (1991) has discussed questioningly the use of consumer satisfaction, that is of the patient and family. Unsolved problems include the timing of outcome measures, since there are long periods of time involved; there are few reliable outcome measures and psychiatric patients have multiple problems. Outcome measures in psychiatry are complex over long time periods; they involve subjective feelings and are greatly dependent on the patient's involvement and motivation (Turner, 1989). Turner (1989) has suggested that it is important to ask "Outcome for whom? – the patient, the patient and family?".

There are problems with the use of outcome measures; many variables, in addition to the process of care itself, may contribute to the final outcome (Tugwell 1979) so that poor outcome does not necessarily imply poor quality of care (Fauman 1989), and, arguably, good outcome does not mean that credit can be apportioned to the health care system. Therefore, risk factors or covariates must be controlled for in any analysis. Confounding is defined as the failure of a crude association to reflect properly the magnitude and direction of an exposure effect because of a different distribution of extraneous risk factors among exposed and unexposed individuals (Datta 1993). A confounder is associated with a disease (outcome) and exposure (process) factor, and is extraneous to two main variables but can distort their relation (Datta 1993). Once a strong cause effect relationship has been established, process can be monitored as a surrogate for outcome of care (Fauman 1989).

Methods of Audit

Robinson (1989) outlines the various methods of audit that exist; some involve process measures and others, outcome. Case note review has been used by the Royal College of Physicians audit in the reaccreditation of training posts. Criterion-based audit is utilised in peer review. Outcome audit is the most sophisticated and valid, but has difficulties. Information-based audit involves a review of aggregated activity and financial data. Topic-based and intermediate outcomes are two other forms of audit. Hatton and Renvoize (1991) also consider the use of a random case note sample that is criterion-based and covers adverse occurrences.

In the USA, audit has been performed by local Professional Standards Review Organisations (PSROs) and the Joint Commission on Accreditation of Hospitals (JCAH). Both were found to be costly and without obvious benefit (Garden et al. 1989). The JCAH focused on diagnosis-related groups (DRG). In Canada and the Netherlands there is a legal requirement to perform quality of care or quality assurance programmes. The JCAH, later known as the Joint Commission on Accreditation of Healthcare Organisations (JCAHO), became involved in monitoring due to public demands for accountability and requirement for institutional accreditation (Fauman 1989). Their new approach involved an emphasis on clinical outcome rather than on delivery of care. Criteria could be classified in relation to structure, process of outcome, they could be implicit or explicit (specified in advance), referents (the problem or diagnosis to which criteria apply or have a normative or empirical source (derived by consensus or by empirical investigation). Indicators, tracers (broadly defined health problems) and thresholds triggering more intensive evaluation could be used in monitoring (Fauman 1989). The JCAHO planned to identify indicators (of outcome) in psychiatry and became the main driving force in the development and application of standards of quality of medical care (Fauman 1990). The JCAHO developed an audit system, the performance evaluation procedure (PEP), which was later discontinued.

There is a conflict between ensuring quality of treatment and controlling expenditures; therefore, attempts are required to link quality assurance with "cost-effectiveness analysis" (Cahn and Richman 1985). There is a distinction between quality assessment and quality assurance; quality assurance means measuring both the level of care and, when necessary, improving it (Cahn and Richman, 1985). The processes of quality assurance include "medical audit" and "PEP".

Benefits and Concerns

There is criticism that little attention is given to patient's desires or perceptions of treatment effects. The Department of Health (1989) acknowledges the inevitable differences between audit in the hospital, community and primary health care. For a satisfactory audit (of representative users), a suitable form of case register is required (Daly 1991). Furthermore, it is important to use doctors time efficiently (Gath, 1991). In order to disseminate the explosion in output of audit reports, in March 1992 the

BMJ Publication Group launched a new journal *Quality in Health Care*. The BMA and BMJ have also set up a joint working group on quality (Moss and Smith 1991). Since 1989, the *Bulletin* of the Royal College of Psychiatrists has regularly carried brief articles on audit. We have reviewed this literature in greater detail in a separate report (Brugha and Lindsay 1994), considering here only those few studies that provide clear findings about the relationship between process and later health status (i. e. outcome).

Quality of Care Studies in Psychiatry

The influence of health care on suicide is uncertain; it has been considered by a number of writers to be an important mental health service outcome indicator (Hawton 1987; Jenkins 1990). Morgan and Priest (1991) have carried out a study following on an initiative by the Royal College of Psychiatrists; in essence it was an audit of unexpected deaths. Demographic and clinical data, including diagnosis and treatment, were collected by means of a questionnaire completed by the responsible consultant. The results pointed to a number of possible risk factors for suicide and other unexpected deaths; the included misleading clinical improvement in the absence of corresponding alleviation of situational problems, and social alienation of the patient. The study was felt to have implications for service development, with major reductions in bed numbers planned; this method of audit would need to be evaluated.

Structure, Process and Outcome Quality Evaluations in Psychiatry

Structure

Education can be considered to be a structural influence on the process of care. Rutz and his colleagues (1992) have carried out a study in which they followed up the long-term development of an educational programme for all general practitioners (GPs) on the prevention and treatment of depression. The educational programme was completed by all GPs on a Swedish island. Process and outcome measures of the quality of care, including the number of referrals, the number of emergencies, sick leave, prescription of psychotropics, inpatient care and suicide frequency, were made before and after the programme. The results of the study have indicated that the effects, strictly related in time to the educational programme, which included a lowered suicide rate, were real and not only a coincidence with local trends. They concluded that the educational programme significantly affected important areas of the health care system. They suggested that such educational programmes should be provided every 2 years. This open study represents one of the most compelling pieces of evidence that suicide can be an outcome of antecedent care, although the results should be cautiously interpreted until similar work is conducted by means of a random allocation design in a more representative setting.

Process

Previous reviewers have noted the small number of studies that have focused on the process of psychiatric care and particularly on aspects of drug treatment (Wells and Brook 1988). The Needs for Care Assessment System referred to earlier has been used in a number of studies evaluating the process of care, particularly for long-term patients (Brewin and Wing 1993). The first such study carried out on 145 long-term users of psychiatric day care showed that benzodiazepine tranquillisers and anticholinergic preparations were being used frequently without their need being reviewed by the responsible clinician; episodes of depression and anxiety disorder were sometimes untreated and psychotic symptoms were often undertreated; deficits in role skills that were being particularly neglected included self-care and literacy skills, for which remedial training or shelter was unlikely to have been offered (Brewin et al. 1988). When a similar methodology was applied to physical health problems in the same population (Brugha et al. 1989) almost half (44%) of those with such problems had not received appropriate assessment or treatment.

In a recent report on a cohort of 119 adults with hospital-treated depression, at 3- to 6-month follow-up, 4 out of 5 of those who were still not recovered had been offered no specific treatment or no change in their previous treatment (Brugha and Bebbington 1992). Two other larger, prospectively assessed cohorts have also documented a fall-off in the use of efficacious treatments after approximately 2 months of active treatment, even in those who have not recovered (Shea et al. 1992; Rogers et al. 1993), as well as a general failure to initiate potentially effective treatments in the first place. Process evaluation has also been used in a primary care based study of quality of care (Sibley et al. 1975), in which depression was one of a list of 10 common indicator conditions evaluated according to detailed predetermined criteria. Although drug treatment was scored as adequate in about 40% of uses, other aspects of the management of depression (frequent follow-up assessments and support) were scored as adequate in about 80% of cases identified.

Outcome

Although there have been observational, outcome studies of community care initiatives and psychotherapy services, in general, there is very little outcome research in relation to the process of psychiatric care. In a recent overview of the strength and quality of evidence for effectiveness of treatments for neurotic, affective and functional psychotic disorders (Wing 1992), no citations were based on well-designed cohort or case-controlled analytic studies (from more than one research group). In one open study evaluating a de-institutionalisation programme, better clinical status appeared to be associated with higher costs (Beecham and Knapp 1992). Schuster (1991) has reported that outcome studies will be critical in preventing further limitations in psychiatric care and its funding. He has suggested that quality and cost should be improved by concentrating on treatment settings and who gives the treatment (i. e. process). The Medical Outcomes Study is a 2-year, prospective, observational study in which depression is one of four chronic conditions under study (Tarlov et al. 1989). In the next section we refer to a key report on the relationship between structure (fee payment), process and outcome of depression.

The Structure-Process-Outcome Paradigm

The structure-process-outcome paradigm provides information from which inferences about quality of care may be made; that is they are not attributes of quality unless they are causally related. It has been argued that, in the future, process and out-come should be measured together (Williamson 1971; Fessel and VanBrunt 1972; Wells and Brook 1988). None of the studies in which the Needs for Care Assessment System, referred to earlier, was used have examined, as an outcome validator, the re-lationship between these very detailed indices of quality of care process and later health status. In a recent report on a cohort of 119 adults with hospital-treated de-pression, outcome at 3–6 months was not explained by prior treatment with medica-tion, even when relevant predictors of outcome such as initial severity of illness were adjusted for (Brugha et al. 1992). Although these workers were unable to find any de-tectable bias in the way treatments were assigned, they have argued that outcome studies of this kind can be interpreted in a misleading way because of the non-ran-domised, observational design employed.

To our knowledge, only one report has appeared to date on predictors of outcome (Rogers et al. 1993) from the Medical Outcomes Study referred to previously. This has shown that a poorer outcome in prepaid services, compared with fee for service financing, is apparently due to an early fall-off in antidepressant treatment in the prepaid-financed service. Arguably this study demonstrates a link between structure (payment procedures), process (drug treatment) and later functioning (outcome), but as the authors point out their non-experimental evidence cannot claim the status of proof. Indeed, the authors were reluctant to report their process-outcome findings as so few of the outpatient cases of depression had received any treatment and there was, not surprisingly, a tendency to treat more actively the more severely ill cases (Wells et al. 1992). However, their study does have the authenticity of patient popula-tion representativeness, a major advantage that cannot be confidently claimed for willing participants in randomised trials (Cross Design Synthesis 1993).

Implementing Change

Glick and his colleagues (1989) discuss the reasons for disparity between the quality of the scientific base and quality of care. They outline the obstacles to quality of care. A central failing of quality assessment is that it is rarely used to change behaviour (Brook, 1977). However, the shortcomings of intervention studies are the lack of in-ternal and external validity of "outcome" measures (Moskowitz, 1993).

Purchasing for Quality

A criticism of recent attempts to reform the management of the NHS has been that *activity* has been the principal measure of performance: the more health care provid-ed the better (Sheldon and Borowitz 1993). Improvement in quality will thus depend on a shift from purchasing activity to purchasing effective technology; but how is this to be achieved?

One suggestion is for purchasers to contract for evidence-based protocols (Shel-don and Borowitz 1993), but with the exception of depression, these have yet to be developed (not to mind evaluated) in psychiatry. Yet there is evidence elsewhere in medicine that some patients receive care they do not need, some are denied care they could benefit from and that these discrepancies occur not only in well-but also in poorly resourced and funded settings (Gill 1993). The way that providers organise and monitor their own activity and thus quality is therefore an important topic. In our companion article (Brugha and Lindsay 1994) we discuss management styles, such as Total Quality Management, which may have a valuable contribution to make to the task of implementing change in the future.

Experimental and Independent Evaluation

Although work has been carried out on the effects of different payment methods on later mental health outcomes (Rogers et al. 1993), we have not been able to obtain any evaluative evidence of the effectiveness of such organisational and management strategies in relation to psychiatric services and outcome. Clearly, if there is any prospect of their widespread acceptance, they should be the subject of experimental evaluation.

There is encouraging evidence already of the beneficial effects of clinical guidelines experimentally introduced locally into medical practice (Grimshaw and Russell 1993). These reviewers have found a number of factors that influence whether guidelines are accepted and implemented. In a limited number of experimentally evaluated studies, evidence in most cases is that when guidelines are adopted in practice, outcomes can be empirically demonstrated by an association between increased adherence to guidelines and subsequent enhanced health status. The durability of such changes in practice is not known.

None of the cited experimental studies has focused on structural or process aspects of psychiatric care, although of possible relevance is separate research showing that when different methods of fee payment are randomised, clinical outcomes are not different (Rogers et al. 1993). Thus, no studies experimentally evaluating the effects of clinical guidelines and protocols on the process and outcome of routine care have been conducted in psychiatric services although we know of unsuccessful attempts to obtain funding support for such work and although such protocols are now beginning to become available (Depression Guideline Panel 1993). We would urge caution about the premature introduction of guidelines in purchaser/payer contracts until their benefits have been empirically tested.

Discussion

Clearly, the difficulties that we encountered in relating process and outcome do not apply to enormous and dramatic effects, such as the effect that inhumane, degrading or punishing environments and regimes clearly have on patients' quality of life. Our difficulties were to do with less substantial and obvious effects, some of them delayed over time, such as the effect of a course of antidepressants, or a series of cognitive behaviour therapy sessions on depressive or anxiety symptoms weeks and months later. It is clearly recognised that it is only for these less substantial effects, which can be difficult to detect and demonstrate in an unbiased way, that sophisticated instruments and research designs are required (NHS Management Executive 1992). Randomised designs are a fundamental part of any such strategy. Before saying anything further about experimental methods, what can be said concerning observational methods, given that most quality assurance activity will be based in some way on these? First, the case against and then the case for observational methods.

If, as some would argue, we cannot be certain that when care is not randomly assigned later status is not due to other antecedent factors that have not been considered or measured (Datta 1993), then later status cannot be relied upon. Arguably, therefore, "outcome measurements cannot be adopted as standard tools to assess the performance of healthcare facilities" (Micossi et al. 1993). For example, having identified post-treatment health status indicators (perhaps erroneously assumed to be outcomes) that are less than optimal, attention may focus logically on the supposedly antecedent factors of structure and process in that order. Whether this is a good or a bad thing depends also on the appropriateness of the targets and the effects on the health care system of any change in focus: "setting inappropriate targets often has the effect of diverting effort from the legitimate activity of the organisation" (Lancet 1993).

In effect, in real world practice settings, if outcome cannot be relied upon then quality can only be judged by assessing the extent to which care that service users are capable of benefiting from is provided according to criterion standards. According to this argument, measurement of quality should be based on the size of the gap between observed and expected (ideal) care actions. This brings the focus back to process and the structural factors (service resources, training and organisation) that underpin care activity. If so, should these criterion standards be determined from scientifically verified evaluations of the efficacy of care actions? Unfortunately, scientifically verified evaluations, which in conventional practice means randomised trials, may not be the perfect "yardstick" for setting down such standards because "the way that patients are recruited for a randomised study can seriously impair the generalisability of results" (see Cross Design Synthesis: A new strategy for Medical Effectiveness Research, US GAO B244808, 1992).

We have gone to great pains to identify reports of prospective data on treatment outcomes in routine practice settings, but mostly to no avail. We share the widely acknowledged reservations about the reliance that can be placed on data on treatments that have not been randomly allocated. However, we are concerned that potentially useful data sets have not been analysed by means of the more advanced and rigorous methods of analysis now available (Cross Design Synthesis 1992). The data available are strikingly inadequate and incomplete; but, where available reveal an unpalatable lesson, which is that existing routine practice has, at best, extremely weak beneficial effects. We could choose to conclude that such existing "routine practice" data are consistently erroneous and that *only* randomised experiments can be relied upon. However, much of the evidence that we accept about the aetiology of disease is based on research using precisely these observational methods: are we being inconsistent if we fail to reject those findings also in their entirety?

Thus, our knowledge of "effective" treatments (again excluding major effects) is based almost exclusively on randomised experiments. These are conducted in unrepresentative ways on unrepresentative and willing subjects. Should it be surprising that, perhaps, the same "good outcomes" might not occur in routine clinical practice (Kupfer and Freedman 1986)? In routine clinical practice, diagnostic and treatment protocols are a rarity, and treatment compliance, which is probably acceptable in 50 % of cases, is not directly monitored through tablet counting or drug metabolite monitoring (Wright 1993); failure to attend for non-tablet treatments (day care, psychotherapy) is unlikely to receive the same urgent attention as it does in treatment trials, unless there is a very real concern of self- or other-directed harm.

How unrealistic is it to demand further experimental evidence? Since traditional randomised clinical trials have tended to furnish data on narrow, unrepresentative subsets of the total population of those attending health services (Cross Design Synthesis 1992), should we be trying to devise new research designs beginning with the aim of minimising patient exclusions that would not occur in day-to-day clinical practice? This may mean randomising structural and process variables, that is ways of treating people, rather than randomising different treatments to each person (as in orthodox treatment trials of the kind that we also continue to need). In this article we referred to encouraging evidence that this approach can lead to improvements in the process and outcome of care (Grimshaw and Russell 1993).

In discussions of quality of psychiatric care, in what way does the process versus outcome debate apply to the major and the commoner psychiatric disorders? First, evidence for potential effectiveness (i. e. efficacy) has been demonstrated, for the most part, in randomised-designed studies in which clinical outcome tends to be assessed over a single or brief period of time. But it is increasingly being recognised that recurrence and chronicity rather than prolonged remission characterises most of these disorders. How should clinical management protocols for depression, already referred to, increasingly define, as targets of intervention, remission maintenance, relapse prevention (Depression Guideline Panel 1993) and altered management for non-responders (Brugha, in press)? If purchasers and payers are to contract for quality based on demonstrable effectiveness, and therefore outcomes, confirming that they are getting what they are paying for, how should this be effected? Will the call for contracts based on treatment protocols (Sheldon and Borowitz 1993) be right for psychiatry (assuming that trials of protocols yet to be commissioned and completed confirm their value (i. e. effectiveness) in routine practice settings)?

So where does this now leave purchasers and providers with responsibility for *assuring quality*? Major changes in the structure, including the management of health services, could act as an ideal opportunity for experimental studies of the kind argued for in the last two paragraphs. For the present, changes in practice should follow the systematic route of adopting process protocols that reflect best clinical practice. This route may be forced upon the medical profession from purchasers and payers unless the profession itself guides its introduction (Horton 1993). But should we also make use of Codman's nineteenth century lesson (Donabedian 1989) that when the end results of health care are less than expected, that is the time to go back and ask why. The case for an outcomes-managed health service is growing on both sides of the Atlantic (Jenkins 1990; Ellwood 1988). How should this be achieved at a local level? There is little evidence to help us answer this question. As contributors to a journal of social psychiatry, it may not surprise readers that we favour exploring solutions that give serious attention to environmental and social aspects. We are less impressed with the arguments for admonishment (try harder, work harder) and more impressed with arguments for changes in the organisation of social systems (management structure). Thus, we suspect a team might do rather better at implementing outcomes management as a working group, whether locally based or at a wider but more removed level. At least this should be experimentally evaluated in relation to process and outcome measures.

When deficiencies in care are identified and localised, we would also endorse the case for a form of clinical supervision based on direct observation and feedback by a recognised expert in the field (Wells and Brook 1988). The educational effectiveness of such direct feedback teaching methods in achieving measurable enhancements in skills has been clearly demonstrated in the area of doctor patient communication and clinical assessment (Maguire et al. 1978); many recent medical graduates are already accustomed to this style of learning and would find it acceptable. Overcoming deficiencies and maintaining improvements may be crucially dependent on a shared clinical information system also. In contrast to these approaches, peer review meetings, for example of audit groups of the kind recently recommended to psychiatrists (The Royal College of Psychiatrists 1989), may be of limited effectiveness (Stocking 1992) (again, effectiveness has yet to be demonstrated).

Until the lessons of a more empirical, scientific approach, which we have attempted to face up to honestly here, begin to be more widely accepted and implemented in practice, we would answer the question we began with by recommending that, in the shorter term, the process of care should be monitored; that monitoring should be particularly pursued when associated outcomes are less than expected. In the longer term we should aim to be able to demonstrate that randomised trial proven technologies do lead to measurable improvements in outcome throughout the population of those capable of benefiting from them. Our ultimate aim for public health should be to base quality of care assessment on outcome. This will only happen through a substantial investment in medical effectiveness technologies (Cross Desing Synthesis 1992; NHS Management Executive 1992) in order to determine the effectiveness of changes in the management of services, the structure and process of care and a rational future for public health policy at local and central levels.

References

Audit Commission for Local Authorities and the National Health Service in England and Wales (1992) Minding the quality. Audit Commission, London

Beerham J, Knapp M (1992) Casting psychiatric interventions. In: Thornicroft G, Brewin CR, Wing J (eds) Measuring mental health needs. Gaskell, London, pp 163–183

Brewin CR, Wing JK (1993) The MRC Needs for Care Assessment: progress and controversies. Psychol Med 23: 837–841

Brewin CR, Wing JK, Mangen SP, Brugha TS, MacCarthy B (1987) Principles and practice of measuring needs in the long-term mentally ill: the MRC Needs for Care Assessment. Psychol Med 17: 971–981

Brewin C, Wing J, Mangen S, Brugha T, MacCarthy B, Lesage A (1988) Needs for care among the long-term mentally ill: a report from the Camberwell High Contact Survey. Psychol Med 18: 457–468

Brook RH (1977) Quality – can we measure it? N Engl J Med 296: 170–171

Brugha TS (in press) Depression undertreatment: lost cohorts, lost opportunities. Psychol Med

Brugha TS, Bebbington PE (1992) The undertreatment of depression. Eur Arch Psychiatry Clin Neurosci 242: 103–108

Brugha TS, Lindsay F (1994) Quality outcomes in Psychiatry – background and policy development. A report for Leicestershire Mental health Services

Brugha TS, Wing JK, Smith B (1989) Physical health of the long-term mentally ill in the community: is there unmet need? Br J Psychiatry 155: 777–781

Brugha TS, Bebbington PE, MacCarthy B, Sturt E, Wykes T (1992) Antidepressives may not work in practice: a naturalistic prospective survey. Acta Psychiatr Scand 86: 5–11

Cahn C, Richman A (1985) Quality assurance in psychiatry. Can J Psychiatry 30: 148–152

Cross Design Synthesis: a new strategy for medical effectiveness research (1992) Report no. B244808 Washington D.C., US GAO

Daly OE (1991) Reading about . . . medical audit. Psychiatr Bull 15: 209–210
Datta M (1993) You cannot exclude the explanation you have not considered. Lancet 342: 345–347
DeLacey G (1992) What is audit? Why should we be doing it? Hosp Update June: 458–466
Department of Health (1989) Working for patients. Medical audit. Working paper 6. HMSO, London
Depression Guideline Panel (1993) Depression in primary care, vol 2. Treatment of major depression.
    Clinical practice guideline number 5. Department of Health and Human Services, Public Health Ser-
    vice, Agency for health Care Policy and Research. AHCPR publication no. 93-0551, Rockville M. D.
Donabedian A (1966) Evaluating the quality of medical care. Milbank Memorial Fund Q 44: 166–206
Donabedian A (1989) The end results of health care: Ernest Codman' contribution to quality assess-
    ment and beyond. Milbank Q 67: 233–256
Donabedian A (1992) The role of outcomes in quality assessment and assurance. Qual Rev Bull 18:
    356–360
Ellwood PM (1988) Outcomes management: a technology of patient experience. N Engl J Med 318:
    1549–1556
Everitt BS (1989) Statistical methods for medical investigations. Oxford University Press, New York
Fauman MA (1989) Quality assurance monitoring in psychiatry. Am J Psychiatry 146: 1121–1130
Fauman MA (1990) Monitoring the quality of psychiatric care. In: Soreff S, Uttermohlen D (eds) Psych-
    iatr Clin North Am 13: 73–88
Feldman MM (1992) Audit in psychotherapy: the concept of Kaizen. Psychiatr Bull 16: 334–336
Fessel WJ, Van Brunt EE (1972) Assessing quality of care from the medical record. N Engl J Med 286:
    134–138
Garden G, Oyebode F, Cumella S (1989) Audit in psychiatry. Psychiatr Bull 13: 278–281
Gath A (1991) Audit. Psychiatr Bull 15: 23–25
Gill M (1993) Purchasing for quality: still in the starting blocks? Quality Health Care 2: 179–182
Glick ID, Showstack JA, Cohen C, Klar HM (1989) Between patient and doctor. Improving the quality
    of care for serious mental illness. Bull Menninger Clin 53: 193–202
Grimshaw JM, Russell IT (1993) Effect of clinical guidelines on medical practice: a systematic review
    of rigorous evaluations. Lancet 342: 1317–1322
Hatton P, Renvoize EB (1991) Psychiatric audit. Psychiatr Bull 15: 550–551
Hawton K (1987) Assessment of suicide risk. Br J Psychiatry 150: 145–153
Holman C (1989) Medical audit in psychiatry. Psychiatr Bull 13: 281–284
Horton R (1993) Data-proof practice. Lancet 342: 1499–1500
Ierodiakonou K, Vandenbroucke JP (1993) Medicine as a stochastic art. Lancet 347: 542–548
Jacyna MR (1992) Audit assesses quality: but what is quality? A clinician's view. Hosp Update Novem-
    ber: 822–824
Janca A, Chandrashekar CR (1993) Catelogue of assessment instruments used in the studies co-ordi-
    nated by the WHO Mental Health Programme. WHO/MNH/92.5, Geneva
Jenkins R (1990) Towards a system of outcome indicators for mental health care. Br J Psychiatry 177:
    500–514
Kupfer DJ, Freeman DX (1986) Treatment for depression. 'Standard' clinical practice as an unexam-
    ined topic. Arch Gen Psychiatry 43: 509–511
Lancet (editorial) (1993) Dicing with death rates. Lancet 341: 1183–1184
Last JM (ed) (1988) A dictionary of epidemiology. Oxford University Press, New York
Maguire P, Roe P, Goldberg D, Jones S, Hyde C, O'Dowd T (1978) The value of feedback in teaching
    interviewing skills to medical students. Psychol Med 8: 695–704
Mental Health Act Commission (1993) Mental Health Act Commission; fifth biennial report 1991–
    1993. HMSO, London
Micossi P, Carbone M, Stancanelli G, Fortino A (1993) Measuring products of health care systems.
    Lancet 341: 1566–1567
McClelland R (1992) The quality issue. Psychiatr Bull 16: 411–413
Morgan HG, Priest P (1991) Suicide and other unexpected deaths among psychiatric in-patients. Br J
    Psychiatry 158: 368–374
Moskowitz JM (1993) Why reports of outcome evaluations are often biased or uninterpretable. Eval
    Program Plann 16: 1–9
Moss F, Smith R (1991) From audit to quality and beyond. BMJ 303: 199–200
NHS Management Executive (1992) Assessing the effects of health technologies. Department of
    Health, London
Quality Assurance Project (1983) A treatment outline for depressive disorders. Aust N Z J Psychiatry
    17: 129–146
Robinson M (1991) Medical audit: basic principles and current methods. Psychiatr Bull 15: 21–23
Rogers WH, Wells KB, Meredith KB, Sturm R, Burnham A (1993) Outcomes for adult outpatients
    with depression under prepaid or fee-for-service financing. Arch Gen Psychiatry 50: 517–525

Roy D (1991) Setting up district audit meetings in psychiatry. Psychiatr Bull 15: 417–418

Royal College of Psychiatrists (1989) Preliminary report on medical audit. Psychiatr Bull 13: 577–580

Royal College of Psychiatrists (1991) Good medical practice in the aftercare of potentially violent or vulnerable patients discharged from in-patient psychiatric treatment. Royal College of Psychiatrists, London

Rutz W, Von Knorring L, Walinder J (1992) Long-term effects of an educational program for general practitioners given by the Swedish Committee for the Prevention and Treatment of Depression. Acta Psychiatr Scand 85: 83–88

Schuster J (1991) Ensuring highest quality care for the cost: coping strategies for mental health providers. Hosp Community Psychiatry 42: 774–776

Shea MT, Elkin I, Imber SD, Sotsky SM et al (1992) Course of depressive symptoms over follow up: findings from the National Institute of Mental Health Treatment of Depression Collaborative Research Program. Arch Gen Psychiatry 49: 782–787

Sheldon T, Borowitz M (1993) Changing the measure of quality in the NHS: from purchasing activity to purchasing protocols. Quality Health Care 2: 149–150

Shepherd G (1988) Evaluation and service planning. In: Lavender A, Holloway F (eds) Community care in practice. Wiley, Chichester, pp 91–114

Sibley JC, Spitzer WO, Rudnick KV, Bell JD, Bethune RD, Sackett DL, Wrigth K (1975) Quality of care appraisal in primary care: a quantitative method. Ann Intern Med 83: 46–52

Stocking B (1992) Promoting change in clinical care. Quality Health Care 1: 56–60

Tarlov AR, Ware JE, Greenfield S, Nelson EC, Perrin E, Zubkoff M (1989) The medical outcomes study. An application of methods for monitoring the results of medical care. JAMA 262: 925–930

Tugwell P (1979) A methodological perspective on process measures of the quality of medical care. Clin Invest Med 2: 113–121

Turner WE (1989) Quality care comparisons in medical/surgical and psychiatric services. Administration Policy Ment Health 17: 79–70

Wells KB, Brook RH (1988) The quality of mental health services: past present and future. Plenum: London

Wells KB, Burnam MA, Rogers W, Hays R, Camp P (1992) The course of depression in adult outpatients. Results from the medical outcomes study. Am J Psychiatry 49: 788–794

Williamson JW (1971) Evaluating quality of patient care. JAMA 218: 564–569

Wing JK (1992) Epidemiologically-based mental health needs assessments. Review of research on psychiatric disorders (ICD-10, F2–F6). Royal College of Psychiatrists Research Unit (Mimeo), London

Wright EC (1993) Non compliance – or how many aunts has Matilda? Lancet 342: 909–913

CHAPTER 8

Measuring Social Disabilities in Mental Health

DURK WIERSMA

Introduction

Mental disorders are in general strongly associated with social dysfunction, particularly in schizophrenia and the major affective disorders. For a long time social dysfunctioning was considered an epiphenomenon and just a part of the disease process. Criteria for the diagnosis of a mental disorder were and still are often derived from the domains of work and social relationship. There are at least two related reasons why social functioning deserves a closer look:

1. There is a increasing trend to treat patients in the community instead of in the hospital: the changing orientation on community care needs careful evaluation with respect to its consequences. To what extent is survival in the community possible and what is the quality of life like there? Are community programs better than hospital treatment, and for whom? Therefore, separate measurement is justified for evaluation of outcome and costs and benefits.
2. There is growing evidence that the courses of symptomatology and social dysfunctioning may vary relatively independently: social disablement of a patient may be characterized much more by social disabilities than by persistent psychiatric symptoms; the former may call for another kind of action than usually available. For example, psychosocial rehabilitation focuses on cognitive and social abilities of the patient which are crucial for a more or less independent life. Therefore, seperate measurement is justified for the sake of the right choice of treatment.

The usual diagnostic systems such as the ICD and the DSM offer no adequate solution to the problem of classification and assessment of social dysfunctioning as a consequence of mental disorder. We have to look for other classification systems such as the International Classification Impairments, Disabilities and Handicaps (ICIDH) of the WHO (1980, 1993) which offers a conceptual model to study the long-term consequences in terms of functional disabilities and experienced social handicaps, and the effectiveness of health care to handle these kind of problems.

Department of Social Psychiatry, University Hospital Groningen, Oostersingel 59, PO Box 30.001, 9700 RB Groningen, The Netherlands

Some Conceptual Models of Disability

The ICIDH has been developed in order to improve the quantity and quality of information on what health care systems do to individuals, and in particular to evaluate the outcome of treatment. This classification distinguishes three levels of experience and consequences for the individual (Fig. 1).

Fig. 1. Consequences of disease (WHO/ICIDH)

Disease or disorder
(Intrinsic, pathological changes in the structure or functioning of the body)
|
Impairment
(Any loss or abnormality of psychological, physiological,
or anatomical structure or function; exteriorization)
|
Disability
(Restriction or lack of ability to perform an activity; objectification)
|
Handicap
(Disadvantage that limits or prevents the fulfillment of a role; socialization)

Disease or disorder refers to an intrinsic situation within the individual and to pathological changes in the structure or functioning of the body.

Impairments (I) are considered as "any loss or abnormality of psychological, physiological or anatomical structure or function"; "I" represents the exteriorization of the pathological state and reflects disturbances at the level of the organ.

Disabilities (D) are defined as "any restriction or lack of ability to perform an activity in the manner or in the range considered normal for a human being"; "D" represents objectification of an "I" and reflects disturbances at the level of the person; "I" and "D" categories are supposed to be value free.

Handicaps (H) represent the disadvantages experienced by the individual as a result of the impairments and/or disabilities and reflect the interaction with the social environment which limit or prevent the fulfillment of social roles. It is supposed to be a classification of circumstances in which disabled people find themselves.

The conceptual model of this classification is rather simple and linear. It is assumed that "I" may cause "D", which in their turn may give rise to "H"; sometimes "I" may directly cause "H" without the intermediate steps of "D", e.g., in case of a social stigma. Although it has, to a certain extent, been recognized as a valuable tool for assessment and research it has already been criticized because of many conceptual problems with respect to the distinction between concepts. There is a lack of internal coherence within the framework with respect to how concepts are defined and used, and how categories are drawn up. There is much overlap between the three classifications.

This is even more so in its application to mental health. In general mental disorders are complex and less precisely defined with disturbances on all three levels. It is therefore difficult to take properly into account factors such as lack of motivation, the psychological reaction of the individual to the disorder, the impact on social functioning, and the reaction of others in the community (stigma).

I will mention a number of problems which are relevant here. The problem that bothers us most is the distinction between role disability and handicap. Both classifications deal with social functioning (in work, household, with partner, children) and use the concept of role in regard to the category disabilities in relationships and to the occupational and social integration handicap. For example, social integration with respect to family, work colleagues, spouse, peers, and other customary social relationships is a one-dimensional concept used on the handicap level ("survival role") while family and marital role functioning are put in several disability categories. In essence, it is a different way of conceptualizing and operationalizing the same thing.

Another problem is that on both levels of disability and handicap social relationships and social functioning are to be assessed against normative standards and expectations, and therefore they are not valuefree, although that is claimed for the disability concept. A third problem is that much terminological confusion about handicap relates to the distinction between physical and social barriers outside the individual versus the inabilities of the person himself. What should be taken into account? The definition of Handicap as a classification of circumstances differs from its actual measurement: the details of the handicap dimensions do not refer to circumstances but explicitly to the individual's abilities and competence.

So, the ICIDH is ambiguous and confusing with respect to social functioning, the use of the concepts of role, values and norms, and the issue of circumstances. Even its triaxial character could be challenged. It remains to be seen whether the concept of Handicap could be kept or that another term should be introduced. Precise conceptual distinction between disabilities is needed on a functional or personal level and disabilities on the level of social relationships. Recently Cooper (1993) made a significant contribution to this by redefining I, D, and H, respectively, as reduction in performance of a function in relation to an isolated task, a reduction in performance as a person in relation to the physical environment (personal disability), and a reduction in performance of a social role in relation to others (role handicap). He will elaborate this further in the next session of the WHO on the Classification and Assessment of disablements.

Further I would like to refer to the conceptual framework of Nagi as an alternative to the ICIDH model which is more coherent and consistent with respect to comparable, but slightly different terms of active pathology (the condition involving interruption of normal processes and simultaneous efforts of the organism to regain a normal stage), impairment (loss or abnormality of anatomical, physiological, mental or emotional nature), functional limitations (functional impairment on the level of the organism as a whole), and disability (inability or limitation in performing socially defined roles and tasks expected within a sociocultural and physical environment, such as those in the family or work/employment, and education, recreation, and selfcare). The word handicap has been left out, primarily because of its felt stigma. Disability in this model is explicitly focused on role functioning and it has become part of an extended model of disability and quality of life proposed by the committee on a national agenda for the prevention of disabilities (Pope 1993). I think it is worthwhile to gear these frameworks to one another (Fig. 2).

Fig. 2. Model of disability (NAGI)

Pathology
(Interruption of normal bodily processes or structure)
|
Impairment
(Loss and/or abnormality of mental, emotional or anatomical structure or
function, not exclusively attributable to active pathology)
|
Functional Limitation
(Restriction or lack of ability to perform an activity)
|
Disability
(Limitation in performing socially defined activities & roles)

Social Role Theory

I will now proceed to the category of social disabilities and social roles because they are of the utmost importance for psychiatry and mental health care. Functioning in social roles signifies the person's integration in his community. Sociologists, psychologists, and anthropologists have used the concept of role to study both the individual as the collective within a single conceptual framework. Anthropologists such as Ralph Linton (1936) have traditionally treated role as a culturally derived blueprint for behavior. In this sense it is an external constraint upon an individual and is a normative rather than a behavioral concept. Roles are always linked to a status or a position in a particular pattern or social structure which consists of a network of social relations and communications. A role represents the dynamic aspect of a status. Linton and other anthropologists have made no distinction, however, between behavioral and normative aspects of role. Actual and ideal behaviors are used to describe the people studied. The assumption is that there exists a uniform mode of behavior with regard to status. Empirical research has shown that these assumption are not valid and that consensus concerning status-role behavior is lacking.

Psychologists such as Newcombe (see Gordon 1966) have leaned heavily on interactional theory and were interested in roles more in relation to the self and to the personality. They treated role and status as a given and not as a variable. Role is defined as the subjective perception of the direct interaction. This comes close to the symbolic interactionism which regards self-consciousness and the continuous interpretations of the actions of others as the motive of human action. The focus is on the individual response based on the meaning attached to certain actions of other people. This interactionistic role concept, however, may not take properly into account the pathological changes in experiences and behavior due to mental disorders.

In contrast, sociologists such as Parsons (1958) and many others, known as the structural functionalists, considered the reciprocal relationship or the socially preconditioned interaction of two or more persons as the core of the analysis. Parsons considered a role as the organized system of participation of an individual in a social system and defined it in terms of reciprocal orientations. Status and role are the building blocks or the means by which individuals are able to engage in the reciprocal relationship. The essential part of such a relationship are expectations which, according to Dahrendorf (1965), could have the character of "can", "should" or "must", implying the application of positive or negative sanctions in order to promote conformity to the prevailing norms and values. Other people are important here to define whether an individual is behaving "normally" or "deviantly" or "maladjusted".

But there is, unfortunately, no clear consensus as to how to define a social role (see also Biddle 1979). The following description composed of common elements found in most of the definitions might be sufficient: A social role is a complex of expectations which people have as to the behavior of a person who takes up a certain position in society.

A position is a location in a social structure which is associated with a set of social norms or expectations held in common by members of a social group. The group consists primarily of people with whom the individual frequently interacts, such as family members, friends, colleagues, and so on. There are many positions in the social structure of a group, an association, a profession, a community or the society as a whole, with a corresponding number of social roles. Role performance refers to the actual behavior of the individual in the context of a particular role.

Therefore, a social disability or a role disability is a deficiency to perform activities and manifest behaviors, as these are expected in the context of a well-defined social role. It is important to understand that someone's behavior should always be assessed against the background of how other people expect the individual to behave. It means that such an assessment, above all, pertains to the individual's capacity for interpersonal functioning.

Social role theory does not produce a standard classification of roles which should be taken into account in order to give an adequate description of the individual's overall functioning or integration in the community. We therefore rely on what researchers put into their schedules.

Classification of Social Functioning or Social Role Performance

The number and content of roles in existing schedules vary. There is an overwhelming number of schedules and instruments, reviewed by Weissman (1975), Weissman et al. (1981), Katschnig (1983), and Wing (1989), or specifically by Hall (1980) in respect of ward behavior, Tyrer (1990) with respect to personality disorders, and Wallace (1984) and Rosen et al. (1989) with respect to schizophrenia. There is nevertheless more or less agreement in various instruments on a number of roles.

A number of instruments are relevant in this respect (Hurry and Sturt 1981). These are all more well-known instruments described in the literature with data on reliability and validity. It is striking that each instrument uses different terms to describe the role behaviors, half of them using terms with a negative connotation (maladjustment, disability) and half neutral terms (adjustment, performance). Nevertheless, their content looks much more the same, although there are large differences as to the precise wording, the description, the assessment, the anchor points, the scaling, etc. Most instruments also measure other concepts such as social support, psychiatric symptomatology, the burden of the illness on the family, or satisfaction. There seems to be a consensus of opinion on the following areas of role behavior:

Fig. 3. Instruments for social functioning or social role performance

Groningen Social Disabilities Schedule (GSDS) (Wiersma et al. 1988/1990)

Psychiatric Disability Assessment Schedule (DAS) (WHO/DAS 1988)

Role Activity Performance Scale (RAPS) (Good-Ellis et al. 1987)

Social Adjustment Scale (SAS) (Weissman et al. 1971; Schooler et al. 1979)

Social Behavior Assessment Schedule (SBAS) (Platt et al. 1980)

Social Role Adjustment Instrument (SRAI) (Cohler et al. 1968)

Standardized Interview to Assess Social Maladjustment (Clare & Cairns 1979)

Structured and Scaled Interview to Assess Maladjustment (SSIAM; Gurland et al. 1972)

Each of these roles delineates and area of expected behaviors which determine to a large extent the level and quality or adequacy of the individual's functioning in his/her community. They describe general domains of roles and status which apply to everybody. Each area could be subdivided into smaller behavioral domains, e.g., in instrumental tasks and affective or attitude aspects.

The description of expected behaviors could, of course, be different in various communities or cultures: e.g., doing nothing is highly undesirable in Western countries but may be less so in Eastern countries. Taking part in the household (e.g, doing some cooking or household chores) may be quite different among men in various European countries. The applicability of the role concept is in principle not limited to time or place. It is very important to notice that the norms and values of the local community or of those with whom the person is interacting are decisive in the assessment. We should not assume general norms and values which apply to everybody. There is no general or objective standard of behavior. Norms and values vary from community to community and the acceptability of particular behavior will sometimes be the result of negotiations between those involved.

So, *ideal norms* with respect to what should be done are not relevant here. Empirical research has shown that their applicability hardly exists in practice. Neither are *statistical norms* sufficient because they do not do justice to the differences between

Fig. 4. Components of social role behaviour

- Occupational role:
  (work, education, household, regular activities)
- Household role:
  (participating and contributing to the household and its economic independence)
- Marital role:
  (emotional, sexual relationship with partner/spouse)
- Parental role:
  (relationship with children, caring)
- Family or kinship role:
  (relationship with parents and siblings, extended family)
- Social role:
  (relationship in the community: friends, acquaintances, neighbors)
- Leisure activities and/or general interests
- Self-care:
  (personal grooming and appearance)

social environments. We prefer the norms of the "reference group" which comprises people who in social or other respect are of great importance to the individual. (Reference group here is not taken in sociological terms, which contains the meaning that a person wants to be member of a group to which he does not belong.) This pertains to people in the close environment, such as the partner and other members of the family and to all those with whom the individual comes into direct contact while performing the different roles: colleagues at work, friends, and neighbors. The composition of the reference group will be dependent partly upon the role to be assessed.

Assessment and Measurement of Social or Role Disability

The following issues are crucial in the assessment of social or role disability and are based on the critical comments of several authors on existing schedules (see Platt 1980; Katschnig 1983; Link et al. 1990) and on our own work (Wiersma 1986; DeJong et al. 1994).

Independence of Psychopathology

Considering the conceptual models of disabilities of WHO/ICIDH or Nagi there should be a clear distinction between signs and symptoms of psychopathology or psychological functioning, and social functioning (such as should be between impairment, functional limitation, disability, and handicap). So, hearing voices or feeling depressed should not automatically lead to the assessment of a disability. Their measurement should be separated and not be mixed like in the "Global Assessment of Functioning Scale (GAFS)" in the DSM-III R. It should, however, also be kept well in mind that social or role disability should demonstrably or plausibly be caused by physical, psychological, and/or psychopathological impairments or functional limitations. The assessment has to take place in the context of health experience or health problem: If no health problem, then no disability. One has to keep in mind that a person may not be working, not be married, have bad relationship with their family, or have financial problems for other reasons than a mental disorder or a personality disorder. The existence of such a problem does not in itself presuppose a mental health problem.

Actual Role Performance

The assessment of social or role disability should be based on the actual performance of activities, actual manifestation of behaviors, or actual execution of tasks over a certain period (e.g., last month). The focus is on observable phenomena and not on inferences from abstract concepts such as competence or abilities which are assumed to be present.

Criteria of Assessment

Each community or society at large has more or less defined criteria of eligibility of sickness benefits, disability pensions, sheltered work or living, and social assistance for entering or exiting social roles, such as the marital role, the work role (disability-pension), or the parental role. These norms and regulations define to a certain extent the level and quality of functioning and are the first guideline for the assessment. Further guidelines are the frequency of contacts, the number of completed tasks, the degree of conflict or depth of involvement or strength of motivation. Important for the assessment of a role disability are criteria of frequency and duration of the deviations, the damage inflicted to the person himself or to others, and the desirability of help. This can mean that not fulfilling/occupying a social role implies a (severe or maximum) disability in role functioning: e.g., not having a job due to mental disorder and therefore exempted from the obligation to look for work, or not fullfilling the parental role because of divesting of parental authority.

Freedom of Action or Available Opportunities

The reduction in or the lack of performance should not result from personal or social circumstances that are beyond the control of the individual. An example is the hospitalized patient who can not demonstrate certain behaviors because of the rules prevailing on the ward (e.g., visiting friends or family). Other examples of limited opportunities are the inaccessibility of the labor market, the stigma attached to mental illness, formal or informal rules precluding an (ex-)patient from normal role fulfillment (civil rights, driving license). It is evident that these factors should not lead to a disability per se. The assessment has to take into account the influence of such a circumstance while assessing the role performance.

Sources of Information

There are three main sources on which the assessment can be based: the patient him- or herself, an informant (the partner or a parent or other family member), and an expert or mental health professional. Each source has its advantages and disadvantages, which influence the validity and reliability of the assessment. In consideration of the proposed assessment of role performance it is preferred that several sources by used and not only one. The patient should always be asked, although the severity of symptoms may negatively influence the report on his/her behavior. Patients' own opinions are of importance in order to get informed about his or her perceptions, feelings, and satisfactions with social situations and the performed activities.

The informant – partner, parent, or friend – is of course also influenced to a certain extent by the patient's symptoms. But factual information on the patient's behavior is of great value in order to see the agreement on the report of the same behaviors or other behaviors not reported by the patient, and the evaluation or judgment of the behaviors. It must be noted that an informant is usually only familiar with some behaviors for some roles. It makes quite a difference whether the informant is the mother or a friend. It is important to find out the normative standards of the people with whom the patient interacts, although that may be difficult for certains groups, e.g., those who live alone. The choice of an expert, i.e., a mental health professional – a nurse or psychiatrist, may be obvious in case of the evaluation of a (hospital) treatment or of a long stay in the hospital. In the latter case they are then in contact with the patient the most, but it should be noted that there are disadvantages in using them as informants: difference in education, opportunity to observe the patient outside the treatment setting, and conception of normal and abnormal social behavior.

From our research on the GSDS we found out the influence of the informant on the ratings is substantial: there is a 8–29 % change in the ratings compared to the ratings based on the patient's report only. It appeared that in most cases greater disability was rated as a result.

Method of Measurement

There are various ways of measuring the disabilities, each with its advantages and disadvantages:

- Self-report (paper and pencil test): easy to administer, no training required, answers, no interview bias, and low costs; but a problem with illiterate or visually handicapped persons; Problems may be underreported as a result of symptomatology, in case of serious mental disorder often no completion or proper understanding of the questions, no allowance for the personal or social context, by definition lack of the opinion of others
- Personal interview: either standardized respondent-based interview schedules or semi-structured investigator-based interview; both rely on an interview at least with the patient; the main differentiating characteristic is that in latter case the interviewer or the investigator determines the rating or score; these methods require training, are time consuming, might suffer from an interviewer bias, and are much more costly. The advantages are the direct observation of the patient's behavior, the possibility of getting more precise information, and the flexibility of taking into account the personal context of the person. For the assessment of social or role disabilities the semi-structured interview is preferred, because it the most flexible method.

Conclusion

Platt (1981) and Katschnig (1983) were rather pessimistic about the state of the art with respect to measuring social adjustment (because of the lack of agreement on social norms, unwarranted assumptions, variability of expectations, number of relevant roles, and lack of validity). Progress in this field seems possible to me in regard to an agreement on the disability concept, on the (minimum) number of social roles, on the allowance for relevant situational factors (freedom of action), and the actual norms of the reference group, the application of criteria for assessment, etc. Therefore, I would like to recall the definition of social or role disability:

- A restriction of the ability to perform activities (tasks) and to manifest behaviors as expected in the context of a social role
- As inferred from violations of or deviations from norms and expectations within the relevant reference group
- Caused by physical, psychological, and/or psychopathological impairments
- *Not* resulting from personal or social circumstances beyond the control of the individual

Our research on social disabilities (DeJong et al. 1994; Kraaijkamp 1992; Wiersma et al. 1988, 1990) has shown that the agreement on the assessment of social disabilities is high, that these assessments can be performed reliably (interrater and test-retest), that they take the sociodemographic background of the patients adequately into account, and that they differentiate between diagnostic and patient groups, that the internal and external validity is very satisfactory, and that they are sensitive to change.

Social role functioning deserves its own place in a classification of consequences of disease. It should not be mingled with other concepts such as social support, adverse social circumstances, or quality of life. The revision of the ICIDM offers a good opportunity to solve a number of conceptual problems.

The extended model of disability (Fig. 5) which combines the conceptual framework of Nagi and the WHO/ICIDH as proposed by the Committee on a national agenda for prevention of disabilities in the US (Pope and Tarlov 1991), may be of some help here.

The model contains, besides the concepts of pathology, impairment, functional limitation and disability described earlier, the notion of risk factors (biological, environmental and lifestyle risk factors) and quality of life, both in interaction with the disabling process. The risk factors may well solve the conceptual problem of Handicap in the ICIDH. For example, some environmental risk factors deal with social expectations and opportunities in specific sociocultural environments, such as paternalism, stigma, access to care, or women work participation, and others with physical circumstances of the design of public places or lead paint. Risk factors of lifestyle refer to smoking, excessive alcohol use, overeating, etc. These risk factors are important for identifying a mechanism for action or a preventive intervention.

The model incorporates further the concept of quality of life which unfortunately is not defined but loosely described as total well-being with reference to the WHO definition of health as a state of complete physical, mental, and social well-being, and not merely the absence of disease. It seems to me that using this concept does not clarify much and might give rise to new conceptual difficulties. The authors described as components of quality of life the performance of social roles, physical and emotional status, social interactions, intellectual functioning, economic status, subjective health status, and also aspects of personal well-being not related to health. Such a description will not help the theoretical formulation of a encompassing classification of disability and may even hinder the process of internal and external val-

Fig. 5. Extended model of disability

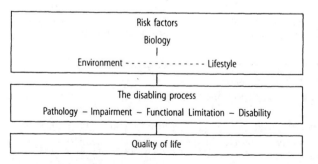

idation. We are in need of a good classification of disability and related factors, not vague concepts which again require the development of new instruments.

Ten years ago social adjustment was said to be an umbrella concept encompassing skills, competence, integration, impairment, disability, inadequacy, etc. Now it seems to have been replaced by the term/concept quality of life, which is treated as a paradigm. It remains to be seen how fruitful this concept will be in theory and practice. I hope this conference will give that discussion a good start.

References

Affleck JW, McGuire RJ (1984) The measurement of psychiatric rehabilitation status. A review of the needs and a new scale. Br J Psychiatry 145: 517–525

American Psychiatric Association (1980) Diagnostic and statistical manual of mental disorders, third edition (DSM-III). APA, Washington

American Psychiatric Association (1987) Diagnostic and statistical manual of mental disorders, third revised edition (DSM-III-R). APA, Washington

Anthony WA, Kennard WA, O'Brien WF, Forbess R (1986) Psychiatric rehabilitation: past myths and current realities. Commun Ment Health J 22: 249–264

Badley EM (1993) An introduction to the concepts and classifications of the international classification of impairments, disabilities and handicaps. Disabil Rehabil 15: 161–178

Biddle B (1979) Role theory: expectations, identities and behaviours. Columbia

Clare AW, Cairns VE (1978) Design, development and use of a standardised interview to assess social maladjustment and dysfunction in community studies. Psychol Med 21: 589–604

Cooper JE (1980) The description and classification of social disability by means of a taxonomic hierarchy. Acta Psychiatr Scand 27: 140–146

Cooper JE (1993) Draft papers of IDH-93. Unpublished manuscript, WHO, Geneva

Dahrendorf R (1965) Homo Sociologicus. Ein Versuch zur Geschichte, Bedeutung und Kritik der Kategorie der sozialen Rolle, 5.
Aufl. Westdeutscher Verlag. Koln und Opladen

Endicott J, Spitzer RL, Fleiss JL, Cohen J (1976) The Global Assessment Scale: a procedure for measuring overall severity of psychiatric disturbance. Arch Gen Psychiatry 33: 766–771

Gordon G (1966) Role theory and illness. A sociological perspective. New Haven

Hall JN (1980) Ward rating scales for long stay patients. A review. Psychol Med 10: 277–288

Hill J, Harrington R, Fudge H, Rutter M, Pickles A (1989) Adult Personality Functioning Assessment (APFA). An investigator-based standardized interview. Br J Psychiatry 155: 24–35

Hurry J, Sturt E (1981) Social performance in a population sample: relation to psychiatric symptoms. In: Wing JK, Bebbington P, Robins LN (eds) What is a case? Grant McIntyre, London, pp 202–213

Jong A de, Giel R, Slooff CJ, Wiersma D (1986) Relationship between symptomatology and social disability. Soc Psychiatry Psychiatr Epidemiol 21: 200–205

Jong A de, Lubbe PM van der (1994) Handleiding van de Groningse Vragenlijst over Sociaal Gedrag (Manual of the Groningen Questionnaire about Social Behaviour). University of Groningen, Department of Social Psychiatry, Groningen

Jong A de, Wiersma D, Lubbe PM van der (in press) Social dysfunction in rehabilitation: classification and assessment. In: Moscarelli M, Rupp A, Sartorius N (eds) The Health Economics of Schizophrenia. John Wiley & Sons

Katschnig H (1983) Methods for measuring social adjustment. In: Helgason T (ed) Methodology in evaluation of psychiatric treatment. Cambridge University Press, Cambridge, pp 205–218

Katz M, Lyerly SB (1963) Methods of measuring adjustment and social behaviour in the community. I. Rationale, description, discriminative validity and scale development. Psychol Rep 13: 503–535

Kraaijkamp HJM (1992) Moeilijke rollen. Psychometrisch onderzoek naar de betrouwbaarheid en validiteit van de Groningse Sociale Beperkingenschaal bij psychiatrische patiënten (Difficult roles. A study into the reliability and validity of the Groningen Social Disabilities Schedule in psychiatric patients). Thesis, University of Groningen

Lewis A (1995) Health as a social concept. Br J Sociol 4: 109–124

Linton R (1936) The study of man. New York

Lubbe PM van der (in press) Over de ontwikkeling van de Groningse Vragenlijst over Sociaal Gedrag: GVSG (On the development of the Groningen Questionnaire about Social Behaviour; GQSB) Thesis, University of Groningen

Morrison RL, Bellack AS (1987) Social functioning of schizophrenic patients: clinical and research is-
    sues. Schizophr Bull 13: 715–725
Nagi SZ (1969) Disability and rehabilitation. Columbus Ohio State University Press
Nagi SZ (1991) Disability Concepts revisited: implications for prevention. In: Pope AM, Tarlov AR
    (eds) Disability in America. Toward a national agenda for prevention. Institute of Medicine, Na-
    tional Academy Press, Washington D.C., appendix A, pp 309–327
Parsons T (1958) Definitions of health and ilness in the light of American values and social structure.
    In: Jaco EG (ed) Patients, physicians, illnesses. Glencoe Ill. Free Press
Platt S (1981) Social adjustment as a criterion of treatment success: just what are we measuring? Psy-
    chiatry 44: 95–112
Platt S, Weyman A, Hirsch SR, Hewett S (1980) The Social Behaviour Assessment Schedule (SBAS):
    rationale, contents, scoring and reliability of a new interview schedule. Soc Psychiatry Psychiatr
    Epidemiol 15: 43–55
Pope AM, Tarlov AR (1991) Disability in America. Toward a national agenda for prevention. Institute
    of Medicine, National Academy Press, Washington D.C.
Remington M, Tyrer PJ (1979) The Social Functioning Schedule. A brief semistructured interview.
    Social Psychiatry Psychiatr Epidemiol 14: 151–157
Rosen A, Hadzi-Pavlovic D, Parker G (1989) The Life-skills Profile: a measure assessing function and
    disability in schizophrenia. Schizophr Bull 15: 325–337
Skodol AE, Link BG, Shrout PE, Horwath E (1988a) The revision of axis V in DSM-III-R: should
    symptoms have been included? Am J Psychiatry 145: 825–829
Skodol AE, Link BG, Shrout PE, Horwath E (1988b) Towards construct validity for DSM-III axis V.
    Psychiatry Res 24: 13–23
Sturt E, Wykes R (1987) Assessment schedules for chronic psychiatric patients. Psychol Med 17: 485–
    493
Tyrer PJ (1990) Personality disorder and social functioning. In: Peck DF, Shapiro CM (eds) Measur-
    ing human problems. A practical guide. Wiley, Chichester, pp 119–142
Wallace CJ (1984) Community and interpersonal functioning in the course of schizophrenic disor-
    ders. Schizophr Bull 10: 233–257
Wallace CJ (1986) Functional assessment in rehabilitation. Schizophr Bull 12: 604–630
Weissman MM (1975) The assessment of social adjustment. A review of techniques. Arch Gen Psychi-
    atry 32: 357–365
Weissman MM, Bothwell S (1976) The assessment of social adjustment by patient self-report. Arch
    Gen Psychiatry 33: 1111–1115
Weissman MM, Shalomskas D, John K (1981) The assessment of social adjustment. An update. Arch
    Gen Psychiatry 38: 1250–1258
Wiersma D (1986) Psychological impairments and social disabilities: on the applicability of the IC-
    IDH to psychiatry. Int Rehabil Med 8: 3–7
Wiersma D, Jong A de, Ormel J (1988) The Groningen Social Disabilities Schedule: development, re-
    lationship with the ICIDH and psychometric properties. Int J Rehabil Res 11: 213–224
Wiersma D, Jong A de, Kraaijkamp HJM, Ormel J (1990) GSDS-II. The Groningen Social Disabilities
    Schedule, second version. Manual, questionnaire and rating form. University of Groningen, De-
    partment of Social Psychiatry, Groningen
Wing JK (1989) The measurement of 'social disablement'. The MRC social behaviour and social role
    performance schedules. Soc Psychiatry Psychiatr Epidemiol 24: 173–178
Wohlfarth TD, Brink W van den, Ormel J, Koeter MWJ, Oldehinkel AJ (1993) The relationship be-
    tween social dysfunctioning and psychopathology among primary care attenders. Br J Psychiatry
    163: 37–44
World Health Organisation (1980) International classification of impairments, disabilities and han-
    dicaps. World Health Organisation, Geneva

SCAN (Schedules for Clinical Assessment in Neuropsychiatry) and the PSE (Present State Examination) Tradition

JOHN WING

Abstract

The development of a series of instruments that has so far culminated in Schedules for Clinical Assessment in Neuropsychiatry (SCAN) version 2.0 began in the late 1950s because of the need for better tools for clinical measurement (including categorization and diagnosis). The basic principles of the Present State Examination (PSE) had long been decided by the time of first publication in 1974 and have remained the same since. Based on the glossary of differential definitions, the aim is to provide comprehensive, accurate and technically specifiable means of describing and classifying clinical phenomena in order to make comparisons. Insofar as it fulfils this aim, SCAN can be used to enhance clinical work and education and advance knowledge through its use in biomedical, epidemiological and psychosocial research.

The Precursors of SCAN

The PSE had its origin in research conducted by the Social Psychiatry Research Unit of the United Kingdom Medical Research Council during the late 1950s and early 1960s. This required a more detailed and reliable method of describing and classifying psychotic symptoms than was then available (Brown et al., 1962; Wing 1960). A simple descriptive categorization of chronic schizophrenia was also constructed based on four symptoms that were commonly seen in long-stay patients in those days – flatness of affect, poverty of speech, incoherence of speech and coherently described delusions and hallucinations (Venables and Wing 1962; Wing 1961, 1962).

Sections dealing with neurotic symptoms were added to produce a further schedule that was designated the third edition of the PSE. This was rapidly developed during intensive studies between 1963 and 1966. The results of wide-ranging tests of the third to fifth editions, based on interviews with patients in ambulatory, day and ward settings, were published in 1967. Reliability on scores, apart from the score on anxiety, was high. Agreement on clinical diagnoses made independently of each other by the five psychiatrists taking part (all trained in the same school) was also high, although no standard definitions of symptoms or algorithms for diagnosis were specific (Wing et al. 1967).

An expanded sixth edition had a very short life because it was adopted and rapidly modified for use in two large international studies – the US-UK Diagnostic Study (Cooper et al. 1972) and the International Pilot Study of Schizophrenia (IPSS;

Research Unit, Royal College of Psychiatrists, 7 Grosvenor Crescent, London SW1X 7EE, UK

WHO 1973, 1979). Reliability was satisfactory in both projects and has remained so in others conducted elsewhere (e.g. Cooper et al. 1977; Kendell et al. 1968; Lesage et al. 1991; Luria and Berry 1979; Luria and McHugh 1974; Rogers and Mann 1986; Wing et al. 1977). Both international projects concentrated on the differential diagnosis of schizophrenia, particularly from affective disorders.

The central result of the US-UK study was that the team of research psychiatrists that examined hospital patients on both sides of the Atlantic diagnosed far fewer schizophrenic disorders than their counterparts in the United States, while agreeing more closely with clinicians in the United Kingdom. The PSE profiles confirmed that New York hospital diagnoses of schizophrenia were substantially broader. This has no implications for validity in the strict sense but does indicate that the boundaries of the disorder were, at that time, drawn so differently that the results of studies into causes, treatments and outcomes would not be comparable between New York and London if based on hospital diagnoses.

The IPSS investigators were a much larger and more diverse group than those of the US-UK study. They came from psychiatric departments in Århus, Agra, Cali, Ibadan, London, Moscow, Taipei and Washington. The result, however, was very similar. When PSE profiles were studied, it was found that centres in Moscow and Washington used a much broader definition of schizophrenia than the other seven.

From the point of view of improving the PSE, three major lessons were learned from these projects:
1. A glossary of differential definitions should be provided as a basis for training courses.
2. Additional schedules would be needed to allow the rating of previous episodes of disorder and possible causes and pathologies.
3. Algorithms for classifying PSE item profiles into ICD-8 diagnostic categories should be provided in order to give a standard of reference in addition to (not as a substitute for) clinical diagnosis. At that time the international diagnostic systems did not provide 'official' algorithms.

These features were incorporated into PSE9, which was short; it contained only 140 items derived from the 500 items of its predecessor. Each was given a differential definition in the glossary. Together with a Syndrome Checklist for previous episodes, an Aetiology Schedule, the CATEGO4 computer program and a laptop version, the new system filled most of the gaps in the old (Wing et al. 1974).

A further innovation was the Index of Definition (ID), which provided a means of differentiating eight levels of confidence that sufficient symptoms were present to allow a diagnosis of one of the 'functional' categories of ICD-8, an important indicator for general population studies (Wing 1976; Wing et al. 1978). Three other modifications were found useful: a change rating scale, using PSE9 items, for monitoring clinical progress over time (Tress et al. 1987); a technique for ascertaining lifetime prevalence (McGuffin et al. 1986); a brief form using only 10 items to identify 'cases' with remarkable success (Cooper and MacKenzie 1981).

Publishing the PSE for the first time in 1974, after 15 years of development, provided an opportunity to state the aims of the system, summarize its limitations and advantages, and specify the relationships between the PSE text and glossary (Wing

1983). These have not changed since. The problems encountered during translation into many different languages have not changed either. The PSE9/CATEGO4 system has been used in numerous studies and translations in most corners of the world, both in sample population surveys and in experimental research (for example: Bebbington et al. 1981; Dean et al. 1983; Henderson et al. 1979; Huxley et al. 1989; Knights et al. 1980; Lehtinen et al. 1990, 1991; Mavreas et al. 1988; Okasha and Ashour 1981; Orley and Wing 1979; Pakaslahti 1994; Sturt 1981; Urwin and Gibbons 1979).

One unexpected problem was appreciated only after long use. There was a tendency to regard the computerized output from PSE9 only in terms of a single diagnosis rather than as a rich and varied psychometric profile. This was far from the authors' intention (Wing 1983, 1994). A central principle was that the system could not 'make a diagnosis' in the straightforward clinical sense. The people who use it are responsible for interpreting the results according to their judgement of the adequacy of the interview, the quality of the data recorded and the choice of outputs from the computer analysis. Most of these last are profiles of scores or prefinal categories. A 'final' category can be derived and interpreted as a diagnosis if the clinician so decides, but that decision is not made by the PSE or by the computer.

Rose (1992) has made the point that diagnosis "splits the world into two"; those who have and those who do not have disorder. However, most problems have continuous distributions. The PSE was not originally designed as a diagnostic instrument but, in the course of its development as comprehensive clinical tool, it came to provide a database capable (in addition to its psychometric properties) of expanding to exploit the more exacting algorithms presented in DSM-III.

Preparation for SCAN

More than 15 years of experience with the PSE9 system has provided a mass of suggestions for improvement. Preparations for a tenth edition were started in 1980 in anticipation of ICD-10 (Jablensky et al. 1983). The major emphasis of correspondents was on broadening the content, both by returning to the larger item-pool of PSE7 and PSE8 and by adding new sections to cover somatoform, dissociative and eating disorders, alcohol and drug use, and cognitive impairments. A second suggestion was that an extra rating point was needed to extend the 0-1-2 scales of severity used for most PSE9 items, providing a mild or 'subclinical' level for population surveys. A third, very obvious, requirement was for a better technique for rating previous episodes of disorder, adding other items relevant to the history and to aetiology, and processing all the resulting information by means of one set of computer programs.

The widespread acceptance and use of DSM-III-R (and subsequently DSM-IV) meant that the database must contain all the clinical and course criteria specified in its manual, as well as those being developed for ICD-10, and that the new CATEGO5 algorithm must contain all three sets of classifying rules. Finally, however, users made it clear that they would wish relevant items in PSE10 to be convertible into PSE9 equivalents so that the CATEGO4 program could be applied to produce output comparable with data from earlier studies.

An early version of SCAN was devised to meet these stringent requirements and has been used in a study of the needs for care and services of long-term attenders at day units in a deprived area of south-east London (Brugha et al. 1988; Wing et al. 1995). This experience, together with suggestions from international reviewers whose opinions were canvassed by the WHO/ADAMHA Task Force, has led to further additions and modifications (Wing et al. 1989). The February 1988 SCAN (version 0) has been used in international field trials to test reliability between interviewer and observer and between two interviewers over time, and to test its general practicality in use across a wide range of disorders. Subsequent changes in the sections dealing with the use of alcohol and other drugs, eating and obsessional disorders, and cognitive impairments have led to further trials (Wing et al. 1996).

SCAN has been redesigned in the light of these experiences. Version 1, in 1992, was different in many respects from version 0 in 1988. However, no sooner had these changes been incorporated and late changes to the Diagnostic Research Criteria of ICD-10 also been assimilated, than DSM-IV began to emerge over the horizon. A further series of changes was undertaken to ensure that all the terms and criteria necessary were included. It was not until September 1994 that a definitive version 2.0 of SCAN was presented at the meeting of the Association of European Psychiatrists in Copenhagen.

Aims, Terminology and Structure of SCAN

The aim of SCAN can be stated very simply in one sentence. It is to provide comprehensive, accurate and technically specifiable means of describing and classifying clinical phenomena, *in order to make comparisons*. Making comparisons is at the heart of all clinical, educational and scientific activities.

The first, clinical, aim is to promote high quality clinical observation. PSE10 is designed to allow a comparison of the respondent's experiences and behaviour against the examiner's glossary-defined concepts by a process of controlled clinical cross-examination. The resulting symptom profiles, scores and rule-based categories of disorder can be compared with each other wherever in the world they are produced, and can be used for clinical audit, needs assessment and monitoring of progress of individual respondents.

The second aim, educational and developmental, is to improve clinical concepts by teaching a common clinical language. This makes it feasible to compare and learn from the usage of different clinical schools. It is not necessary to agree with a common standard of reference to appreciate its value as a basis for communication, quantification and comparison. Different clinical schools of thought *do* exist and *are* taught. Comparison between them by means of a common standard of reference provides a basis for informed development. SCAN, itself, must benefit from such comparisons. New item-concepts will be added and old ones improved. However, modifications should be made in carefully designed stages following periods long enough to provide a substantial basis for change.

The third, scientific, aim is to accelerate the accumulation of knowledge. Using standard technical procedures in research projects makes the results more precise and comparable, thus leading to more rapid agreement on useful theoretical lines for further research. This is true of all types of scientific research – biological, epidemiological and psychosocial. The three aims together facilitate the accumulation of knowledge for clinical purposes of all kinds, including primary, secondary and tertiary prevention and high quality health service management and planning.

The Structure of SCAN

The components of SCAN version 2 needed to achieve the aims are its tools:
1. The SCAN manual or text, which comprises: the Present State Examination, tenth edition (PSE10); section 26, Item Group Checklist (IGC); section 27, Clinical History Schedule (CHS); recording booklets
2. The SCAN glossary
3. The computer-assisted PSE10 (CAPSE10)
4. The SCAN training materials
5. The SCAN reference manual

Present State Examination, tenth edition

PSE10 is the largest part of the SCAN manual, taking up the first 25 sections. Each section is devoted to a particular type of symptom or sign or other clinical feature, covering the symptoms and signs of disorders in subchapters F0–F5 of ICD-10 and their equivalents in DSM-III-R and DSM-IV (F0 dementia, including symptomatic mental disorders; F1 mental and behavioural disorders due to psychoactive substance use; F2 schizophrenia, schizotypal and delusional disorders; F3 mood disorders; F4 neurotic, stress-related and somatoform disorders; F50–51 eating disorders, non-organic sleep disorders). Some sections have optional checklists attached, covering items related to disorders that require specific time relationships, for example to psychosocial trauma, as in the stress and adjustment disorders. Other checklists allow a more extended list of items to be rated than is provided in the main text, for example in an extra list of somatoform symptoms.

The Item Group Checklist

The IGC provides a simple means of rating information obtained only from case-records and/or informants other than the respondent. The Item Groups are not diagnostic syndromes. They do not contain all the items necessary for algorithms for ICD-10 disorders, and the resulting classification is approximate compared with that from the PSE, but it is a useful supplement to PSE information and can substitute in situations where the PSE cannot be fully completed.

Users of the IGC must have been trained in the use of the PSE and its glossary, and be completely familiar with the structure of SCAN. This provides a substantial degree of operationalization for rating items groups, each of which is composed of designated PSE10 items.

The Clinical History Schedule

The main headings in subchapter F6 of ICD-10, for personality disorders, are included as a list in the CHS for direct rating. An independent instrument, the International Personality Disorder Examination, has been developed under the auspices of WHO and ADAMHA, and is recommended for use in association with SCAN if a full assessment is required. Subchapters F7 (mental retardation), F8 (developmental disorders) and F9 (disorders with an onset in childhood) are also not covered in detail, since the interview format is not generally suited to eliciting the problems associated with these disorders. However, provision is made for direct rating in the CHS.

When people with F6–F9 disorders also suffer from the problems listed in F0–F5 and can be interviewed using SCAN, the data will be relevant to their main condition. Moreover, behavioural problems and social impairment common to disorders in the autistic spectrum (F84.0, F84.1) are covered. In the form known as Asperger's syndrome, those afflicted are often able to take part in the examination and enjoy doing so. However, a developmental history, which is essential for full diagnosis, is not covered.

The CHS is optional, but is recommended because of the opportunity it offers to match the information against data recorded elsewhere in SCAN. A simple statistical package is provided with the computer software that enables the user, after collecting a series of cases, to examine profiles of diagnoses or scores against age, sex, personality, disablement, physical illness, etc, since co-morbidity is a prominent feature of mental illness.

The SCAN Glossary

The glossary is at the heart of the SCAN system. It consists of differential definitions of items in the SCAN text, i.e. not only a definition of what the item is but of what it is not. This 'item concept' is carried in the examiner's mind. Virtually every item in SCAN is defined in the glossary, not only those representing symptoms and signs, but those concerned with the clinical course, attribution of cause and so on. It provides a common clinical language in which users, whatever their own school of thought and wherever in the world they are working, can communicate with each other and make comparisons.

Computer Applications

Computer programs are provided to facilitate data entry, data analysis and output of the results for individual respondents. Data analysis is both 'top down', in terms of rule-based categories such as the disorders in ICD-10, DSM-III-R or DSM-IV, and also 'bottom up', in the sense that the items and item-groups, and the dimensional scores, provide alternative descriptive profiles. CAPSE10.1 was designed by G. Glover and is still in use for SCAN version 1. CAPSE10.2, designed by A. Tien and S. Chatterji, is available from September 1995. Both laptop applications can provide an immediate output as each interview is completed. CAPSE10.2 will also provide a standard statistical output from a series of cases and allow downloading into statistical packages. PSE9 is still in use. PSE10 can be converted to PSE9 items, which can then be analysed using CATEGO4 for an ICD-8 diagnosis and comparison with profiles derived from earlier studies.

SCAN Training

Training centres, recognized by WHO because they have a critical mass of staff experienced in the use of SCAN for clinical and research purposes and are knowledgeable about translation problems, have been set up worldwide, for example in China, Denmark, Luxembourg, Germany, India, Russia, Spain the United Kingdom and the United States. A core element is standard in all centres, but details are adapted to local circumstances. Further information can be obtained from the Division of Mental Health, WHO, Geneva.

Further Work

Because of the changes in SCAN from version 1 to version 2, several further studies are planned or are being undertaken to establish current reliability, structure and usefulness. One project nearing completion in the United Kingdom is part of a survey of mental health needs, in which SCAN is used to interview people screened from a first stage national sample to identify people with possibly severe mental illness (Meltzer and Jenkins 1994). A further study compares a lay-administered diagnostic interview (Composite International Diagnostic Interview) with part one of SCAN, the target disorders being current anxiety, depressive and obsessional disorders. International projects are coordinated from Geneva. Other developments will include the preparation of versions dedicated to particular diagnostic systems or diagnoses, testing an Index of Definition for PSE10, developing a short form equivalent to that of PSE9 and a more efficient 'psychosis screen', and psychometric analysis of the scoring system.

Acknowledgements. The SCAN system has been developed in the framework of the WHO and NIH Joint Project on Diagnosis and Classification of Mental Disorders, Alcohol and Drug Related Problems (principal investigator, N. Sartorius, WHO). The development was funded by WHO, NIH and Institutes employing collaborators who took part in the project.

The manuals for SCAN versions 1 and 2 contain lists of the centres and individuals taking part in the field trials and other developments. The international editorial group supervising current work on SCAN comprises: T. Babor, P. E. Bebbington, A. Bertelsen, T. S. Brugha, S. Chatterji, W. Compton III, G. Harrison, V. Mavreas, A. J. Romanoski, N. Sartorius, A. Y. Tien and J. K. Wing (Chair); for WHO: T. B. Üstün and A. Janca.

References

Bebbington PE, Hurry J, Tennant C, Sturt E, Wing JK (1981) Epidemiology of mental disorders in Camberwell. Psychol Med 11: 561–580
Brown GW, Monck E, Carstairs GM, Wing JK (1962) Influence of family life on the course of schizophrenic illness. Br J Prev Soc Med 16: 55–68
Brugha TS, Wing JK, Brewin CR, MacCarthy B, Mangen S, Lesage A, Mumford J (1988) The problems of people in long-term psychiatric day-care. An introduction to the Camberwell High Contact Survey. Psychol Med 18: 443–456
Cooper JE, McKenzie S (1981) The rapid prediction of low scores on a standardized psychiatric interview (PSE). In: Wing JK, Bebbington P, Robins LN (eds) What is a case? Grant McIntyre, London
Cooper JE, Kendell RE, Gurland BJ, Sharpe L, Copeland JRM, Simon R (1972) Psychiatric diagnosis in New York and London. Oxford University Press, Oxford
Cooper JE, Copeland JRM, Brown GW, Harris T, Gourlay J (1977) Further studies on interviewer training and inter-rater reliability of the PSE. Psychol Med 7: 517–523
Dean C, Surtees PG, Sashidharan SP (1983) Comparison of research diagnostic systems in an Edinburgh community sample. Br J Psychiatry 142: 247–256
Henderson S, Duncan-Jones P, Byrne DG, Scott R, Adcock S (1979) Psychiatric disorder in Canberra. A standardized study of prevalence. Acta Psychiatr Scand 60: 355–374
Huxley P, Raval H, Korer J, Jacob C (1989) Psychiatric morbidity in the clients of social workers. Clinical outcome. Psychol Med 19: 189–198
Jablensky A, Sartorius N, Hirschfeld R, Pardes H (1983) Diagnosis and classification of mental disorders and alcohol- and drug-related problems. A research agenda for the 1980s. Psychol Med 13: 907–921

Kendell RE, Everitt B, Cooper JE, Sartorius N, David ME (1968) Reliability of the PSE. Psychiatry 3: 123–129

Knights A, Hirsch SR, Platt SD (1980) Clinical change as a function of brief admission to hospital in a controlled study using the PSE. Br J Psychiatry 137: 170–180

Lehtinen V, Lindholm T, Veijola J, Väisänen E (1990) The prevalence of PSE-CATEGO disorders in a Finnish adult population cohort. Soc Psychiatry Psychiatr Epidemiol 25: 187–192

Lehtinen V, Joukamaa M, Jyrkinen T, Lahtela K, Raitasalo R, Maatela J, Aromaa A (1991) Mental health and mental disorders in the Finnish adult population. Social Institute, Helsinki, pp 308–342

Lesage AD, Cyr M, Toupin J (1991) Reliable use of the PSE by psychiatric nurses of psychotic and non-psychotic patients. Acta Psychiatr 83: 121–124

Luria RE, Berry R (1979) Reliability and descriptive validity of the PSE syndromes. Arch Gen Psychiatry 36: 1187–1195

Luria RE, McHugh PR (1974) Reliability and clinical utility of the Wing PSE. Arch Gen Psychiatry 30: 866–871

Mavreas VG, Bebbington PE (1988) Greeks, British Greek Cypriots and Londoners. A comparison of morbidity. Psychol Med 18: 433–442

McGuffin P, Katz R, Aldrich J (1986) Past and present state examination. The assessment of 'lifetime ever' psychopathology. Psychol Med 16: 461–466

Meltzer H, Jenkins R (1994) The national survey of psychiatric morbidity in Great Britain. Int Rev Psychiatry 6: 349–356

Okasha A, Ashour A (1981) Psycho-demographic study of anxiety in Egypt. The PSE in its Arabic version. Br J Psychiatry 139: 70–73

Orley J, Wing JK (1979) Psychiatric disorders in two African villages. Arch Gen Psychiatry 36: 513–520

Pakaslahti A (1994) Predictors of working disability in first admission schizophrenic patients. Psychiatr Fenn 25: 150–168

Rogers B, Mann SA (1986) The reliability and validity of PSE assessments by lay interviewers. A national population survey. Psychol Med 16: 689–700

Rose G (1992) The strategy of preventive medicine. Oxford University Press, Oxford

Sturt E (1981) Hierarchical patterns in the distribution of psychiatric symptoms. Psychol Med 11: 783–794

Tress KH, Bellenis C, Brownlow JH, Livingston G, Leff JP (1987) The PSE change rating scale. Br J Psychiatry 150: 201–207

Urwin P, Gibbons JL (1979) Psychiatric diagnosis in self poisoning patients. Psychol Med 9: 501–507

Wing JK (1960) The measurement of behaviour in chronic schizophrenia. Acta Psychiatr Neurol 35: 245–254

Wing JK (1961) A simple and reliable subclassification of chronic schizophrenia. J Ment Sci 107: 862–875

Wing JK (1962) Institutionalism in mental hospitals. J Soc Clin Psychol 1: 38–51

Wing JK (1976) A technique for studying psychiatric morbidity in in-patient and out-patient series and in general population samples. Psychol Med 6: 665–671

Wing JK (1983) Use and misuse of the PSE. Br J Psychiatry 143: 111–117

Wing JK (1994) Relevance of psychiatric epidemiology to clinical psychiatry. Int Rev Psychiatry 6: 259–264

Wing JK, Birley JLT, Cooper JE, Graham P, Isaacs AD (1967) Reliability of a procedure for measuring and classifying 'present psychiatric state'. Br J Psychiatry 113: 499–515

Wing JK, Cooper JE, Sartorius N (1974) The description and classification of psychiatric symptoms. An instruction manual for the PSE and CATEGO system. Cambridge University Press, Cambridge

Wing JK, Nixon JM, Mann SA, Leff JP (1977) Reliability of the PSE (ninth edition) used in a population survey. Psychol Med 7: 505–516

Wing JK, Mann SA, Leff JP, Nixon JM (1978) The concept of a 'case' in psychiatric population surveys. Psychol Med 8: 203–217

Wing JK, Babor T, Brugha T, Burke J, Cooper J, Giel R, Jablensky A, Regier D, Sartorius N (1989) SCAN: Schedules for Clinical Assessment in Neuropsychiatry. Arch Gen Psychiatry 47: 589–593

Wing JK, Sartorius N, Üstün TB (eds) (1996) Diagnosis and clinical measurement in psychiatry. An instruction manual for the SCAN system. Cambridge University Press, Cambridge

World Health Organization (1973) The International Pilot Study of Schizophrenia. WHO, Geneva

World Health Organization (1979) Schizophrenia. An international follow-up study. WHO, Geneva

CHAPTER 10

Mental Health Care Costs: Paucity of Measurement

Paul McCrone and Scott Weich

Abstract

For an evaluation of a mental health care programme to be comprehensive, it should include an economic component. However, very few cost instruments appear to exist, and only one has been fully described in the literature. This paper seeks to review the studies where costs have been calculated. For this exercise to be facilitated the different elements which make up overall cost are described. A number of areas have experienced economic evaluations, and the more important studies are described. The paper concludes that all too often evaluations either fail to measure costs or do so in an incomplete and inappropriate way.

Introduction

Resources in an economy are limited. However, the demand for these resources is unlimited. This is clearly the case with health care; if the technology and expertise to treat people exist, then there will be a demand for such resources. If the technology and expertise do not exist then there will be a demand for their provision.

In health care, scarcity of resources leads to competing alternatives. Policy makers and clinicians are confronted with having to decide how health care resources should be allocated. This is particularly relevant given the high cost of health care. However, the measurement of economic cost should not be concerned with simply cutting costs. Rather, good quality cost data should be combined with good quality outcome data to indicate which of the competing options under scrutiny is to be chosen. It may be that the more expensive option is in fact associated with the best outcome. If an evaluation does not include a cost component then inefficient services may go undetected, and resources will be used inappropriately. High quality outcome and cost data are required to advise policy makers and clinicians as to the best use of their limited resources. This paper examines the extent to which costs have been calculated in an appropriate way in mental health care evaluations.

P. McCrone
PRiSM, Institute of Psychiatry, De Crespigny Park, Denmark Hill, London SE5 8AF, UK

S. Weich
Section of Epidemiology and General Practice, Institute of Psychiatry, De Crespigny Park, Denmark Hill, London SE5 8AF, UK

Cost measurement has been undervalued in many evaluations. Sometimes costs have been omitted. In other cases not all relevant, and some irrelevant costs have been collected. Costs are frequently measured incorrectly or not interpreted correctly. When costs have been measured it has often been in an ad hoc fashion. Hardly any costing instruments have been published and described. One exception in the United Kingdom is the Client Service Receipt Interview (Beecham and Knapp 1992). This is unfortunate as costs are one of the few measures that have regularly exhibited variations among treatment interventions.

We need to be sure that the cost data being collected are appropriate. Although cost measurement has been performed imperfectly in many evaluations, a number of programmes and projects have sought to incorporate a cost-benefit or cost-effectiveness analysis into their study. Without an adequate measurement of cost the usefulness of such analyses will not be fully realised. Indeed the very term 'cost-effective' has often been poorly understood and misused (Doubilet et al. 1986). This paper examines evaluations that have included an economic element. From these studies we can deduce what services were considered as relevant for the purposes of costing.

Cost

Definition

It is important to have an understanding of the concept of cost prior to calculating it. Cost is often referred to as *opportunity cost,* which is the value of resources in their best alternative use. This is a definition used by economists in general. Health economists are no exception: 'The cost of a unit of a resource is the benefit that would be derived from using it in its best alternative use' (Drummond 1980). For many products and services it is assumed that an appropriate proxy for opportunity cost is the market value of the product. However, for some products there is no market price and, therefore, an opportunity cost must be imputed.

How Should Cost be Measured?

Cost can refer to an entire service or to the cost of any one individual using the service. It would be advantageous to know the cost of one more person using the service. If there is spare capacity (such as unused hospital beds) this cost might be small. Higher costs are associated with a service operating a full capacity. Considering these *marginal costs* is intrinsically correct. They are also difficult to calculate. However, in the long run (the period in which the structure of a service can alter) *average costs* tend to approximate marginal costs. Most studies in this area focus upon potential policy changing schemes and, therefore, examining average costs is acceptable.

The time scale during which costs are measured is crucial. It is important to choose a length of time that would be a representative example of the users service receipt. Three to six months could be acceptable, although this would depend on the particular programme being evaluated. In addition, different service components require particular costing procedures. For an outline of such costing procedures, the reader is referred to Allen and Beecham (1993).

Components of Cost Packages

All relevant costs should be examined to assess the economic impact of a mental health care intervention (Knapp and Beecham 1990; Rubin 1982; Clark et al. 1993; Weisbrod 1981; Drummond 1980; Glass and Goldberg 1977). It is rare for mental health service users to only have contact with one particular agency, and services often will have effects on each other via inter-agency cooperation, and substitution and complementation effects. For example, the implementation of a mental health programme could potentially decrease costs to the mental health service but increase costs to social services departments or general practitioners, indeed overall costs may be higher than initially. However, if only direct service costs were calculated the results would show that the new programme was less costly. Thus, not only is it important to capture the economic effect of the direct service intervention, but also of great relevance is the effect of secondary services. There may also be hidden effects of a mental health care intervention. Thus, we have direct costs, indirect costs and hidden costs to calculate. A fourth category, non-measured costs, includes aspects of care that are either impossible to cost or inappropriate to cost on the grounds of ethics.

A cost instrument, should capture information that would enable comprehensive costs to be calculated. It is realised, though, that there are limits as to how comprehensive a cost evaluation should be. Collecting data on every possible cost may result in accuracy of measurement being sacrificed. It may sometimes be preferable to ensure that the major costs are measured with utmost accuracy with perhaps less emphasis being placed upon minor services (Challis et al. 1993).

Direct Costs

When contacts are made with the specialist mental health providers direct costs are incurred. The range of direct costs is indicated in Table 1. They are often hospital-based services or community psychiatric services. Many studies only calculate direct costs. This can sometimes appear reasonable. Patients in hospital will often not be using many services that are not provided by the hospital. In addition, staff conducting the research may only be concerned with the costs that fall to their service. These costs are relatively straightforward and less time consuming to calculate than full costs. However, there will inevitably be other cost implications of mental health care programmes, particularly when they are based in the community. To ignore these other costs reduces the impact and usefulness of an economic evaluation, and can make conclusions regarding cost-effectiveness invalid.

Table 1. Elements of direct cost

Psychiatric hospital:	Community:
Inpatient	Community psychiatric nurse
Outpatient	Psychiatric home visit
Day patient	Community mental health centre
Depot clinic	Crisis house
Emergency clinic	Respite house
Psychologist	Drop-in
Occupational therapy	Day centre

Indirect Costs

Indirect costs can refer to lost production caused by mental health problems. We prefer to define this as a hidden cost (see below). Indirect costs should be regarded as those that are due to contacts with services that are not primarily part of the mental health care programme. They are services that are used by a wide range of individuals. Table 2, not an exhaustive list, reveals that the range of indirect services is extensive. Indirect costs have been disaggregated into seven categories: other health services, law and order agencies, social services, educational training, employment training, the voluntary sector and accommodation settings.

Hidden Costs

Hidden costs are by definition not readily observable. Three main types are identified (Table 3). The burden on families is reflected by the cost of *informal care*. Time may need to be taken off work to care for a family member with a mental health problem, or leisure time may need to be given up.

Table 2. Elements of indirect cost

Family health services:	**Employment:**
General practitioner (GP)	Job centre
GP home visit	Job club
Optician	Disablement rehabilitation officer
Chiropodist	Careers advice
Gynaecologist	
Family-planning clinic	**Vountary services:**
Nurse	Counselling
Domiciliary nurse	Bereavement service
Dentist	Samaritans
	Voluntary day centres
General hospital services:	Churches
Inpatient	
Outpatient	**Accommodation:**
Day patient	Supported residential care
Accident and emergency	Private accommodation
Physiotherapy	
Dental services	
Law and order:	
Police	
Probation service	
Court	
Solicitor	
Legal aid	
Prison	
Social services:	
Field social worker	
Field social worker home visit	
Home help	
Meals on wheels	
Social security officer	
Counsellor	

Table 3. Elements of hidden cost

Informal care: Lost employment of friends and relatives Lost leisure time of friends and relatives
User time: Travelling Waiting
Lost employment: Time off work due to mental health problem Foregone potential employment Lost production to economy

Many users are also unemployed. There are clear costs associated with this *lost employment*. From the point of view of the user there is the absence of earnings. The whole of society suffers from reduced production. The degree of this depends on the workings of the labour market. It may be that lost employment opportunities are not included in cost evaluations as they will be the same whatever the intervention, i.e. ill clients remain unemployed. This would be inappropriate. The aim of many involved in mental health care is to help people to become rehabilitated, which should increase their employment prospects; thus, the costs of lost employment are indeed relevant. The financial gains made from employment, in the form of earnings, are often included in cost-benefit analyses (where outcomes are monetised).

Finally, the costs of time and travelling, which are incurred when services are used, should be part of a cost evaluation. The cost of travelling is partly determined by what the user would have been doing if not travelling (the opportunity cost of his/her time).

Welfare Benefits

Welfare benefits are not essentially a cost, that is a means of production, but a transfer payment from one group of economic agents (taxpayers) to another (recipients). The cost to taxpayers is exactly offset by the gain to recipients and hence there is no residual cost (excluding the costs of administrating the benefits system). However, to the individual service user welfare benefits are a definite gain, and to the rest of society they are a cost. The level of benefits may also be an indication of the cost of living (Knapp 1991).

Areas in which costing has been undertaken

Many areas of mental health care have undergone evaluation, and costs have frequently been reported. It should be stressed that reporting costs alone is as dangerous as omitting them altogether – the cost element should be viewed in the context of a full evaluation. However, here we are concerned with those costs that have been collected, and actual cost figures are not reported. Table 4 summarises the studies. No one evaluation covers all relevant areas of cost. The more sophisticated evaluations are dicussed below. Readers are advised to refer to these papers when un-

Table 4. Summary of studies including economic evaluation

Study	Indirect costs								Hidden costs					
	DC	OHS	CJ	SS	ED	EMP	VOL	ACC	IC	LEM	TT	WB	OTH	W
Hospital discharge:														
Beecham et al. (1991)	✓	✓	✓	✓	✓		✓	✓	✓					
Knapp et al. (1990)	✓	✓	✓	✓	✓		✓	✓		✓				✓
Haefner and an der Heiden (1989)	✓					✓								
Muller and Caton (1983)	✓	✓		✓							✓			
Murphy and Datel (1976)	✓	✓		✓				✓	✓			✓		✓
Cassell et al. (1972)	✓													
Residential/Home-based care:														
Beecham et al. (1993)	✓	✓	✓	✓				✓						
Bedell and Ward (1989)	✓							✓						
Bond et al. (1989)	✓							✓						
Hyde et al. (1987)	✓	✓	✓	✓				✓						✓
Rappaport et al. (1987)	✓							✓						
Wherley and Bisgaard (1987)	✓							✓						
Dickey et al. (1986)	✓	✓	✓	✓				✓						
Linn et al. (1985)	✓							✓						
Weisman (1985)	✓							✓						
Mosher et al. (1975)	✓							✓						
Sheehan and Atkinson (1974)	✓							✓						
Aftercare:														
Cardin et al. (1985)	✓	✓	✓	✓				✓				✓		✓
Linn et al. (1979)	✓													
Alternative hospital based services														
Grizenko and Papineau (1992)	✓													
Moscarelli et al. (1991)	✓													
Marinoni et al. (1988)	✓	✓		✓					✓					
Dick et al. (1985)	✓	✓									✓			
Gudeman et al. (1983)	✓							✓	✓					
Schulz et al. (1983)	✓													
Goldberg and Jones (1980)	✓	✓		✓		✓	✓		✓			✓		✓
Jones et al. (1980)	✓	✓		✓		✓	✓		✓			✓		✓
Endicott et al. (1978)	✓			✓										
Levenson et al. (1977)	✓													
Washburn et al. (1976)	✓													
Glick et al. (1974)	✓													
May (1971)	✓													
Case management/assertive outreach:														
McCrone et al. (1994)	✓	✓	✓	✓	✓	✓	✓	✓				✓		
Burns et al. (1993)	✓	✓		✓										
Muijen et al. (1992)	✓													
Burns and Raftery (1991)	✓	✓												
Kivlahan et al. (1991)	✓													
Hu and Jerrell (1991)	✓	✓	✓	✓				✓	✓		✓			
Wiersma et al. (1991)	✓	✓												
Bond et al. (1988)	✓	✓	✓	✓				✓				✓		✓

Table 4 continues on p. 137

Table 4. Continued

Franklin et al. (1987)	✓							
Fenton et al. (1984)	✓							
Hoult et al. (1983)	✓							
Mueller and Hopp (1983)	✓							
Weisbrod et al. (1980)	✓	✓	✓	✓	✓		✓		✓	✓
Others:								
Scott and Freeman (1992)	✓							
Ginsberg et al. (1984)	✓	✓		✓			✓✓	
Mangen et al. (1983)	✓	✓					✓	✓	✓

DC, direct costs; OHS, other health service; CJ, criminal justice system; SS, social services; ED, education; EMP, employment; VOL, voluntary costs; ACC, accomodation costs; IC, informal care; LEM, lost employment; TT, time and travelling; WB, welfare benefit receipt; OTH, other.

dertaking similar studies. Some studies that just examine direct costs are sometimes valuable in their costing of such services, and these can also be of use. It should be pointed out that there is a cost to costing – research time is itself limited by scarce resources.

Hospital Closure and Discharge Studies

There is a trend towards deinstitutionalisation in the United Kingdom and other nations (Thornicroft and Bebbington 1989). This has major economic implications. As hospitals close and people are placed in the community the cost burden on local agencies may rise. This necessitates cost comparisons between long-stay hospital care and community provision.

In the United Kingdom the closure of the Friern and Claybury hospitals and discharge of patients into the community has been evaluated. The economic component (Knapp et al. 1990; Beecham et al. 1991) was comprehensive in its costing. It involved the calculation of direct mental health service costs and many indirect service costs. Client travel costs were also calculated and benefit receipt information was recorded. Informal care and lost employment were not costed. This latter cost is important. In a discharge study from the United States (Muller and Caton 1983) the costs of forgone employment were calculated, and these proved to be extremely high.

An attractive aspect of costing reprovision programmes is the possibility of extrapolating cost for other potential dischargees. A number of studies have sought to do this (Knapp et al. 1992; Murphy and Datel 1976). Clearly, an accurate and comprehensive calculation of cost is a precondition for the gains of this exercise to be realised.

Residential and Home-Based Treatment as Alternatives

Recently there has been a reluctance to admit patients to hospital. This has been reflected by the introduction of alternative residential placements for potential inpatients. Evaluation is required to ascertain whether these alternatives are more efficient than traditional hospital care.

An evaluation of crisis housing stands out in its comprehensive approach to costing. The 'Quarterway House' was a residential alternative to inpatient care for patients with chronic schizophrenia deemed to be unsuitable for normal community placement. A 2-year cost evaluation of the project was undertaken (Dickey et al. 1986). Cost data were collected for direct, and a wide range of indirect services. Omitted were costs associated with education, employment and voluntary services. Hidden costs were not included. An examination of domus care in two different facilities also explored a wide range of costs (Beecham et al. 1993). However, due to the nature of residential provision, few outside services were required.

Aftercare

Often, choices regarding aftercare provision must be made. Some relevant studies are also discussed in the section on hospital closure. The economic costs of 50 schizophrenic patients randomised to day treatment or standard aftercare has been evaluated (Wiersma et al. 1991). Though not described in detail, day treatment included case management, day hospital and short-term domiciliary care. Cost data were limited to average primary and secondary treatment costs.

The cost-effectiveness of behavioural family therapy in the aftercare of patients discharged from hospital following an acute schizophrenic illness has been studied by Cardin et al. (1985). Patients at high risk of relapse were randomly allocated to receive either family therapy or individual supportive psychotherapy. Costs were measured relatively comprehensively, and included welfare benefits and the value of earnings gained.

Alternative Hospital Based Services

It may still be appropriate to treat people in hospital for mental health problems. However, the particular way in which hospital provide care need not be fixed, and different methods should be explored. Again, careful cost examination must be undertaken.

Psychiatric units based in general hospitals have been considered as an alternative to traditional mental hospitals. One prominent study has compared these two possibilities in the Manchester area (Jones et al. 1980; Goldberg and Jones 1980). The authors gathered direct costs and also a number of indirect costs.

Day treatment and outpatient contacts have also been compared to inpatient episodes for non-psychotic psychiatric patients in a randomised trial at three Scottish centres (Dick et al. 1985). In addition to directs costs, general practitioner (GP) costs and travelling costs were measured. However, many others were overlooked.

A study in Boston has reported on the reorganisation of acute hospital services with the aim of reducing admission and increasing day hospital use by introducing a dormitory for homeless patients (Gudeman et al. 1983). Monetary costs were measured for accommodation and all mental health services, and costs to families were estimated.

The Italian mental health care system underwent major reforms during the late 1970s. From 1978, psychiatric hospitals were not allowed to admit patients – inpatients would be cared for in general hospitals. An evaluation measured the costs of managing psychotic patients in the community (Marinoni et al. 1988). Cost comparisons were made between patients in contact with the mental health services and those who had dropped out of care. Direct costs and some indirect costs were measured, as well as informal care contacts.

Case Management/Assertive Outreach

Often the move to community provision has taken the form of implementing case management programmes. This is a method of allowing for the continuation and co-ordination of care. Usually an individual will act as the case manager for a number of users. Case management is not rigidly defined and it takes many forms. Consequently, its cost implications are unpredictable and should be examined.

One of the more thorough cost evaluations of a case management system was that carried out on a community mental health service in Wisconsin (Weisbrod et al. 1980). The community initiative, which included assertive home based care, was compared with traditional provision. Cost information was gathered for the direct service, indirect services and informal care. This study has been replicated in a number of countries (Fenton et al. 1984; Hoult et al. 1983; Muijen et al. 1992), but with far less comprehensiveness.

A number of other forms of case management have been implemented and evaluated. The problem of applying model programmes to other settings that are not identical has been illustrated by Bond et al. (1988). Patients at risk of re-hospitalisation in three centres were randomised to home-based assertive case management or to a control condition consisting of all other public mental health services. The range of costs measured was relatively comprehensive. They included direct psychiatric service costs, residential costs and law enforcement costs.

Community psychiatric nurses became case managers in Greenwich, London. This was a departure from generic community psychiatric nursing (CPN) care. The evaluation of the new service (McCrone et al. 1994) involved the assessment of patients who were randomly allocated to the new community support team or to the traditional team acting as a control. Costs were measured for direct services and a wide range of indirect services. Hidden costs were not calculated.

In two randomised cost-effectiveness studies in California, Hu and Jerrell (1991) set out a method for comparing different models of case management and public capitation funding, coupled with assertive community treatment. Comprehensive cost measures were described for both studies covering direct treatment costs and a range of indirect cost areas. Additionally, informal care and travelling time were costed.

In an area of London, home-based community outreach has been compared to standard care for psychiatric referrals (Burns et al. 1993). However, some relevant costs were not included, with the emphasis being on primary and secondary health care and social worker costs. In a previous study (Burns and Raftery 1991) the social worker costs were not included.

Other Alternatives to Traditional Care

Outpatients in south London with diagnoses of neurosis or personality disorder were allocated to continued outpatient care or to CPN treatment (Mangen et al. 1983). Costs were measured widely, and included direct services, social service input, travel time and welfare benefits. CPN care was cheaper than outpatient care. Cost measurement excluded forgone earnings on the grounds that no differences were found on measures of social functioning.

Ginsberg et al. (1984) have evaluated patients with specific neurotic disorders referred by their GP as suitable for psychotherapy. They were randomly allocated to immediate nurse led treatment or to a waiting list control group. Cost data were derived concerning forgone earnings and family burden, as well as medical and social support costs.

Conclusions

Cost information is vital for a complete and worthwhile evaluation of a mental health care intervention. However, cost calculations have, with the exceptions discussed earlier, been poorly performed and many areas of service provision that are effected have been neglected. Clearly, there is a need for a stringent methodology towards costing. Indeed, well thought out costing frameworks have been proposed (Knapp and Beecham 1992; Drummond et al. 1987; Weisbrod 1981). Few cost instruments have been described - in the United Kingdom only one (Beecham and Knapp 1992). However, many of the recommendations put forward have not as yet been accepted. Ignoring the relevance of economic evaluation can, at best, reduce the impact of wider evaluation and, at worse, provide wrong information to policy makers which would be to the detriment of all.

References

Allen C, Beecham J (1993) Costing services: ideals and reality. In: Netten A, Beecham J (eds) Costing community care: theory and practice. Ashgate, Aldershot, pp 25–42

Bedell J, Ward J (1989) An intensive community-based treatment alternative to state hospitalization. Hosp Community Psychiatry 40: 533–535

Beecham J, Knapp M (1992) Costing psychiatric interventions. In: Thornicroft G, Brewin C, Wing J (eds) Measuring mental health needs. Gaskell, London, pp 163–183

Beecham J, Knapp M, Fenyo A (1991) Costs, needs, and outcomes. Schizophr Bull 17: 427–439

Beecham J, Cambridge P, Hallam A, Knapp M (1993) The costs of domus care. Int J Geriatr Psychiatry 8: 827–831

Bond GR, Miller LD, Krumwied RD, Ward RS (1988) Assertive case management in three CMHCs: a controlled study. Hosp Community Psychiatry 39: 411–418

Bound GR, Witheridge TF, Wasmer D, Dincin J, McRae SA, Mayes J, Ward RS (1989) A comparison of two crisis housing alternatives to psychiatric hospitalization. Hosp Community Psychiatry 40: 177–183

Burns T, Raferty J (1991) Cost of schizophrenia in a randomized trial of home-based treatment. Schizophr Bull 17: 407–410

Burns T, Raftery J, Beadsmoore A, Mcguigan S, Dickson M (1993) A controlled trial of home-based acute psychiatric services. II: Treatment patterns and costs. Br J Psychiatry 163: 55–61

Cardin V, McGill C, Falloon I (1985) An economic analysis: costs, benefits, and effectiveness. In: Falloon I (ed) Family management of schizophrenia: a study of clinical, social, family, and economic benefits. John Hopkins, Baltimore, pp 115–123

Cassell WA, Smith CM, Grunberg F, Boan JA, Thomas RF (1972) Comparing costs of hospital and community care. Hosp Community Psychiatry 23: 17–20

Challis D, Chesterman J, Traske K (1993) Case management: costing the experiments. In: Netten A, Beecham J (eds) Costing community care: theory and practice. Ashgate, Aldershot, pp 143–162

Clark RE, Drake RE, Teague GB (1993) The costs and benefits of case management. In: Harris M, Bergman HC (eds) Case management for mentally ill patients. Harwood, Langorne, pp 217–235

Dick P, Cameron L, Cohen D, Barlo M, Ince A (1985) Day and full time psychiatric treatment: a controlled comparison. Br J Psychiatry 147: 246–250

Dickey B, Cannon NL, McGuire TG, Gudeman JE (1986) The Quarterway House: a two-year cost study of an experimental residential program. Hosp Community Psychiatry 37: 1136–1143

Doubilet P, Weinstein MC, McNeil BJ (1986) Use and misuse of the term "cost effective" in medicine. N Engl J Med 314: 253–256

Drummond M (1980) Principles of economic appraisal in health care. Oxford University Press, Oxford

Drummond M, Stoddart G, Torrance G (1987) Methods for the economic evaluation of health care programmes. Oxford University Press, Oxford

Endicott J, Herz MI, Gibbon M (1978) Brief verses standard hospitalization: the differential costs. Am J Psychiatry 135: 707–712

Fenton FR, Tessier L, Struening EL, Smith FA, Benoit C, Contandriopoulos A-P, Nguyen H (1984) A two-year follow-up of a comparative trial of the cost-effectiveness of home and hospital psychiatric treatment. Can J Psychiatry 29: 205–211

Franklin JL, Solovitz B, Mason M, Clemons JR, Miller GE (1987) An evaluation of case management. Am J Public Health 77: 674–678

Ginsberg G, Marks I, Waters H (1984) Cost-benefit analysis of a controlled trial of nurse therapy for neuroses in primary care. Psychol Med 14: 683–690

Glass NJ, Goldberg D (1977) Cost-benefit analysis and the evaluation of psychiatric services. Psychol Med 7: 701–707

Glick ID, Hargreaves WA, Goldfield MD (1974) Short vs long hospitalization. Arch Gen Psychiatry 30: 363–369

Goldberg D, Jones R (1980) The costs and benefits of psychiatric care. In: Robins L, Clayton P, Wing J (eds) The social consequences of psychiatric illness. Brunner/Mazel, New York, pp 55–70

Grizenko N, Papineau D (1992) A comparison of the cost-effectiveness of day treatment and residential treatment for children with severe behaviour problems. Can J Psychiatry 37: 393–400

Gudeman JE, Shore MF, Dickey B (1983) Day hospitalization and an inn instead of inpatient care for psychiatric patients. N Engl J Med 308: 749–753

Haefner H, Heiden W an der (1989) Effectiveness and cost of community care for schizophrenic patients. Hosp Community Psychiatry 40: 59–63

Hoult J, Reynolds I, Charbonneau-Powis M, Weekes P, Briggs J (1983) Psychiatric hospital verses community treatment: the results of a randomised trial. Aust N Z J Psychiatry 17: 160–167

Hu T-W, Jerrall J (1991) Cost-effectiveness of alternative approaches in treating severely mentally ill in California. Schizophr Bull 17: 461–468

Hyde C, Bridges K, Goldberg D, Lowson K, Sterling C, Faragher B (1987) The evaluation of a hostel ward: a controlled study using modified cost-benefit analysis. Br J Psychiatry 151: 805–812

Jones R, Goldberg D, Hughes B (1980) A comparison of two different services treating schizophrenia: a cost-benefit approach. Psychol Med 10: 493–505

Kivlahan DR, Heiman JR, Wright RC, Mundt JW, Shupe JA (1991) Treatment cost and rehospitalization rate in schizophrenic outpatients with a history of substance abuse. Hosp Community Psychiatry 42: 609–614

Knapp M (1991) The direct costs of the community care of chronically mentally ill people. In: Freeman H, Henderson J (eds) Evaluation of comprehensive care of the mentally ill. Gaskell, London

Knapp M, Beecham J (1990) Costing mental health services. Psychol Med 20: 893–908

Knapp M, Beecham J, Anderson J, Dayson D, Leff J, Margolius O, O'Driscoll C, Wills W (1990) The TAPS project. 3. Predicting the community costs of closing psychiatric hospitals. Br J Psychiatry 157: 661–670

Knapp M, Beecham J, Gordon K (1992) Predicting the community cost of closing psychiatric hospitals: national extrapolations. J Ment Health 1: 315–325

Levenson AJ, Lord CJ, Sermas CE, Thornby JI, Sullender W, Comstock BS (1977) Acute schizophrenia: an efficacious outpatient treatment approach as an alternative to full-time hospitalization. Dis Nerv Syst 38: 242–245

Linn MW, Caffey EM, Klett CJ, Hogarty GE, Lamb R (1979) Day treatment and psychotropic drugs in the aftercare of schizophrenic patients. Arch Gen Psychiatry 36: 1055–1066

Linn MW, Gurel L, Williford WO, Overall J, Gurland B, Laughlin P, Barchiesi A (1985) Nursing home care as an alternative to psychiatric hospitalization. Arch Gen Psychiatry 42: 544–551

Mangen SP, Paykel ES, Griffith JH, Burchell A, Mancini P (1983) Cost-effectiveness of community psychiatric nurse or out-patient psychiatric care of neurotic patients. Psychol Med 13: 407–416

Marinoni A, Grassi M, Ebbli D, Brenna A, Silva S, Torer E (1988) Cost-effectiveness of managing chronic psychotic patients: Italian experience under the new psychiatric law. In: Schwefel D, Zöllner H, Potthoff P (eds) Costs and effects of managing chronic psychotic patients. Springer, Berlin Heidelberg New York

May PRA (1971) Cost efficiency to treatments for the schizophrenic patient. Am J Psychiatry 127: 118–121

McCrone P, Beecham J, Knapp M (1994) Community psychiatric nurses in an intensive community support team: cost-effectiveness comparisons with generic CPN care. Br J Psychiatry 165: 218–221

Moscarelli M, Capri S, Neri L (1991) Cost evaluation of chronic schizophrenic patients during the first 3 years after the first contact. Schizophr Bull 17: 421–426

Mosher LR, Menn A, Matthews SM (1975) Soteria: evaluation of a home-based treatment for schizo-phrenia. Am J Orthopsychiatry 45: 455–467

Mueller J, Hopp M (1983) A demonstration of the cost benefits of case management services for dis-charged mental patients. Psychiatr Q 55: 17–24

Muijen M, Marks IM, Connolly J, Audini B, McNamee G (1992) The Daily Living Programme: preli-minary comparison of community verses hospital-based treatment for the seriously mentally Ill facing emergency admission. Br J Psychiatry 160: 379–384

Muller CFR, Caton CLM (1983) Economic costs of schizophrenia: a postdischarge study. Med Care 21: 92–104

Murphy JG, Datel WE (1976) A cost-benefit analysis of community verses institutional living. Hosp Community Psychiatry 27: 165–170

Rappaport M, Goldman H, Thornton P, Stegner B, Moltzen S, Hall K, Gurevitz H, Attkisson C (1987) A method for comparing two systems of acute 24-hour psychiatric care. Hosp Community Psy-chiatry 38: 1091–1095

Rubin J (1982) Cost measurement and cost cata in mental health settings. Hosp Community Psychia-try 33: 750–754

Schulz RI, Greenley JR, Peterson RW (1983) Management, cost, and quality of acute inpatient psy-chiatric services. Med Care 21: 911–928

Scott AIF, Freeman CPL (1992) Edinburgh primary care depression study: a treatment outcome, pa-tient satisfaction, and cost after 16 weeks. BMJ 304: 883–887

Sheehan D, Atkinson J (1974) Comparative costs of state hospital and community-based inpatient care in Texas: who benefits most? Hosp Community Psychiatry 25: 242–244

Thornicroft G, Bebbington P (1989) Deinstitutionalisation – from hospital closure to service develop-ment. Br J Psychiatry 155: 739–753

Washburn S, Vannicelli M, Longabaugh R, Scheff B-J (1976) A controlled comparison of psychiatric day treatment and inpatient hospitalization. J Consult Clin Psychol 44: 665–675

Weisbrod BA (1981) A guide to benefit-cost analysis, as seen through a controlled experiment in treating the mentally ill. J Health Polit Policy Law 808–845

Weisbrod BA, Test MA, Stein LI (1980) Alternative to mental hospital treatment: II. economic benefit-cost analysis. Arch Gen Psychiatry 37: 400–405

Weisman G (1985) Crisis-orientated residential treatment as an alternative to hospitalization. Hosp Community Psychiatry 36: 1302–1305

Wherley M, Bisgaard S (1987) Beyond model programs: evaluation of a countywide system of resi-dential treatment program. Hosp Community Psychiatry 38: 852–857

Wiersma D, Kluiter H, Nienhuis FJ, Ruphan M, Giel R (1991) Costs and benefits of day treatment with community care for schizophrenic patients. Schizophr Bull 17: 411–419

Uses and Limits of Randomised Controlled Trials in Mental Health Service Research

RUTH TAYLOR and GRAHAM THORNICROFT

Introduction

This chapter begins by outlining the theoretical requirements which must be fulfilled in an adequate evaluation of any medical intervention. The Randomised Control Trial (RCT) fulfils these requirements. The power of this experimental design in overcoming methodological difficulties, and its consequent value in assessing alternative clinical interventions are summarized. There are, however, important differences between the paradigms in medicine, where the RCT has been most extensively used and developed, and its use in evaluating psychiatric care. These differences are due to the nature of that which is being evaluated, and they produce both conceptual and technical problems in using the RCT design.

Conceptual problems arise from the social and political context of mental health services. Whilst researchers in mental health service provision have had to tackle technical problems, they have often failed to recognise difficulties at the conceptual level. RCT designs have been attempted in other fields of public services research; however in these fields, for example, in the penal system, the conceptual difficulties have been recognised and extensively discussed. These conceptual problems can place specific limitations on the information which an RCT can yield about alternative methods of psychiatric care.

Methodological Issues in Evaluative Research

Theoretical Aspects of Evaluation

Evaluation is essentially a process which aims to reach a conclusion about the value of an intervention, and in the field of mental health services it involves considering the effectiveness of a particular treatment or type of service. There are two basic aspects to the evaluation of any system: (1) the identification of the goals of the system and (2) the method used to determine to what extent a particular intervention achieves these goals. In evaluating community mental health services, both of these components give rise to particular methodological problems.

Essentially what the researcher wants to show is that there is a causal association between the intervention used and a specific outcome. Ideally, a closed system should be designed which comprises intervention, specified outcome and a knowledge of all other factors which might be relevant to the outcome, all of which are

PRiSM, Institute of Psychiatry, De Crespigny Park, Denmark Hill, London SE5 8AF, UK possible confounding factors. To determine a causal connection, an evaluation must fulfil the following criteria in its design:

1. The patient group should be characterised.
2. The intervention must be standardised and clearly described.
3. The outcome must be clearly identified in advance and measurable.
4. Intervening variables must be known and controlled for.

The Randomised Controlled Trial

The method of evaluation which best fulfills the requirements listed above and which is widely used in medical research is the RCT. In critically examining RCT studies it is important to consider internal and external validity (Braun et al. 1981; Haefner and an der Heiden 1989). Internal validity is defined as the extent to which the study design ensures that changes in one variable can be explained by changes in another variable; external validity refers to the applicability of the results to conditions outside the study setting. An advantage of the RCT design is that, if properly conducted, its internal validity is high.

The current prevailing view on RCTs within the field of medicine as a whole is illustrated by the opening statement in a paper on RCTs in the Lancet: "Randomised clinical trials are the sine qua non for evaluating treatment in man" (Korn and Baumrind 1991). In the field of psychiatry there is now a substantial amount of literature which testifies to the fact that the RCT is regarded as the "gold standard" for answering questions about treatment efficacy (Kraemer and Pruyn 1987; Leber 1991).

The RCT design has been extensively used in drug trials comparing two treatments. Pocock (1983) gives a detailed account of the use, design and analysis of RCTs. This design is extremely powerful, and one of its major advantages is that it controls for the many confounding variables which may exist. It also eliminates the problematic effects of spontaneous remission, regression to the mean and the placebo effect, all of which can produce an improvement that might be incorrectly attributed to the treatment. A further important advantage provided by the RCT is that, if blindness is maintained, the results are independent of any bias from the clinicians involved in administering the treatment or from the researchers conducting the study. The RCT methodology in medicine as a whole, and in psychiatry in particular, has been applied to the evaluation of the efficacy of new drugs. Leber (1991) states that in the view of the Food and Drug Administration in the USA there is simply no acceptable alternative to the randomised controlled trial in assessing drug efficacy. However, the methodology has also been enthusiastically applied to the evaluation of other treatments, for example psychotherapy (Andrews 1989), and to the evaluation of alternatives to hospital treatment in psychiatry.

Technical limits of Randomised Controlled Trials in Community Mental Health Service Evaluation

Achieving Random Allocation

A difficulty occurs when random allocation of patients is not possible. An example of this is a patient who is potentially suicidal or homicidal where clinicians involved in the trial may feel it is unsafe to allocate such a patient to a community rather than a hospital treatment. This problem may be dealt with by stipulating exclusion criteria, but this ensures that only a particular and selected patient population is included in such RCTs and that the more challenging patients are never studied. The results of RCTs may not therefore be generalised to the true wider population of patients in need of psychiatric care.

Most of the earlier community care evaluation studies reported in the international literature used an RCT design. Although important in demonstrating the value of community care, the careful review by Braun et al. (1981) of these early studies of alternatives to hospitalisation illustrates well many of the technical difficulties in using RCTs in this setting. The majority of studies did claim to have randomly allocated patients, but this was often achieved by resorting to exclusion criteria which removed from the study patients who would present problems for random allocation. All except two of the studies excluded important patient groups. The major exclusions were patients exhibiting homicidal or suicidal behaviour, patients with severe or chronic disorders, and those with no family or surrogate family support. In addition, many studies excluded patients with organic brain disorder or a diagnosis of primary drug or alcohol misuse.

Another review by Kiesler (1982) reveals similar limitations, with only two of ten RCTs of alternative care having no exclusion criteria, and many studies, for example that carried out by Pasamanick et al. (1967), having very restrictive inclusion criteria or excluding a high proportion of patients prior to randomization (78 % of the total pool was excluded in one study!). The population of patients included in such studies are therefore far from representative of the general population of patients with psychiatric disorder. The external validity of these RCTs can be considered to be extremely low and their claims that community care approaches are superior may only apply to a rather select group of less challenging patients.

More recently, the three most important studies of alternatives to hospital care which have tried to overcome the methodological deficiencies of earlier work are those by Stein and Test in Madison in the USA, the evaluation by Hoult and Reynolds in Sydney and the evaluation of the Daily Living Program in London. For example, the comparison by Stein and Test (1980) of an intensive community treatment model (the Training in Community Living (TCL) model) with hospital care using a RCT is widely quoted because it seems to have overcome many of the obstacles to RCTs in this field. It achieved complete random allocation, and the authors specifically comment that no patients were excluded on the basis of severity of illness. However, although the exclusion criteria are few there is no mention of how patients requiring compulsory detention or homicidal or suicidal patients were managed, and there was a lack of data on the frequency of various diagnoses thus constraining the generalisability of the study.

In another UK study, reported by Burns et al. (1993) a RCT compared home based with hospital based acute psychiatric care for all patients referred. No patients were excluded on grounds of diagnosis or severity of illness; however, there was a very high rate of exclusion after random allocation with 48 % failing to become study subjects. The authors comment that their eventual sample had an under-representation of long-term, severely disabled patients.

Studies of day hospital versus inpatient care further illustrate potentially serious problems in conducting RCTs. Platt et al. (1980) found met with such difficulties in using an RCT design to compare day hospital and inpatient care that they abandoned their project. The problem was that doctors would allow only 10 % of patients to be randomly allocated, many patients being regarded as mandatory inpatients because they were too ill or suicidal. Creed et al. (1990) reported a prospective RCT of day patient versus inpatient psychiatric treatment for all acutely ill patients presenting for admission. Although they did not have major exclusion criteria they found that 42 % of patients could not be allocated. Another RCT of day hospital care compared to inpatient care (Dick et al., 1985) was also plagued by the difficulty in achieving a random allocation. In this case, although only a rather select group of non-psychotic patients were considered, out of 242 patients, 101 were deemed too ill for allocation to the study.

"Intention to Treat" Analysis

A problem related to the difficulty in achieving random allocation is that some patients initially included in a study subsequently withdrawn from the study (for example if they require formal admission because of the nature of their disturbance). Newell (1992) draws attention to this problem and suggests that it can be solved by using an "intention to treat" analysis. This concept, which is widely accepted but not always applied in practice, involves the inclusion of all patients who were allocated to a particular treatment option in the analysis, even if they were subsequently withdrawn from, or dropped out of, the treatment. This is frequently relevant in comparing alternative care settings, for example the hospitalization, and therefore withdrawal from the community treatment group, of patients who become a risk to self or to others.

Patient Consent and Motivation

Prior to participation in RCTs, patients need to be informed about the study and give their consent to enter it. The most disabled patients give their consent less often and so, out of their own choice, they are excluded from such studies. This is another problem which may bias evaluative studies by increasing the proportion of less severely ill patients participating in these studies and so limit our ability to generalise from them. A related issue is that of patient motivation which, in the RCTs discussed so far, was never taken into account. Brewin and Bradley (1989) draw attention to the importance of a patient's preference for a particular treatment in what they call "participative" interventions. These include, for example, de-institutionalisation programmes for the chronically mentally ill where clearly the patients' motivation will influence outcome. They argue that it is vital that patients are fully informed about both treatment options. Even if the patients still agree to random allocation, they may prefer one treatment over the other, and this will influence the enthusiasm with which they participate in the treatment. Brewin and Bradley consequently criticise research which designs participative treatments trials as though they were drug trials ignoring the psychological processes involved.

Blindness

We have seen that blindness of the subjects, of the clinicians giving the treatment and of the researcher rating the outcome is a crucial component in the design of a

RCT. As the intervention in mental health evaluation usually consists of a specific approach to service provision, it is usually impossible for patients, their relatives or the researchers to remain blind with respect to the type of intervention used in treating the patient. This is particularly important because it means that such research is prone to researcher and clinician bias. Since this field is subject to close political and public scrutiny, there is a danger that ideologically committed clinicians may pursue research with a view to confirming their preconceived convictions about the value of alternatives to hospitalisation. A related difficulty is that since both experimenters and patients will always know which group they are in, the Hawthorne effect may operate whereby patients and their relatives benefit from non-specific factors associated with being studied and therefore the results may be biased towards the experimental intervention condition.

Nature of the Experimental Condition

In other areas of medicine or psychiatry the "treatment" is a specifiable single intervention, be it simply a particular drug or a more complex but nevertheless known and quantifiable therapy. In contrast, the interventions in community mental health usually consist of a particular innovative service provision, e.g., the provision of out-patient care instead of hospital admission. There is a tendency in evaluating different service provisions to overlook this complexity and treat the alternatives as if they were simple, unified entities. This is flawed becaus the multi-faceted nature of the interventions creates two problems for the RCT design. Since there is no one single intervention, patients receive a care package appropriate to their needs. Hence, there are many different factors which could contribute to a particular outcome and which often the identification of ingredients of a care package.

Nature of the Control Condition

The review by Braun et al. (1981) clearly illustrates the number of studies which failed to adequately describe the interventions used and the control condition. In the Daily Living Progrmme study (Muijen et al. 1990), precise details of the interventions used by staff are not given, though there is mention of family sessions, and an emphasis on practical help. No details are given of the care actually provided in the control condition other than that the patients received "standard hospital care". Indeed there may often be far less homogeneity between control conditions than between experimental conditions of similar interventions, thus reducing the comparability of studies for the purposes of meta-analysis.

Measuring Outcomes

A major requirement in using a RCT design is that the outcomes be specified and measurable. Since "mental health" is neither operationally defined nor an easily measurable domain, it is therefore necessary to choose indicators of mental health to use as outcome measures. In severe mental illness, the goal of achieving mental health may not be valid and more realistic aims may be to lessen symptoms (impairment), to improve a patient's functions (lessen disability) or to improve quality of life. Many of the early studies in this area used indicators of outcome which reflect these aims, e.g. lengths of stay in hospital and re-admission rates to hospital (Hafner and an der Heiden 1991). With the evolution of evaluative research, there has been a shift towards measures of symptomatology and social function. Recently, more subjective patient-centred outcome measures such as quality of life (Oliver 1991) and satisfaction with services (Ruggeri 1993) have become more prominent. Other chapters in this volume summarise many of the relevant outcome measures available.

Ethical Aspects

RCTs in any setting pose a range of ethical issues. Some researchers in the field maintain that random allocation of patients to what are presumed inferior or placebo treatments is becoming increasingly difficult to justify (e.g. Hafner and an der Heiden 1991). In the evaluation of mental health services it could be argued that it for humanitarian reasons patients should be treated in the least restrictive settings, it is unethical for the purposes of research to offer some patients care in an institution when it is already known that for the majority of patients it is possible to offer community-based care. This issue may lead staff in community mental health teams not to co-operate in some research projects. The counter argument is that it is in fact unethical to proffer treatments to patients unless they have been subject to scrutiny using the most possible rigorous methods of scientific evaluation.

Internal and External Validity

There is often a tendency to trade-off internal validity for external validity and vice versa. In order to achieve the rigour demanded by the RCT design (i.e., to achieve high internal validity), the resulting study may apply only to a rather select group of patients under particular experimental circumstances (i.e., low external validity). Newcombe (1988) discusses the practical difficulties which psychiatric treatments present in the execution of a RCT; he believes that these are merely technical difficulties that can be overcome with sufficient ingenuity and dedication. Even if an ideal RCT could be conducted in the field of service evaluation it would involve conducting an experiment within what is essentially a social situation, and this gives rise to further conceptual issues which are addressed below.

Conceputal Issues in Randomised Controlled Trials for Mental Health Services

In addition to the limitations of RCTs which are due to specific technical difficulties in achieving the rigour demanded by their design, other limitations arise because of factors quite specific to the evaluating systems of psychiatric care which are intrinsically social and political in nature. Minimal attention has been drawn to the fundamental difference between mental health service evaluation and the evaluation of a particular drug or surgical technique. Similar problems are most frequently encountered in sociological research where they have long been recognised.

Randomised Controlled Trials in Institutional Settings

In discussing an evaluation of a new treatment regime in an approved school for adolescents using a randomised controlled trial, Clarke and Cornish (1972) outline the numerous difficulties encountered which they regard as inevitable when attempting such a trial within an institutional setting, and most of these are germane to the mental health services setting. They suggest that any penal treatment setting is not an isolated system but exists as part of a wider social system. Thus the isolated system where inputs, outputs, and intervening variables are all known or controlled for, on which the RCT depends, is often not achievable in such real life settings. For example, they noted that the selection criteria for inclusion of boys in the new treatment regime led to a "creaming-off" of less challenging boys into the study, and that this had an impact on both staff and the boys' morale in the control house, and on the way this house was run. The success of the new treatment may be offset by negative effects such as increasing staff tensions and turnover, which may make it impossible to complete the evaluation. Similar considerations may apply to experimental programmes of mental health services in which a particular group of less difficult patients is selected, as illustrated in the previous section. In addition more enthusiastic might be selected for the experimental setting, thereby producing disruptive effects on the morale and resources in the standard service.

Another problem which Clarke and Cornish encountered was enlisting the co-operation of practitioners whose fears of losing prestige, power and responsibility, or of being found to be ineffective or inefficient. Thus the experiment may be viewed as a personal or professional threat. It is conceivable that in the field of psychiatry, similar concerns may exist. Professionals working in institutional settings may fear the consequences of having their work examined very closely or the loss of power which a shift of mental health services to community provision may bring.

The Limits of Innovative Mental Health Service Systems

The RCT has a central role in mental health research; its high internal validity can lend scientific weight to assertions that a particular new alternative treatment strategy works. However its limitations, which arise from the nature of the system within which it is being used, must not be ignored.

Firstly, many of the experimental programmes utilised in the RCTs which have been described were intensive and demanded extremely high levels of dedication and commitment from the staff involved. However, because of their experimental nature they were time-limited. The staff were able to provide the high level of care demanded over the short, defined period of time. They often benefited from charismatic understanding, and the goal of proving an experimental point maintained moral. This level of performance may be more difficult to achieve in an ongoing routine service. This point may only be countered by evidence which proves that community care works when it is provided as an ongoing part of a standard psychiatric service. The RCT methodology is not able to provide such evidence.

Secondly, the experimental approach makes the assumption that a closed system can be created in which all factors influencing the outcome can be either eliminated in their effect by randomisation or controlled for in study design or analysis. This assumption often does not hold since in reality patients live in a wider society and factors in that society such as housing policy and unemployment can have a profound influence on mental health.

Thirdly, as Goldberg (1991) has pointed out, RCTs alone do not create a new health policy, but only allow us to compare existing alternative interventions. Leber (1991), in the context of the use of RCTs to evaluate psychiatric drugs, makes a similar point. He argues that if the goal is the generation of new ideas and hypotheses, RCTs can limit inventiveness; furthermore the importance of controls is not as great as when specific questions about existing alternative drugs need to be answered.

Finally, and importantly, the experimental approach to evaluation is expensive. It requires the setting up of a specific intervention and the employment of an independent research team to evaluate it. The intervention often has to be terminated at the end of the sutdy for financial reasons. This can be demoralizing for the staff and patients involved, particularly if the intervention was shown to be successful. The wait for results to filter through to planners and politicians can be frustrating for all concerned.

Conclusion

This chapter has illustrated that although the RCT is often seen within evidence based medicine as the ultimate test of treatment efficacy, there are important technical and conceptual problems which limit its use in evaluating alternative mental health service provisions. In spite of this, it has facilitated good quality research, and has provided evidence that psychiatric care can be successfully provided outside hospital settings for substantial numbers of patients. The problems produced in trying to conduct these trials have also thrown some light on the types of patients for whom such alternative treatment settings are not possible. In considering the results of such studies it is important to be aware that even if they have achieved a reasonable degree of internal validity through their rigourous design, their external validity may be limited. This is because they have been forced to include a rather select group of patients. Furthermore the nature of the intervention may have been atypical in its quality and the enthusiasm with which it was applied may have been greater than usual. Even if an increasingly sophisticated study design overcomes some of the technical difficulties, the problems posed by evaluating something which is part of and interacts with a wider social system will remain.

The RCT will undoubtedly continue to have an important part to play, particularly in establishing a strictly causal connection between a specific intervention and an outcome. However, other study designs should be considered in order to better examine the complexity of processes involved in providing mental healt care. An alternative strategy to the RCT is to use what Hafner and an der Heiden (1991) describe as more naturalistic studies which offer a way of dealing with the complexity of factors involved in such systems. These new approaches will not provide direct information about an intervention and its outcome, but may enable us to take a realistic look at how community services work for different groups of patients. Furthermore, they may help us to gain some understanding of the complex but important blend of factors involved, and so enhance generalisability.

References

Andrews G (1989) Evaluating Treatment Effectiveness. Australian and New Zealand Journal of Psychiatry 23: 186

Braun P, Kochansky G, Shapiro R, Greenberg S, Gudeman JE, Johnson S, Shore MF (1981) Overview: Deinstitutionalisation of Psychiatric Patients, A Critical Review of Outcome Studies. American Journal of Psychiatry, 138 (6): 736–749

Brewin C, Bradley C (1989) Patient preferences and randomised controlled trials. British Medical Journal 299: 313–315

Burns T, Beadsmoore A, Bhat AV, Oliver A, Mathers C (1993) A Controlled Trial of Home-Based Acute Psychiatric Services. I: Clinical and Social Outcome. British Journal of Psychiatry 163: 49–54

Clarke RVG, Cornish DB (1972) The Controlled Trial in Institutional Research – paradigm or pitfall for penal evaluators. London: HMSO

Creed F, Black D, Anthony P et al (1989) Day Hospital and Community Treatment for Acute Psychiatric Illness. A Critical Appraisal. British Journal of Psychiatry 154: 300–310

Creed F, Black D, Anthony P et al (1990) Randomised Controlled Trial of Day Patient Versus Inpatient Psychiatric Treatment. British Medical Journal 300: 1033–1037

Dean C, Phillips J, Gadd EM, Jospeh M, England S (1993) Comparison of community based service with hospital based service for people with acute, severe psychiatric illness. British Medical Journal 307: 473–476

Dick P, Cameron L, Cohen D, Barlow M, Ince A (1985) Day and Full Time Psychiatric Treatment: A controlled comparison. British Journal of Psychiatry, 147, 246–250

Goldberg D (1991) Cost effectiveness studies in the treatment of schizophrenia: A review. Social Psychiatry and Psychiatric Epidemiology, 26, 139–142

Hafner H, an der Heiden W (1991) Evaluating Effectiveness and Cost of Community Care for Schizophrenic Patients. Schizophrenia Bulletin, 17(3) 441–451

Hafner H, an der Heiden W (1989) The Evaluation of Mental Health Care Systems. British Journal of Psychiatry, 155, 12–17

Hoult J, Rosen A, Reynolds I (1984) Community Orientated Treatment Compared to Psychiatric Hospital Orientated Treatment. Soc Sci Med 18(11) 1002–1010

Kiesler CA (1982) Mental hospitals and alternative care: non institutionalisation as a potential public policy for mental patients. American Psychologist, 37, 349–360

Korn EL, Baumrind S (1991) Randomised clinical trials with clinician-preferred treatment. The Lancet, 337, 149–153

Kraemer HC, Pruyn JP (1990) The Evaluation of Different Approaches to Randomized Clinical Trials. Archives of General Psychiatry, 47, 1163–1169

Leber P (1991) The Future of Controlled Clinical Trials. Psychopharmacology Bulletin, 27(1) 3–8

Muijen M, Marks I, Connolly J, Audini B (1992) Home based care and standard hospital care for patients with severe mental illness: a randomised controlled trial. British Medical Journal, 304, 749–754

Newell DJ (1992) Intention-to-Treat Analysis: Implications for Quantitative and Qualitative Research. Int J Epidemiol 21(5) 837–841

Newcome RG (1988) Evaluation of treatment Effectiveness in Psychiatric Research. British Journal of Psychiatry, 152, 696–697

Oliver JPJ (1991) The Social Care Directive: Development of a Quality of Life Profile for Use in Community services for the Mentally Ill. Social Work and Social Sciences Review 3(1) 5–45

Pasamanick B, Scarpitti FR, Dinitz S (1967) Schizophrenics in the community: An experimental study in the prevention of hospitalisation. New York Appleton Century Crofts

Platt SD, Knights AC, Hirsch SR (1980) Caution and conservatism in the use of psychiatric day hospital: evidence from a research project that failed. Psychiatry Research, 3. 123–132

Pocock SJ (1983) Clinical Trials: A Practical Approach. New York: Wiley

Ruggeri M, DallÁgnola R (1993) The development and use of the Verona Expectations for Care Scale (VECS) and the Verona Service Satisfaction Scale (VSSS) for measuring expectations and satisfaction with community-based psychiatric services in patients, relatives and professionals. Psychological Medicine, 23, 511–524

Stein LI, Test MA (1980) Alternative to Mental Hospital Treatment: 1. Conceptual model, treatment program and clinical evaluation. Archives of General Psychiatry, 37, 392–397

CHAPTER 12

Psychiatric Assessment Instruments Developed by the World Health Organization

Norman Sartorius and Aleksandar Janca

Abstract

Over the past 30 years the World Health Organization (WHO) has produced a number of assessment instruments intended for national and cross-cultural psychiatric research. WHO instruments have been tested and used in many collaborative studies involving more than 100 centres in different parts of the world. This article reviews the main WHO instruments for the assessment of (a) psychopathology, (b) disability, quality of life and satisfaction, (c) services, and (d) environment, and risks to mental health. The principles used in the development of WHO instruments, their translation and their use across cultures and settings are discussed.

The World Health Organization (WHO) occupies a unique position in the field of health care and represents a neutral platform that can be used to bring about international collaboration in research. Over the years WHO has gained experience in the management of international collaborative research projects and has produced reliable methods for their conduct in different cultures and settings (Sartorius 1989).

The development of cross-culturally applicable and reliable methods for the assessment of problems related to mental health has been one of the major activities in the WHO Mental Health Programme[1]. Many of these methods have been described in scientific publications, released for general use and applied in various research projects worldwide (Sartorius 1993). This chapter outlines the basic characteristics of the main instruments produced and used in the studies coordinated by the WHO Mental Health Programme.[1] The specific characteristics of the instruments described – such as their format, area of assessment, main users, training requirements and available translations – are summarized in Tables 1–4.

---

[1] More details about these and other WHO instruments can be found in the *Catalogue of assessment instruments used in the studies coordinated by the WHO Mental Health Programme* (Janca and Chandrashekar 1993), available from WHO on request.

N. Sartorius
Department of Psychiatry, University of Geneva, Boulevard de la Cluse 51, CH-1205 Geneva, Switzerland

A. Janca
Division of Mental Health and Prevention of Substance Abuse, World Health Organization, CH-1211 Geneva 27, Switzerland

Table 1. World Health Organization instruments for the assessment of psychopathology

Instrument	Format	Area	User	Training	Languages
Alcohol Use Disorder Identification Test	Structured	Harmful alcohol use	Health or research worker	Not required	English, Japanese, Norwegian, Romanian, Spanish
Composite International Diagnostic Interview	Structured	ICD-10, DSM-III-R and DSM-IV mental disorders	Lay interviewer	Essential	Arabic, Chinese, Dutch, English, French, German, Icelandic, Italian, Japanese, Kannada, Russian, Serbian, Spanish
ICD-10 Symptom Checklist for Mental Disorders	Semi-structured	ICD-10 mental disorders	Psychiatrist or psychologist	Not required	Chinese, English, Estonian, German, Italian, Japanese, Kannada, Portuguese, Russian, Spanish
International Personality Disorder Examination	Semi-structured	ICD-10, DSM-III-R and DSM-IV personality disorders	Psychiatrist or psychologist	Essential	Dutch, English, Estonian, French, German, Hindi, Japanese, Kannada, Norwegian, Swahili, Tamil
Schedules for Clinical Assessment in Neuropsychiatry	Semi-structured	Symptoms and signs of mental disorders	Psychiatrist or psychologist	Essential	Chinese, Danish, Dutch, English, French, German, Greek, Italian, Kannada, Portuguese, Spanish, Turkish, Yoruba
Standardized Assessment of Depressive Disorders	Semi-structured	Depressive disorders	Psychiatrist or psychologist	Essential	Bulgarian, Farsi, French, German, Hindi, Japanese, Polish, Turkish
Schedules for Clinical Assessment o Acute Psychotic States	Semi-structured	Acute psychotic states	Psychiatrist or psychologist	Essential	Czech, Danish, English, Hindi, Yoruba
Social Description	Semi structured	Social history	Social worker or psychologist	Essential	Chinese, Czech, Danish, English, Hindi, Russian, Spanish, Yoruba
Self-Reporting Questionnaire	Questionnaire	Neurotic and psychotic symptoms	Self-administered	Not applicable	Amharic, Arabic, Bahasa (Malaysia), Bengali, English, French, Hindi, Italian, Kiswahili, Njanja Lusaka, Portuguese, Spanish, Tagalog

ICD, International classification of diseases; DSM, Diagnostic and statistical manual).

Table 2. World Health Organization instruments for the assessment of disability, of illness, and quality of life

Instrument	Format	Area	User	Training	Languages
WHO Psychiatric Disability Assessment Schedule	Semi-structured	Disability due to mental and often disorders	Psychiatrist or psychologist	Essential	Arabic, Bulgarian, Chinese, Croatian, Danish, English, French, German, Hindi, Japanese, Russian, Serbian, Spanish, Turkish, Urdu
Psychological Impairments Rating Schedule	Semi-structured	Psychological and behavioural deficits	Psychiatrist or psychologist	Essential	Arabic, Bulgarian, Croatian, English, French, German, Serbian, Turkish
WHO Disablement Scale	Rating scale	Disablement due to mental and/or physical disorders	Psychiatrist or psychologist	Not required	Arabic, Chinese, Czech, Danish, Dutch, English, German, Hindi, Italian, Japanese, Kannada, Portuguese, Romanian, Russian, Spanish
Broad Rating Schedule	Semi-structured	Psychotic symptoms and related disability	Psychiatrist or psychologist	Not required	Bulgarian, Chinese, Czech, Danish, English, German, Hindi, Japanese, Russian, Yoruba
Family Interview Schedule	Structured	Family perception of patient	Psychiatrist or psychologist	Essential	Bulgarian, Chinese, Czech, Danish, English, German, Hindi, Japanese, Russian, Yoruba
Social Unit Rating	Semi-structured	Burden of mental illness on the family	Lay interviewer	Essential	Arabic, English, French, Hindi, Portuguese, Spanish
WHO Quality of Life Assessment Instrument	Questionnaire	Quality of life	self-administered	Not applicable	Croatian, Dutch, English, French, Russian, Shona, Spanish, Tamil
Subjective Well-Being Inventory	Questionnaire	Feelings of wellbeing	Self-administered	Not applicable	English, Hindi

WHO, World Health Organization.

Table 3. World Health Organization instruments for the assessment of services

Instrument	Format	Area	User	Training	Languages
Pathways Interview Schedule	Semi-structured	Sources of care	Health or research worker	Not required	Arabic, Bahasa (Indonesia), Chinese, Czech, English, French, Japanese, Kannada, Korean, Portuguese, Spanish, Turkish, Urdu
Quality Assurance in Mental Health Care Checklists:					
Mental Health Policy Checklist	Semi-structured	Mental health care (policy)	Health or administrative worker	Not required	Chinese, English, French, Italian, Portuguese, Spanish
Mental Health Programme Checklist	Semi-structured	Mental health care (programme)	Health or administrative worker	Not required	Chinese, English, French, Italian, Portuguese, Spanish
The Primary Health Care Facility Checklist	Semi-structured	Mental health care (primary care facility)	Health or administrative worker	Not required	Chinese, English, French, Italian, Portuguese, Spanish
The outpatient Mental Health Facility Checklist	Semi-structured	Mental health care (outpatient facility)	Health or administrative worker	Not required	Chinese, English, French, Italian, Portuguese, Spanish
The Inpatient Mental Health Facility Checklist	Semi-structured	Mental health care (inpatient)	Health or administrative worker	Not required	Chinese, English, French, Italian, Portuguese, Spanish
The Residential Facility for the Elderly Mentally Ill Checklist	Semi-structured	Mental health care (residential facility for the elderly mentally ill)	Health or administrative worker	Not required	Chinese, Czech, Danish, English, Hindi, Russian, Spanish, Yoruba
WHO Child Care Facility Schedule	Semi-structured	Quality of child care facility	Health or administrative worker	Not required	English, French, Greek, Portuguese

WHO, World Health Organization.

Table 4. World Health Organization instruments for the assessment of environment, risks and qualitative research

Instrument	Format	Area	User	Training	Languages
Axis III Checklist	Semi-structured	Contextual factors	Psychiatrist or psychologist	Not required	Arabic, Chinese, Czech, Danish, Dutch, English, German, Hindi, Italian, Japanese, Kannada, Portuguese, Romanian, Russian, Spanish
Interview Schedule for Children	Semi-structured	Child's psychosocial environment	Psychiatrist or psychologist	Not required	English, German, Portuguese, Slovenian, Spanish
Parent Interview Schedule	Semi-structured	Child's psychosocial environment	Psychiatrist or psychologist	Not required	English, German, Portuguese, Slovenian, Spanish
Home Risk Card	Semi-structured	Child's home risk factors	Health or research worker	Not required	English, Hindi
Qualitative Research Instruments					
A. Exploratory Translation and Back-translation Guidelines	Guide	Linguistic equivalence	Health or research worker	Not required	English, Greek, Kannada, Korean, Romanian, Spanish, Turkish, Yoruba
B. Key Informant Interview Schedule	Semi-structured	Cultural aspects of mental health	Anthropologist or ethnographer	Essential	English, Greek, Kannada, Korean, Romanian, Spanish, Turkish, Yoruba
C. Focus Group Interview Guide	Guide	Cultural aspects of mental health	Anthropologist or ethnographer	Essential	English, Greek, Kannada, Korean, Romanian, Spanish, Turkish, Yoruba

WHO, World Health Organization.

Instruments for the Assessment of Psychopathology

Alcohol Use Disorders Identification Test (AUDIT)

AUDIT (Babor et al. 1989) is a brief structured interview aimed at identifying people whose alcohol consumption has become harmful to their health. It consists of ten questions: three questions on the amount and frequency of drinking, three on drinking behaviour and four on problems or adverse psychological reactions related to alcohol. The instrument can be interviewer- or self-administered, and the average administration time is 1–2 minutes. If the respondent is defensive or uncooperative, the clinical screening procedure (CSP) may be used to complement AUDIT. CSP contains a listing of indirect questions and clinical signs likely to indicate the harmful consequences of alcohol use.

AUDIT has been tested in a WHO collaborative project on the early detection of people with harmful alcohol consumption. High reliability of the constituent scales, as well as high face validity and the ability to distinguish light drinkers from those with harmful drinking has been reported (Saunders and Aasland 1987; Saunders et al. 1993a, b).

Composite International Diagnostic Interview (CIDI)

Composite International Diagnostic Interview (CIDI; WHO, 1993a) is a highly standardized diagnostic instrument for the assessment of mental disorders according to the definitions and criteria in the ICD-10 *Classification of mental and behavioural disorders* (WHO 1992) and the revised third edition of the *Diagnostic and statistical manual of mental disorders* (DSM-III-R; APA 1987). A version of CIDI that will accommodate DSM-IV criteria (APA 1994) will be released in 1995.

CIDI is primarily intended for use in epidemiological studies of mental disorders in general populations. The instrument consists of fully spelled-out questions and of a probing system aimed at assessing the clinical significance and psychiatric relevance of reported phenomena. No clinical judgement is required in coding and recording respondents' answers, and the schedule can be competently administered by a lay or clinician interviewer after 1-week's training. The average administration time of CIDI is 90 min. CIDI is accompanied by a set of supporting materials that includes manuals and computer programs for data entry, cleaning and scoring of ICD-10 and DSM-III-R diagnoses.

A number of versions and modules of CIDI have been produced for specific research purposes (Janca et al. 1994a); of these only two, a computerized version of CIDI (CIDI Auto; WHO 1993c) and the Substance Abuse Module (Robins et al. 1990), have so far been formally adopted as parts of CIDI by the WHO CIDI Advisory Committee. CIDI has been extensively tested in two fields trials involving 20 centres, 12 languages and about 1200 respondents. The field trials results show that the instrument is generally acceptable, appropriate and a reliable diagnostic tool for use across cultures and settings (Robins et al. 1988; Wittchen et al. 1991; Cottler et al. 1991; Janca et al. 1992).

ICD-10 Symptom Checklist for Mental Disorders

The ICD-10 Symptom Checklist for Mental Disorders (Janca et al. 1994b) is a semi-structured instrument intended for clinicians' assessment of psychiatric symptoms and syndromes in the F0–F6 categories of ICD-10. The instrument requires the clinician user to examine the patient or case notes in order to be able to rate the presence or absence of symptoms that are necessary to make a firm diagnosis in the ICD-10 system. The Checklist also lists symptoms and states that, according to ICD-10 criteria, have often been found to be associated with the syndrome (e. g. alcohol abuse in patients with mania) or should be assessed independently from the syndrome (e. g. mental retardation in patients with organic mental disorder). The symptom lists are accompanied by instructions intended to help the user in considering differential diagnoses. The possibility of recording onset, severity and duration of the syndrome, as well as number of episodes (where applicable), is also provided. The Checklist is accompanied by the ICD-10 Symptom Glossary for Mental Disorders (Isaac et al. 1994). The Glossary provides brief definitions of the symptoms and terms used in the Checklist.

The ICD-10 Symptom Checklist for Mental Disorders has been used at one of the sites participating in the field trials of ICD-10, and preliminary results have shown good psychometric properties for the instrument. The average administration time is 15 min, and the interviewer/observer reliability is acceptable (kappa 0.72; Janca et al. 1993).

International Personality Disorder Examination

The International Personality Disorder Examination (IPDE; WHO, 1993b) is a semi-structured interview schedule designed for the assessment of personality disorders according to ICD-10 and DSM-III-R criteria. It is designed for use by clinicians who have also received training in the use of the IPDE. The IPDE covers the following six areas of the respondent's personality and behaviour: work, self, interpersonal relationships, affects, reality testing and impulse control. The last six items in the schedule are scored without questioning and are based on the interviewer's observation of the respondent during the interview. The IPDE requires that behaviour or a trait be present for at least 5 years before it should be considered a manifestation of personality or a symptom of personality disorder and that at least one criterion of personality disorder be fulfilled before the age of 15 years. The information about the respondent obtained by reliable informants can also be recorded and is used in the final scoring of the diagnosis. The final scoring, which may be done clerically or by computer, is used in making ICD-10 and/or DSM-III-R diagnoses; a dimensional score can also be calculated.

Because of the length of the interview (2–3 h) the IPDE has recently been produced in two versions, one for ICD-10 and the other for DSM-IV diagnoses. Both versions of the instrument are accompanied by the user manual, screener, hand-scoring sheets and computer-scoring programs.

The IPDE has been tested in a WHO-coordinated field trial in which 14 centres from 11 countries participated. The field trial results indicate good acceptability, high inter-rater reliability and satisfactory temporal stability for the criteria and diagnoses assessed by the interview (Loranger et al. 1991, 1994).

Schedules for Clinical Assessment in Neuropsychiatry

Schedules for Clinical Assessment in Neuropsychiatry (SCAN; WHO, 1994) is a semi-structured clinical interview schedule designed for clinicians' assessment of the symptoms and course of adult mental disorders. SCAN comprises an interview schedule, i. e. the 10th edition of the Present State Examination (PSE; Wing et al. 1974), Glossary of Differential Definitions, Item Group Checklist (IGC) and Clinical History Schedule (CHS). The SCAN schedule consists of part 1, which covers non-psychotic symptoms such as physical health, worrying, tension, panic, anxiety and phobias, obsessional symptoms, depressed mood and ideation, impaired thinking, concentration, energy, interests, bodily functions, weight, sleep, eating disorders, and alcohol and drug abuse; part 2 covers psychotic and cognitive disorders, as well as abnormalities of behaviour, speech and affect. When using SCAN, the clinician interviewer (e. g. psychiatrist or clinical psychologist) decides whether a symptom has been present during the specified time and to what degree of severity. One or two periods are selected to cover the main phenomena necessary for diagnosis. The periods usually include the "present state" (i. e. the month before examination) and the "lifetime before" (i. e. any time previously). Another option is to rate the "representative episode", which may be chosen because it is particularly characteristic of the patient's illness. The average administration time of SCAN is 90 min. The SCAN glossary is an essential part of SCAN and provides differential definitions of SCAN items and a commentary on the SCAN text.

A set of computer programs (CATEGO) is used for processing SCAN data and for the scoring and diagnoses according to ICD-10 and DSM-IV criteria. A computerized version of SCAN (CAPSE) is also available. It assists the interviewer in applying SCAN and allows direct entry of ratings at the time of the interview. Questions and ratings are displayed on the screen; if needed, SCAN glossary definitions can also be referred to.

SCAN has been tested in WHO-organized field trials involving 20 centres in 14 countries. The field trials results indicate good feasibility and reliability of the instrument comparable to those obtained in testing the PSE-9 (Wing et al. 1990).

Standardized Assessment of Depressive Disorders

Standardized Assessment of Depressive Disorders (SADD) is a structured clinical interview schedule aimed at assessing the symptoms and signs of depressive disorders. Part 1 of the instrument covers the basic sociodemographic data about the patient. Part 2 contains a checklist of 39 symptoms and signs characteristic of depression and is accompanied by a glossary that provides definitions of symptoms and signs to be assessed, a listing of possible probes and examples of answers for each symptom. The checklist also includes a number of open-ended questions for recording rare or culture-specific symptoms of depression, as well as items related to the past history of the patient (e. g. number of previous episodes, precipitating factors, presence of mental disorders in relatives). Part 3 of the instrument serves to record the diagnosis and severity of the patient's condition. The ratings in SADD refer to the week preceding the interview and to any other time prior to the current episode. The administration of the instrument takes a short time if the clinician has examined the patient previously. If the case is "fresh", the time taken to obtain the necessary information and rate it is longer (i. e. 45–60 min).

SADD has been tested in the WHO Collaborative Study on the Standardized Assessment of Depressive Disorders and has been found to be easy to use and acceptable to both psychiatrists and patients. The reliability of the sociodemographic, symptom checklist and past history sections of the instrument has been found to be high (Sartorius et al. 1980, 1983).

Schedule for Clinical Assessment of Acute Psychotic States

Schedule for Clinical Assessment of Acute Psychotic States (SCAAPS) is a semistructured interview schedule for clinicians' recording of information about patients with acute psychotic states. Such information is collected from different sources, such as the clinical interview of the patient, key informants and medical records. The instrument also offers the possibility of recording the follow-up diagnostic evaluation of the patient.

SCAAPS consists of six parts. Part A contains the screening criteria for acute psychotic states (e.g. onset of symptoms within 3 months of the initial assessment); part B comprises items related to the psychiatric history and social description of the patient; part C contains a 19-item symptom checklist covering symptoms from worrying and anxiety to symptoms reflecting stressful life events; part D serves to record the initial diagnostic evaluation and the results of the 1-year follow-up assessment; part E covers the treatment, course and outcome of the disorder; part F is intended for narrative summaries of the initial examination, and 3-month and 1-year follow-up. The average duration of the SCAAPS interview is 120 min.

The instrument has been used in the WHO Collaborative Studies on Acute Psychoses and has been found to be a cross-culturally appropriate tool for collecting data about acute psychotic states in different parts of the world (Cooper et al. 1990).

Social Description

The Social Description (SD) is a schedule with open-ended questions aimed at collecting information in a systematic manner about the social history of the psychiatric patient. The schedule is intended for research purposes, and can be used by social workers or clinicians. It covers the following areas: residence and household; education of the patient; work activities of the patient; children; marital status; education and occupation of the spouse; education and occupation of the parents; education and occupation of the head of the current household; religion; patient's childhood setting; daily and leisure activities; birth order of the patient and siblings; a thumbnail sketch by the interviewer who has to rate on a 5-point scale the current socioeconomic status of the patient, the patient's family background and the patient's current social isolation within the framework of his/her respective culture. The average administration time of the instrument is 120 min.

The SD has been used in the WHO International Pilot Study of Schizophrenia and has been found to be a useful means for collecting the social history of patients in different cultures and settings (WHO, 1973). It has been used in a modified form in several other WHO studies such as the Collaborative Determinants of Outcome of Severe Mental Disorders (Jablensky et al. 1992).

Self-Reporting Questionnaire

The Self-Reporting Questionnaire (SRQ) is an instrument designed for screening the presence of psychiatric illness in patients contacting primary health care settings. It can be self-administered or interviewer-administered with illiterate or semi-literate patients, and its administration time is 5–10 minutes. The questionnaire consists of 24 questions, 20 of which are related to neurotic symptoms and 4 of which relate to psychotic symptoms. Each of the 24 questions is scored 1 or 0: a score of 1 indicates that the symptom was present during the past month; a score of 0 indicates that it was absent. Depending on the criteria, culture and language, different cut-off scores are selected in different studies, but most often the cut-off is 7. A score of 7 or above indicates the existence of a probable psychological problem. The SRQ is accompanied by a recently produced user's guide (Beusenberg and Orley 1994) that describes the instrument, its use and scoring, and also summarizes its results of reliability and validity studies.

The SRQ has been tested in over 20 studies, (including the WHO Collaborative Study on Strategies for Extending Mental Health Care and the WHO Study on Mental Disorders in Primary Health Care), and has been found to be an appropriate, reliable and valid case-finding tool for use in primary health care settings, particularly in developing countries (Harding et al. 1980, 1983; WHO 1984).

Instruments for the Assessment of Disability and Burden

World Health Organization Psychiatric Disability Assessment Schedule

World Health Organization Psychiatric Disability Assessment Schedule (WHO/DAS) is a semi-structured instrument designed for the evaluation of the social functioning of patients with mental disorders. Such an evaluation can be done by a psychiatrist, psychologist or social worker. The information about the functioning of the patient is collected from the patient, key informant(s) or written records. The instrument has been developed in accordance with the principles underlying the WHO *International classification of impairments, disabilities and handicaps* (WHO 1980).

WHO/DAS consists of 97 items grouped in five parts. Part 1 comprises items related to the patient's overall behaviour, and includes ratings of self-care, underactivity, slowness and social withdrawal. Part 2 serves to assess the patient's social role performance, and covers participation in household activities, marital role, parental role, sexual role, social contacts, occupational role, interests and information, and behaviour in emergencies or out-of-the ordinary situations. Part 3 of WHO/DAS is intended for the assessment of the patient's social functioning in the hospital, including ward behaviour, nurses' opinions, occupations and contact with the outside world. Part 4 covers modifying factors related to the patient's dysfunction (specific assets, specific liabilities, home atmosphere and outside support). Parts 5 and 6 serve for a global evaluation of the patient and a summary of the ratings and scoring, respectively. Items in parts 1 and 2 of DAS are rated on a 6-point scale, i.e. no dysfunction, minimal dysfunction, obvious dysfunction, serious dysfunction, very serious dysfunction and maximum dysfunction. The patient's current functioning (past month) is to be rated against the presumed "average" or "normal" functioning of a person of the same sex, comparable age and similar socioeconomic background. The average administration time of WHO/DAS is 30 min. A guide to the use of WHO/DAS and an explanation of certain key terms (e.g. psychological burden, social skills, impairment, etc.) accompany the instrument.

WHO/DAS has been tested and used in the WHO Collaborative Study on the Assessment and Reduction of Psychiatric Disability and has been found to be a reliable and valid tool for the assessment and cross-cultural comparison of psychiatric disability (Jablensky et al. 1980).

World Health Organization Psychological Impairments Rating Schedule

The World Health Organization Psychological/Impairments Rating Schedule (WHO/PIRS) is a semi-structured instrument intended for clinicians' assessment of selected areas of psychological and behavioural deficits in patients with functional psychotic disorder. The main areas covered by the instrument concern negative symptoms, social skill and communication, and an overall impression of the patient and his/her personality. WHO/PIRS should be administered after a PSE interview, preferably by the same clinician. The average administration time is 25 min.

The instrument consists of 97 items grouped in 10 sections. Part A includes items and scales for rating observed behaviour of the patient. Part B includes a pattern assembly, three Rorschach cards and a letter-deletion test aimed at eliciting the patient's performance when presented with standard tasks.

WHO/PIRS has been used in the WHO Collaborative Study on Impairments and Disabilities Associated with Schizophrenic Disorders and has been found to be a reliable assessment tool (test-retest reliability kappa: 0.79; Jablensky et al. 1980).

World Health Organization Disablement Scale

The WHO Disablement Scale (DS) has been developed as a component of the multi-axial presentation of the ICD-10 *Classification of mental and behavioural disorders*. It is a simple scale intended for the recording of the clinicians' assessment of disablement caused by mental and physical disorders. The ratings refer to specific areas of functioning, such as personal care (e.g. personal hygiene, dressing, feeding), occupation (e.g. function in paid activities, studying, home-making), family and household (e.g. interaction with spouse, parents, children and other relatives), and the broader social context (e.g. performance in relation to community members, participation in leisure and other social activities). The scale provides anchor-point definitions for six ratings ranging from 0 (no dysfunction) to 5 (maximum dysfunction). The administration time of WHO DS takes 5 min if the clinician knows the patient and has examined him or her.

WHO DS has been tested in WHO-coordinated field trials of the ICDIO Multiaxial Classification that involved about 70 centres from more than 25 countries. The field trials results indicate good acceptance of the instrument by clinicians belonging to different psychiatric schools and traditions (Lopez-Ibor et al. 1994).

Broad Rating Schedule

The Broad Rating Schedule (BRS) has been developed for use in a long-term follow-up study of patients given the diagnosis of schizophrenia, and serves to summarize the follow-up findings. The schedule uses information from all available sources, including the patient, informant and medical or other records. The severity of psychotic symptoms and disabilities is rated for the previous month on a scale ranging from absent to severe. Symptoms, as well as disabilities, are also rated on a modified version of the DSM-III-R Global Assessment of Functioning (GAF) Scale, which ranges from 1 (persistent danger of severely hurting oneself or others, or persistent inability to function in almost all areas) to 90 (absent or minimal symptoms, or good functioning in all areas, interested and involved in a wide range of activities, etc.). The instrument also contains sections on subjects lost to follow-up and deceased subjects. The ratings of these sections are based on the best judgement of the clinician using all available information. The BRS should be rated after completion of the interview of the patient and informant and a review of the records. Clinicians do not need specific training in the use of the schedule.

Family Interview Schedule

The Family Interview Schedule (FIS) is a structured instrument for the assessment of family members' perception of the patient's psychiatric problems and their consequences for the patient and his or her family. It is also an instrument developed for use in the WHO Long-Term Follow-Up Study of Schizophrenia. The source of information for this schedule should be a permanent member of the patient's family. The schedule is divided into the following sections: I – symptoms and social behaviour; II – impact; III – stigma; IV – service providers; V – attribution. The section on symptoms and social behaviour covers the day-to-day behaviour and responsibilities of the patient in the past month (e. g. helping with household chores). The section on impact ascertains involvement of family members in helping the patient as well as their difficulties in managing and coping with problems caused by the patient's psychiatric problems. The section on stigma consists of a list of experiences the family member has had because of the patient's psychiatric problems (e. g. that neighbours treated him or her differently). The service providers section of the instrument is aimed at assessing the help provided to the patient and the family by doctors, nurses and other relevant care-givers. The section on attribution is intended for recording the family member's views (based on the information obtained from care-givers) on causes of the patient's psychiatric problems.

The FIS is accompanied by a "visual analogue" measure, i. e. a graphic presentation of the scale ranging from "almost never or not at all" to "almost always or a lot". The administration time of the FIS is 30–45 min. The user (psychiatrist, psychologist, social worker or nurse) should be trained in the administration of the instrument.

Social Unit Rating

The Social Unit Rating (SUR) is a semi-structured interview aimed at recording the effect of a patient's illness on his/her immediate living group. The instrument consists of 20 items including basic sociodemographic information about the patient (e.g. occupation, education, employment), time residing in a given area, time residing in the present household, composition of the social unit, main sources of income, total weekly income and sources of help for the social unit. The rest of the items in the instrument relate to the pre-illness status of the social unit and to the effect of the patient's illness on the social unit.

Any lay interviewer can administer the SUR after appropriate training. The administration time of the instrument is 30–45 min. The SUR has been used in the WHO Collaborative Study on Strategies for Extending Mental Health Care and has been found to be a useful means for the assessment of the effects of mental illness on the family or household of the patient (Giel et al. 1983).

Instruments for the Assessment of Quality of Life

World Health Organization Quality of Life Assessment Instrument

The WHO Quality of Life Assessment Instrument (WHOQOL) is an assessment instrument that allows an enquiry into the perception of individuals of their own position in life in the context of the culture and value systems in which they live and in relation to their goals, expectations, standards and concerns. The instrument covers the following six broad domains of the quality of life: physical domain, psychological domain, level of independence, social relationships, environment and spiritual domain. Within each domain a series of facets of the quality of life summarizes that particular domain. For example, the psychological domain includes the facets positive feelings; thinking, learning, memory and concentration; self-esteem; body image and appearance, negative feelings. Response scales in the instrument are concerned with the intensity, frequency and subjective evaluation of states, behaviour and capacities. The WHOQOL provides a quality of life profile that consists of an overall quality of life score, scores for each of the broad domains of the quality of life, scores for individual facets of the quality of life and within facets, separate scores for the recording of the subject's perception of his or her condition and quality of life.

The WHOQOL is being developed in the framework of a WHO collaborative project on quality of life measures involving numerous centres in different cultural settings. One of the main goals of the project is to assess the psychometric properties of the instrument such as its reliability, validity and cross-cultural sensitivity (The WHOQOL Group 1994).

Subjective Well-Being Inventory

The Subjective Well-Being Inventory (SUBI) is a questionnaire for the assessment of subjective well-being. It can be self- or interviewer-administered and is designed for research purposes. The questionnaire consists of 40 items designed to measure feelings of well-being (or lack of it) as experienced by an individual in relation to concerns such as their health or family. The items in SUBI represent the following factors in the structure of subjective well-being: general well-being – positive effect; expectation-achievement congruence; confidence in coping; transcendence; family group support; social support; primary group concern; inadequate mental mastery;

perceived ill-health; deficiency in social contacts; general well-being – negative effect. SUBI is accompanied by the "stepwise ethnographic exploration" procedure that can be used to assess that SUBI is appropriate for use in the cultural setting in which the study will take place.

The instrument has been used in research projects carried out by the WHO Regional Office for South-East Asia and has been found to be culturally applicable for the quantitative measurement of subjective well-being (Sell and Nagpal 1992).

Instruments for the Assessment of Services

Pathways Interview Schedule

This Pathways Interview Schedule is a semi-structured instrument designed for the systematic gathering of information on the routes and sources of care used by patients before seeing a mental health professional. The instrument can be administered by a psychiatrist, psychologist, social worker or nurse, and its average administration time is 10 min. An instruction manual describing how to use the instrument is available.

The Pathways Interview Schedule consists of seven sections. Section A covers basic information about the centre and the mental health professional. In Section B the basic information about the patient is recorded (e.g. age, sex, marital status, social position, past history of care by any mental health service). Section C covers the details of the first carer (e.g. who he/she was, who suggested that care, what was the main problem presented, when it began, what was the main treatment offered, duration of patient's journey to first carer). Sections D, E and F cover similar details of the second, third and fourth carers. Section G is intended for the diagnosis of the patient according to the assessment by the mental health professional.

The instrument has been used in the WHO Study on Pathways to Psychiatric Care and has been found to be a simple and inexpensive method of studying a psychiatric service and routes followed by patients seeking care for psychiatric disorders (Gater et al. 1990, 1991).

Checklists for Quality Assurance in Mental Health Care

Checklists for Quality Assurance in Mental Health Care are a set of checklists accompanied by glossaries designed to assist in the development of programmes of quality assurance in mental health care. The checklists are based on recommendations of a group of experts in the field of mental health care and have been tested in a field trial that included 10 countries in all the WHO regions (Bertolote 1994).

The following checklists and glossaries are available:

1. The Mental Health Policy Checklist is an instrument aimed at assessing national mental health policies and assisting in the development of country programmes of quality assurance in mental health. The checklist has 21 items enquiring about issues such as the existence of a written mental health policy and operational programmes. The rest of the items are grouped into the following categories: decentralization, in-

tersectoral action, comprehensiveness, equity, continuity, community participation and periodic reviews of mental health policy. The average administration time is 75 min. The instrument can also be used to assess the policy of smaller population units (e. g. a federal state).

2. The Mental Health Programme Checklist is an instrument aimed at assessing the countries' mental health programmes and assisting in the development of programmes of quality assurance in mental health. The checklist consists of 32 items covering several main areas such as whether there are written national, regional and local mental health programmes, the range of actions for promotion of mental health, treatment, rehabilitation and prevention of mental disorders, etc. The rest of the items are grouped into the following sections: plan of work, monitoring and evaluation, and community participation in the planning, implementation and evaluation of mental health actions/programmes. A glossary provides descriptions of these items. The average administration time of the checklist is 30 min.

3. The Primary Health Care Facility Checklist is an instrument for the assessment of primary health care facilities delivering mental health care and for assistance in the development of programmes of quality assurance of mental health care in such facilities. The instrument consists of a checklist, glossary, scoring instructions and list of references. The checklist has 42 items covering physical environment (e. g. reasonable space available, adequate supply of basic drugs, etc.); administrative arrangements (e. g. written procedures available for the protection of confidentiality of patients and staff records); care process (e. g. treatment plans are written down for each patient and followed by all staff); interaction with families (e. g. family members are encouraged to be involved in the patient's treatment programme); outreach (e. g. contact is regularly made with other health facilities, social agencies, patients' employers, etc.). The average administration time is 60 min.

4. The Outpatient Mental Health Facility Checklist is an instrument used to assess outpatient mental health facilities in a given country or set-up, and to assist in the development of programmes of quality assurance in mental health in such facilities. The instrument consists of a checklist, glossary and scoring instructions. The checklist comprises 53 items and covers areas such as physical environment (e. g. the facility has been officially inspected and needs local standards for the protection of the health and safety of patients and staff); administrative arrangements (e. g. a written policy on philosophy and model of care is available and priorities have been defined); care process (e. g. every patient is evaluated in terms of biological, psychological and social functioning); interaction with families (e. g. home visits for improving caring and coping skills of families of selected patients are carried out); outreach (e. g. a standard information form is always sent to another facility whenever a patient is referred to it). The average administration time is 60 min.

5. The Inpatient Mental Health Facility Checklist is an instrument used to assess inpatient mental health facilities in a given country or set-up, and to assist in the development of programmes of quality assurance in mental health in such facilities. The instrument consists of 77 items covering areas such as physical environment, ad-

ministrative arrangements, staffing, care process, interaction with families, discharge and follow-up. A glossary provides descriptions of items to be assessed. Scoring instructions are also available. The average administration time is 20 min.

6. The Residential Facility for Elderly Mentally Ill Patients Checklist is an instrument used to assess residential facilities for the elderly mentally ill in a given set-up and assist in the development of programmes of quality assurance in mental health in such facilities. The checklist consists of 69 items that cover the physical environment, administrative arrangements, care process, and interaction with families and community. The glossary provides a description of these items and instructions for their scoring are also given. The average administration time is 75 min.

World Health Organization Child Care Facility Schedule

The WHO Child Care Facility Schedule (WHO CCFS; WHO, 1990a) is an observer rating schedule aimed at assessing the quality of child care in day-care programmes for children. It can be administered by a research or administrative worker who should be familiar with recording and rating procedures. The average administration time is 90 min.

The instrument consists of 80 items covering the following areas that define quality child care: (1) physical environment (e.g. the indoor environment is spacious enough for the number of children present and is attractive and pleasant); (2) health and safety (e.g. the facility meets local standards for protection of the health and safety of children in group settings); (3) nutrition and food service (e.g. meal times are used by staff to promote good nutrition); (4) administration (e.g. at least annually, staff conduct a self-study to identify strengths and weaknesses of the programme); (5) staff-family interaction (e.g. parents and other family members are encouraged to be involved in the programme in various ways and there are no rules prohibiting their unannounced visits); (6) staff-children interaction (e.g. staff respect the cultural backgrounds of the children and adopt the learning situation to preserve their heritage and acquaint other children with the cultural legacy of all members of the group); (7) observable child behaviour (e.g. children respect the needs, feelings and property of others, i.e. take turns, share toys); (8) curriculum (e.g. the daily schedule is planned to provide a variety of activities, including those that are indoor/outdoor, quiet/active, etc.).

WHO CCFS contains a glossary which defines each of the items to be observed and rated. The instrument is also accompanied by the user manual and a list of relevant references. Field studies of WHO CCFS have been carried out in Greece, the Philippines and Nigeria and the instrument has been found to be cross-culturally acceptable and reliable in terms of a level of percentage agreement between raters (Tsiantis et al. 1991).

Instruments for the Assessment of Environment and Risks

Axis III Checklist

The Axis III Checklist instrument has been produced in the framework of the development of the ICD-10 multiaxial schema and is intended for clinicians' assessment of Axis III, i. e. contextual (environmental/circumstantial and personal lifestyle/life management) factors contributing to the presentation or course of the ICD-10 mental and/or physical disorder(s) recorded on Axis I of the schema. The contextual factors listed under Axis III represent a selection of ICD-10 Z00–Z99 categories, i. e. Factors Influencing Health Status and Contact with Health Services (Chapter XXI of ICD-10). The following groups of contextual factors are covered by Axis III and assessed by the Checklist: negative events in childhood (e. g. removal from home in childhood, Z61.1); problems related to education and literacy (e. g. underachievement in school, Z55.3); problems related to the primary support group including family circumstances (e. g. disruption of family by separation or divorce, Z63.5); problems related to the social environment (e. g. social exclusion and rejection, Z60.4); problems related to housing or economic circumstances (e. g. homelessness, Z59.0); problems related to (un)employment (e. g. change of job, Z56.1); problems related to physical environment (e. g. occupational exposure to risk factors, Z57); problems related to psychosocial or legal circumstances (e. g. imprisonment or other incarceration, Z65.1); problems related to a family history of diseases or disabilities (e. g. family history of mental or behavioural disorders, Z81); lifestyle and life management problems (e. g. burn-out, Z73.0).

The Axis III Checklist is included in the ICD-10 Multiaxial Diagnostic Formulation Form, and the clinician is required to tick all applicable categories of Z factors and specify Z codes for each. A listing of contextual factors and the respective ICD-10 Z codes is given as an appendix to the form. The average administration time of the Axis III Checklist is 10 min. The instrument has been tested in the multicentre international field trials of the multiaxial presentation of ICD-10 and has been found to be useful and easy to use by clinicians in different parts of the world (Janca et al. 1994c).

Interview Schedule for Children

The Interview Schedule for Children (ISC; WHO, 1991) is a semi-structured instrument for the systematic collection of information on a child's psychosocial environment. The instrument has been developed as a companion to the psychosocial axis (Axis V) of the WHO *Multiaxial classification of child and adolescent psychiatric disorders* (WHO 1988). The ISC is accompanied by a glossary that provides descriptions of items and diagnostic guidelines for Axis V (associated abnormal psychosocial situations). However, to ensure the smooth flow of the interview, the items in the ISC are in a different order from that of the glossary. The items in the schedule are as follows: abnormal immediate environment; stressful events/situations resulting from child's disorder/disability; societal stressors; chronic interpersonal stress associated with school/work; acute life events; abnormal qualities of upbringing; abnormal intrafamilial relationships; inadequate or distorted intrafamilial communication; mental disorder, deviance or handicap in the child's primary support group.

The relevant codes for each category have to be inserted into each individual section and the results are transferred to the summary page. It is, however, recommended that the coding and scoring should not be done until the interview has been completed. The instrument is intended for psychiatrists, psychologists, social workers or nurses, and its administration takes 60 min (van Goor-Lambo et al. 1990).

Parent Interview Schedule

The Parent Interview Schedule (PIS; WHO, 1990b) is a semi-structured instrument for the systematic collection of information about the child's psychosocial environment so that appropriate codings can be made on the psychosocial axis (Axis V) of the WHO *Multiaxial classification of child and adolescent psychiatric disorders* (WHO 1988). The instrument is accompanied by a glossary and diagnostic guidelines for the assessment of items. As in the ISC, the relevant codes have to be inserted in each individual section and the results should be transferred to the summary page after the interview. Items in the PIS are identical with those in the ISC, and their order in the schedule and glossary is different to ensure the smooth flow of the interview.

The instrument is intended for psychiatrists, psychologists, social workers or nurses, and its administration takes 60 min. The preliminary results of the Axis V field trials (van Goor-Lambo et al. 1990) were used in the preparation of the PIS version which is being tested at present.

Home Risk Card

The Home Risk Card is a listing of risk factors that, if present at the home of a child, may indicate that such a child and home need extra help and special attention. The risk factors covered by the instrument include: mother's age (under 17 years); number of children under 3 years (more than two); mother/carer ignorant about the child's needs and unresponsive to health messages (e.g. cannot answer questions about the child that mothers normally can answer); mother/carer mentally disordered or severely depressed (e.g. looks desperate, hopeless, cries easily); mother/carer neglectful or uninterested in the well-being/development of the child (e.g. shouts or hits the child for trivial reasons during home visit); disorganized, uncleaned house; father known to be delinquent (e.g. arrested by police), alcoholic or otherwise mentally disordered; severe marital discord (e.g. physical violence between parents); abject poverty (e.g. no change of clothing).

The Home Risk Card guides the user in noting facts about the child and household that may adequate intervention measures. The recorded information should also be inserted into require the child's weight card and serve as a reminder to the health professional about the child's need for extra help and attention.

A brief set of instructions helps the user in the application of the Card, which usually takes 5–10 min. The Home Risk Card has been used in a project organized by the WHO Regional Office for South-East Asia and has been found to be a useful guide for the assessment of home risk factors in this region (Sell and Nagpal 1992).

Instruments for Qualitative Research

A guide providing a general overview of the concepts, methods and tools commonly used in qualitative research has recently been produced by WHO (Hudelson 1994). It is an introductory guide for programme managers, project directors, researchers and others who need to make decisions concerning when and how to conduct research for programme development purposes. This guide gives an overview of qualitative research and its potential uses; provides descriptions of the most common data collection methods used in qualitative research, specifying their strenghts and weaknesses; discusses issues of sampling, study design and report-writing in qualitative research; gives examples of several qualitative research designs used by health programmes.

For the WHO Cross-cultural Applicability Research (CAR) study on diagnostic criteria and instruments for the assessment of alcohol and drug abuse and dependence, a set of qualitative research methods and instruments has been developed (Room et al. in press). These include the following:

1. The Exploratory Translation and Back-translation Guidelines is a set of specified procedures for conducting a careful translation and back-translation of an instrument so as to ensure its equivalence in different languages and cultures. The exploratory translation and back-translation used in the WHO CAR study comprises a series of step-by-step procedures summarized in Table 5.

2. The Key Informant Interview Schedule is a semi-structured, exploratory, ethnographic interview schedule that covers phenomena relevant to ICD-10 and DSM-III-R definitions and criteria for substance use disorders (e.g. withdrawal, tolerance, loss of control, etc.). The questions in the interview schedule follow a "funnel-type structure", i.e. general topics are first discussed and then more detailed questions about specific issues are asked.

Table 5. Steps in the development of equivalent versions of instruments in different languages

Step 1	Establishment of a (bilingual) group of experts belonging to the culture in which the instrument was developed and the culture in which it will (also) be used.
Step 2	Examination of the conceptual structure of the instrument by the expert group.
Step 3	Translation of items into the target language (or formulation of items in both languages if the instrument is produced anew).
Step 4	Examination of translation by bilingual group.
Step 5	Examination of the translation in unilingual groups (i.e. a group of individuals who do not know the source language of the instruments and therefore cannot guess the meaning of badly formulated items. The unilingual groups are usually moderated by a member of the billingual expert group.
Step 6	Back-translation of the text, possibly amended by the unilingual group.
Step 7	Examination of back-translation by bilingual group informed by its members about the contents of discussion in the unilingual groups. Participation of members of the bilingual group in the designing of the studies to establish the metric properties (e.g. validity, reliability, sensitivity) of the instrument.

The informant's answers are noted on the schedule verbatim. However, to ensure accuracy of the notes, the key informant interviews should be tape-recorded whenever possible or an observer should be present while the interviewer asks questions and both should take notes.

The Key Informant Interview Schedule developed for the WHO CAR study has been applied in nine centres representing distinct cultures and has been found to be an appropriate method for eliciting information on culture-specific characteristics of substance use and abuse in different parts of the world (Bennett et al. 1993).

3. The Focus Group Interview Guide is a brief interview guide specifying the main topics for discussions on various aspects of culture-specific characteristics of psychoactive substance use and abuse. According to the WHO CAR study protocol the following topics have been explored by this method what is normal and abnormal use of alcohol or drugs; what are the meanings of the various diagnostic terms related to the concept of alcohol or drug dependence; what are the similarities and differences between alcohol and drug abuse and alcohol and drug addiction; which prevention and intervention strategies are most likely to be effective against alcohol- or drug-related problems in the culture?

A set of instructions for the selection, composition and moderation of focus groups accompanies the list of discussion topics. Techniques of recording, reconstructing, managing and analysing the information obtained through the focus groups are also specified.

Discussion

All the WHO instruments have been developed in the context of collaborative and cross-cultural studies. In some instances an instrument that was already in use in one cultural setting was selected as the initial draft, which was then developed further; in other instances the development of the instrument started from a draft produced by an international group of experts representing several cultural settings and disciplines. All the instruments exist in more than one language and the vast majority have been used in more than one country. This was not accidental: WHO has in fact made it its aim to produce instruments for cross-cultural and collaborative work that will serve as a part of a common language helping researchers and other experts from different countries to understand one another, to work together and to compare the results of their studies even when these are not performed at a particular time following a commonly agreed protocol.

The decision to develop instruments suitable for international, cross-cultural and collaborative work had several consequences. *First*, the development of the instruments took more time than it would take to develop an instrument for use in a single country or language. *Second*, certain characteristics of patients, their sociocultural surroundings and the health services that they receive are so different that it is not possible to assess them using the same instrument. In such instances guidelines about the assessment were provided, while the formulation of specific items and other measurement tasks were entrusted to groups of experts who were fully acquainted with the circumstances.

Third, the development of instruments required additional funds for face-to-face meetings of the experts involved in the development of the instruments. These meetings (usually conducted at the centres participating in the development of an instrument) proved to have important consequences and benefits for the process of instrument development. The discussions of the results of the field trials and other aspects of the research necessary to produce the instrument and assess its metric characteristics gave invaluable insights into the differences between cultures and into the feasibility of investigations in different settings. The meetings also served as an important motivator to continue the often tedious work required over a long period of time. An effort was made on each occasion to bring together the centre heads and younger investigators for whom attendance at such meetings was of particular importance.

Fourth, certain constraints were imposed on the instruments by the structure of the languages in which the instruments were produced. Certain concepts have no natural "home" in other languages and enquiring about them can therefore become very time-consuming and difficult. In such instances it is usually best to sacrifice an item or section rather than to make part of the instrument awkward to use and complicate the training of interviewers. When this is not acceptable, it is usually necessary to return to the beginning and consider whether it is possible to obtain information about the topic of interest in another manner, not using assessment instruments of the type described here.

Fifth, cross-cultural differences can best be overcome if the assessments are carried out by individuals who are familiar with the culture and well trained in the use of the instruments. Most of the instruments that WHO has developed are therefore semi-structured and have been proposed for application by a well-trained member of the same culture. The use of semi-structured interviews, however, requires a considerably more intensive training than is the case for fully standardized instruments. This is a disadvantage that is less grave than the much more intensive training necessary when non-structured assessment methods are chosen. Furthermore, semi-structured instruments share some of the advantages of the fully structured instruments (e.g. the systematic coverage of all areas of interest, simpler data processing). *Sixth*, issues such as copyright, translation rights and modification procedures have to be designed with a view to covering the different centres and languages in which the instrument has been produced.

The WHO instruments have been developed in collaboration with groups of experts in many countries. Their contribution to the production of the instruments has been invaluable, and it is certain that without their selfless and enthusiastic collaboration it would not have been possible to develop the many materials – instruments and results of scientific investigations – that have been made available over the years. In the course of this work over the past 3 decades most of the centres that have participated in this work have made many international contacts, gained new insights about other cultures, increased their expertise in cross-cultural work and learned about the most convenient ways of international collaboration. The network of centres that has come into existence and that continues to work on instruments (and collaborate in research) has been an excellent by-product of the work on instrument development.

Another by-product of the work on instruments and of other WHO-coordinated international and cross-culturalcollaborative research has been the formulation of guidelines concerning ethical aspects of collaboration in the field of mental health across national borders (Sartorius 1990). One of the principles developed is that collaboration in research – in view of the high investments and various potential disadvantages of short-term international collaborative projects – should be structured in a manner that will make it highly probable that collaboration in the collaborative network will continue after the project that started the network has been completed. This has been realized in the instance of the WHO network that continues its existing collaborative links among all centres – including those that are at present not actively involved in any particular studies.

The technology of translation used in the development of WHO instruments deserves a brief mention. The method that has been developed rests on various previous methods used to ensure equivalence of translation in collaborative mental health research (Sartorius 1979) but has parts that have not been systematically used before. The steps used to produce equivalent versions in different languages are shown in Table 5. The procedure shown in this table is an approximation of the process described in more detail elsewhere (Sartorius 1995; Sartorius and Kuyken 1994). The features that deserve attention at this point are the decision to incorporate an examination of the translation by a unilingual group and the existence of bilingual/bicultural groups that can guide the process of producing equivalent versions of the instrument in different languages.

The instruments described in this paper cover the needs for data collection in a number of areas of psychiatric investigation. Other areas, however, also require attention, and it is to be hoped that WHO will continue working on the development of instruments for these. Among them are

1. The instruments that could be used to assess *the stigma of psychiatric illness* and its changes under the influence of various interventions that the health services or the society as a whole might undertake to diminish it
2. Instruments that would be useful to measure the *tolerance* of individuals for their own diseases and the diseases in those who surround them
3. Instruments that might help us to better assess conditions and states such as *"burn-out"* and *"malaise"* and their impact on the productivity of the individuals who suffer from them and of the community as a whole
4. Instruments that could help us to assess *features of the community* relevant to the provision of mental health care (e.g. the capacity of the community to accept sick and disabled members)
5. Instruments that could better describe the *needs of individuals and communities*
6. Instruments we could use in the assessment of states that are at the borderline of normality (e.g. mild cognitive disorders, subthreshold mental disorders)
7. Instruments that could be used in international studies of *impairments, disabilities and handicaps* defined in terms of the second revision of the *International classification of impairments, disabilities and handicaps*

The difficulties of producing an instrument satisfying all the metric requirements and dealing with an area of assessment that should be investigated because of its public health importance pale in comparison with the difficulty of ensuring that the instrument is well known, properly updated, sufficiently well learned and widely applied. It is probably to this second task that the majority of efforts should be directed if we are to contribute to a better understanding among all those concerned with mental illness and with ways of helping them, their families and communities.

References

American Psychiatric Association (1987) Diagnostic and statistical manual of mental disorders 3rd edn, revised (DSM-III-R). APA, Washington, DC

American Psychiatric Association (1994) Diagnostic and statistical manual of mental disorders, 4th edn (DSM-IV). APA, Washington, DC

Babor TF, de la Fuente JR, Saunders JB, Grant M (1989) AUDIT, the Alcohol Use Disorders Identification Test. Guidelines for use in primary health care. WHO, Geneva

Bennett LA, Janca A, Grant BF, Sartorius N (1993) Boundaries between normal and pathological drinking: a cross-cultural comparison. Alcohol Health Res World 17: 190–195

Bertolote J (1994) Quality assurance in mental health care: checklists and glossaries, vol 1. WHO, Geneva

Beusenberg M, Orley J (1994) A user's guide to the Self-Reporting Questionnaire (SRQ). WHO, Geneva

Cooper JE, Jablensky A, Sartorius N (1990) WHO collaborative studies on acute psychoses using the SCAAPS schedule. In: Stefanis CN et al (eds) Psychiatry: a world perspective, vol. 1. Classification and psychopathology, child psychiatry, substance use. (International congress series) Excerpta Medica, Amsterdam, pp 185–192

Cottler LB, Robins LN, Grant BF, Blaine J, Towle LH, Wittchen HU, Sartorius N, Altamura AC, Andrews G, Burke JD, Dingemans PR, Droux A, Farmer A, Helzer JE, Janca A, Lepine JP, Miranda CT, Pull C, Regier DA, Rubio-Stipec M, Sandanger I, Smeets R, Tacchini G, Tehrani M, Tipp JE, Allgulander C, Halikas J, Ingebrigsten G, Isaac M, Jenkins PL, Kuehne GE, Lyketsos G, Maier W, Kraus J, Liang Shu (1991) The CIDI-Core substance abuse and dependence questions: cross-cultural and nosological issues. Br J Psychiatry 159: 653–658

Gater R, Goldberg D, Sartorius N (1990) The WHO Pathways to Care Study. In: Stefanis CN et al (eds) Psychiatry: a world perspective, vol 4. (International congress series) Excerpta Medica, Amsterdam, pp 75–78

Gater R, De Almeida E, Sousa B, Barrientos G, Caraveo J, Chandrashekar CR, Dhadphale M, Goldberg D, Alkathiri AH, Mubbashar M, Silhan K, Thong D, Torres-Gonzales F, Sartorius N (1991) The pathways to psychiatric care: a cross-cultural study. Psychol Med 21: 761–74

Giel R, de Arango MV, Babikir AH, Bonifacio M, Climent CE, Harding TW, Ibrahim HHA, Ladrido-Ignacio L, Srinivasa Murthy R, Wig NN (1983) The burden of mental illness on the family. Results of observations in four developing countries. Acta Psychiatr Scand 68: 186–201

Harding TW, de Arango MV, Balthazar J, Climent CE, Ibrahim HHA, Ladrido-Ignacio L, Srinivasa Murthy R, Wig NN (1980) Mental disorders in primary health care: a study of their frequency and diagnosis in four developing countries. Psychol Med 10: 231–41

Harding TW, Climent CE, Diop M, Giel R, Ibrahim HHA, Srinivasa Murthy R, Suleiman MA, Wig NN (1983) The WHO collaborative study on strategies for extending mental health care. II. The development of new research methods. Am J Psychiatry 140: 1474–80

Hudelson PM (1994) Qualitative research for health programmes. WHO, Geneva

Isaac M, Janca A, Sartorius N (1994) The ICD-10 symptom glossary for mental disorders. WHO, Geneva

Jablensky A, Schwarz R, Tomow T (1980) WHO collaborative study on impairments and disabilities associated with schizophrenic disorders. A preliminary communication: objectives and methods. In: Strömgren E et al (eds) Epidemiological research as basis for the organization of extramural psychiatry. Acta Psychiatr Scand 62: (suppl. 286): 152–159

Jablensky A, Sartorius N, Ernberg G, Anker M, Korten A, Cooper JE, Day R, Bertelsen A (1992) Schizophrenia: manifestations, incidence and course in different cultures: a World Health Organization ten-country study. Psychol Med [Monograph Suppl 20]

Janca A, Chandrashekar CR (1993) Catalogue of assessment instruments used in the studies coordinated by the WHO Mental Health Programme. WHO, Geneva

Janca A, Robins LN, Cottler LB, Early TS (1992) Clinical observation of assessment using the Composite International Diagnostic Interview (CIDI): an analysis of the CIDI field trials-wave II at the St. Louis site. Br J Psychiatry 160: 815–818

Janca A, Üstün TB, Early TS, Sartorius N (1993) The ICD-10 symptom checklist – a companion to the ICD-10 classification of mental and behavioural disorders. Soc Psychiatry Psychiatr Epidemiol 28: 239–242

Janca A, Üstün TB, Sartorius N (1994a) New versions of World Health Organization instruments for the assessment of mental disorders. Acta Psychiatr Scand 90: 73–83

Janca A, Üstün TB, van Drimmelen J, Dittmann V, Isaac M (1994b) The ICD-10 symptom checklist for mental disorders, version 2.0. WHO, Geneva

Janca A, Mezzich JE, Kastrup MC, Katschnig H, Lopez-Ibor JJ, Sartorius N (1994c) The multiaxial presentation of the ICD-10 classification of mental and behavioural disorders. Presented at the 7th European Symposium of the Association of European Psychiatrists, Vienna

Lopez-Ibor JJ, Sartorius N, Janca A, Kastrup M, Katschnig M, Mezzich J (1994) The ICD-10 multiaxial system: preliminary results of field trials. In: Beigel A, Lopez-Ibor JJ, Costa e Silva JA (eds) Past, present and future of psychiatry: IX World Congress of Psychiatry, vol I. World Scientific, Singapore, pp 157–168

Loranger A, Hirschfield R, Sartorius N, Regier D (1991) The WHO/ADAMHA international pilot study of personality disorders: background and purpose. J Pers Disord 5: 296–306

Loranger AW, Sartorius N, Andreoli A, Berger P, Bucheim P, Channabasavanna SM, Coid B, Dahl A, Diekstra R, Ferguson B, Jacobsberg LB, Mombour W, Pull C, Ono Y, Regier DA (1994) The international personality disorder examination (IPDE): the WHO/ADAMHA international pilot study of personality disorders. Arch Gen Psychiatry 51: 215–224

Robins LN, Wing JE, Wittchen H-U, Helzer JE, Babor TF, Burke JD, Farmer A, Jablensky A, Pickens R, Regier DA, Sartorius N, Towle LH (1988) The composite international diagnostic interview: an epidemiologic instrument suitable for use in conjunction with different diagnostic systems and in different cultures. Arch Gen Psychiatry 45: 1069–1077

Robins LN, Cottler LB, Babor T (1990) CIDI substance abuse module. Department of Psychiatry, Washington University School of Medicine, St Louis, Mo

Room R, Janca A, Bennett LA, Schmidt L, Sartorius N (in press) WHO cross-cultural applicability research on diagnosis and assessment of substance use disorders: an overview of methods and selected results. Addiction

Sartorius N (1979) Cross-cultural psychiatry. In: Kisker KP, Meyer JE, Muller C, Stromgren E (eds) Psychiatrie der Gegenwart, vol I/1, 2nd edn. Springer, Berlin Heidelberg New York, pp 711–737

Sartorius N (1989) Recent research activities in WHO's mental health programme. Psychol Med 19: 233–244

Sartorius N (1990) Cultural factors in the etiology of schizophrenia. In: Stefanis CN et al (eds) Psychiatry: a world perspective, vol 4. Social psychiatry ethics and law: history of psychiatry, psychiatric education. (International congress series) Excerpta Medica, Amsterdam, pp 33–44

Sartorius N (1993) WHO's work on the epidemiology of mental disorders. Soc Psychiatry Psychiatr Epidemiol 28: 147–155

Sartorius N (1995) SCAN translation. In: Wing JK, Sartorius N, Ustun TB (eds) Diagnosis and clinical measurement in psychiatry – an instruction manual for the SCAN system. Cambridge University Press, London

Sartorius N, Kuyken W (1994) Translation of health status instruments. In: Orley J, Kuyken W (eds) Quality of life assessment: international perspectives. pp 3–18

Sartorius N, Jablensky A, Gulbinat W, Ernberg G (1980) WHO collaborative study: assessment of depressive disorders. Preliminary communication. Psychol Med 10: 743–749

Sartorius N, Davidian H, Ernberg G, Fenton FR, Fujii I, Gastpar M, Gulbinat W, Jablensky A, Kielholz P, Lehmann HE, Naraghi M, Shimizu M, Shinfuku N, Takahashi R (1983) Depressive disorders in different cultures. Report on the WHO collaborative study on standardized assessment of depressive disorders. WHO, Geneva

Saunders JB, Aasland OG (1987) WHO collaborative project on the identification and treatment of persons with harmful alcohol consumption. Report on phase I. Development of a screening instrument. WHO, Geneva

Saunders JB, Aasland OG, Arundsen A, Grant M (1993a) Alcohol consumption and related problems among primary health care patients. WHO collaborative project on early detection of persons with harmful alcohol consumption. I. Addiction 88: 339–352

Saunders JB, Aasland OG, Babor TF, de la Fuente JR, Grant M (1993b) Development of the Alcohol Use Disorders Identification Test (AUDIT). WHO collaborative project on early detection of persons with harmful alcohol consumption. II. Addiction 88: 617–629

Sell H, Nagpal R (1992) Assessment of subjective well-being. The subjective well-being inventory (SUBI). WHO Regional Office for South-East Asia, New Delhi

The WHOQOL Group (1994) The development of the WHO Quality of Life Assessment Instrument (The WHOQOL). In: Orley J, Kuyken W (eds) Quality of life assessment: international perspectives. Springer, Berlin, Heidelberg New York pp 41–57

Tsiantis J, Caldwell B, Dragonas T, Jegede RO, Lambidi A, Banaag C, Orley J (1991) Development of a WHO child care facility schedule (CCFS): a pilot collaborative study. Bull WHO 69: 51–57

Van Goor-Lambo G, Orley J, Poustka F, Rutter M (1990) Classification of abnormal psychosocial situations: preliminary report of a revision of a WHO scheme. J Child Psychol Psychiatry 31: 229–241

Wing JK, Cooper JE, Sartorius N (1974) Measurement and classification of psychiatric symptoms: an instruction manual for the PSE and CATEGO programme. Cambridge University Press, London

Wing JK, Babor T, Brugha T, Burke J, Cooper JE, Giel R, Jablensky A, Regier D, Sartorius N (1990) SCAN: schedules for clinical assessment in neuropsychiatry. Arch Gen Psychiatry 47: 589–593

Wittchen H-U, Robins LN, Cottler L, Sartorius N, Burke J, Regier D, Altamura AC, Andrews G, Dingemanns R, Droux A, Essau CA, Farmer A, Halikas J, Ingebrigsten G, Isaac M, Jenkins P, Kühne GE, Krause J, Lepine JP, Lyketsos G, Maier W, Miranda CT, Pfister H, Pull C, Rubio-Stipec M, Sandanger I, Smeets R, Tacchini G, Tehrani M (1991) Cross-cultural feasibility, reliability and sources of variance of the Composite International Diagnostic Interview (CIDI) – results of the multicentre WHO/ADAMHA field trials (wave I). Br J Psychiatry 159: 645–653

World Health Organization (1973) Report on the international pilot study of schizophrenia, vol. 1. WHO, Geneva

World Health Organization (1980) International classification of impairments, disabilities and handicaps. WHO, Geneva

World Health Organization (1984) Mental health care in developing countries: a critical appraisal of research findings. Report of a WHO study group. WHO, Geneva

World Health Organization (1988) Draft multiaxial classification of child psychiatric disorders. Axis V. Associated abnormal psychosocial situations including glossary descriptions of items and diagnostic guidelines. WHO, Geneva

World Health Organization (1990a) WHO child care facility schedule with user manual. WHO, Geneva

World Health Organization (1990b) Parent interview schedule. Draft for comments and field testing. WHO, Geneva

World Health Organization (1991) Interview schedule for children. Draft for comments and field testing. WHO, Geneva

World Health Organization (1992) The ICD-10 classification of mental and behavioural disorders: clinical descriptions and diagnostic guidelines. WHO, Geneva

World Health Organization (1993a) The composite international diagnostic interview, core version 1.1. American Psychiatric Press, Washington, DC

World Health Organization (1993b) International personality disorder examination. WHO, Geneva

World Health Organization (1993c) Computerized CIDI (CIDI-Auto). WHO, Geneva

World Health Organization (1994) Schedules for clinical assessment in neuropsychiatry (SCAN). American Psychiatric Research, Washington, DC

The Composite International Diagnostic Interview: An Instrument for Measuring Mental Health Outcome?

HANS-ULRICH WITTCHEN and CHRISTOPHER B. NELSON

Introduction: History and General Characteristics of the Composite International Diagnostic Interview

The World Health Organization (WHO) Composite International Diagnostic Interview (CIDI; WHO 1990) is a comprehensive, fully standardized diagnostic instrument developed for use in epidemiological studies by an international group of researchers under the patronage of the US National Institutes of Health and the WHO. Based on two predecessors, the National Institute of Mental Health (NIMH) Diagnostic Interview Schedule (DIS; Robins et al., 1981) and the Present State Examination (PSE; Wing et al., 1974), the CIDI is designed for the assessment of pyschiatric diagnoses according to the revised third edition of the *Diagnostic and Statistical Manual of Mental Disorders* (DSM-III-R; American Psychiatric Association (APA), 1987) and the *International Classification of Diseases,* 10th edn. ICD-10 Diagnostic Criteria for Research (DCR; WHO, 1993). Although initially developed for large-scale general population research (e. g., National Comorbidity Survey (NCS); Early Developmental Stages of Psychopathology (EDSP; Kessler et al., 1994, Wittchen et al. in press), the CIDI can also be used for clinical and health service research (see review: Wittchen 1994).

The CIDI instrument has several advantages, the most important of which may be that it is a fully standardized and structured interview with established reliability an validity (for a review see Wittchen, 1994). These characteristics ensure that results from different studies are directly comparable, that the interview can be repeatedly administered in a uniform style and that non-clinical interviewers can administer the interview. (This last point is of particular importance for researchers interested in studies involving from several hundred to several thousand interviews.) Because of the comprehensive nature of the instrument, which allows the assessment of up to 75 diagnostic categories in both the DSM and ICD classification systems, its flexible, modular format allows researchers to use only those sections which are relevant to their objectives. It may also be used in the assessment of lifetime or 12-month prevalence and can therefore be applied to etiological as well as health service research. Availability of the CIDI in a Computer-Assisted Personal Interview (CAPI) format (Andrews et al., 1993) and in several language are further advantages of this WHO-sanctioned instrument.

This chapter briefly describes the main features of the WHO CIDI core version as well as those of some of the more frequently used modifications. These include the Primary Care version of the CIDI (CIDI-PMC) developed by WHO (Üstün and Sar-

Clinical Institute, Clinical Psychology Unit, Max Planck Institute for Psychiatry, Kraepelinstr. 2, D-80804 München, Germany

Table 1. Examples of CIDI questions and other information extractable from the CIDI Core

Domain	Example	Coding
Questions regarding symptoms with probing	C.7 Have you ever had a lot of trouble with excessively painful menstrual periods? Doctors diagnosis: .... Other attributions:	Probing for doctor and his diagnosis, other health professional, a lot of interference, relatedness to physical illness (Codes: PRB: 1 2 4 5)
Series of explicit questions regarding help-seeking and interference	D27 Did you tell a doctor about your fears of ...? 1. Did you tell any other professional about any of them? 2. Did you take medication more than once because of these fears? 3. Did these fears interfere with your life or activities a lot?	NO YES NO YES NO YES NO YES
Questions on frequency	E41 In your lifetime how many spells like that have you had that lasted two weeks or more?	–/– no of spells
Questions on onset and recency	E37 When was the first time you had a period of two weeks or more, when you had several of these problems and also felt low, uninterested or depressed? And when was the last time ...?	ONS: 1 2 3 4 5 6 AGE ONS: –/– REC: 1 2 3 4 5 6 AGE REC: –/– 1 = within the past 2 weeks 2 = within the past months 6 = more than a year ago

ONS, onset; REC, recurrence, PRB, Probe; CIDI, Composite International Diagnostic Interview

torius, 1995), the University of Michigan CIDI (UM-CIDI; Wittchen and Kessler, 1994) and the more recent Munich-CIDI (M-CIDI; Wittchen et al., 1995a,b,c). Particular emphasis will be placed upon those instrument features which are potentially relevant for the measurement of mental health outcomes.

The CIDI Core Version

Characteristics

The CIDI Core consists of 276 questions related to symptoms, arranged as stem and probe questions; not all need to be asked because of skip rules. Many of the symptoms are probed according to a differentiated probe flow chart (see examples in Table 1). The following information can be collected using the chart: whether the symptom was present, whether the respondent (R) talked with a medical doctor or another mental health professional about the symptom, whether R took medication because of the symptom and whether the symptom has caused significant impairment. Furthermore, whether the symptom occurred in conjunction with substance use or physical illness can also be recorded. Similar information can be collected separately for key syndromes (somatoform, anxiety,

psychotic and affective syndromes). The syndrome-related questions for these domains are, however, always coded for a lifetime peak episode. Thus, there is no
cross-sectional current rating possible for those cases who have partially or fully
remitted.

The coding of all answers in the CIDI is strictly categorical, that is, the standardized symptom and impairment questions can only be coded yes and no; no dimensional ratings are possible. Another set of questions assess the length of an episode
for key syndromes (General anxiety disorder and affective disorders) and the frequency of the episodes (e.g., affective disorders). The CIDI core version is accompanied by a computerized diagnostic program that facilitates the classification of R's
symptoms according to the DSM-III-R or the ICD-10 Criteria for Research. Besides reporting diagnoses, the program prints out the times at which criteria were first an last
time met. The coding options for this are: within the past 2 weeks, 2 weeks to one
month, one month to six months, 6 months to one year and more than a year in the
past. For the latter coding option, the age of the respondent at that time is registered.

Use of CDI Core in Mental Health Outcome and Service Research

Despite the lack of any dimensional measures this version of the CDI, similar to the
DIS (Robins et al., 1991) has been used for outcome measurement in several ways
(Kessler et al., 1995):

1. Measures of remission for each diagnosis can be derived by examining whether as
   specific episode is currently still present. This judgment is based on the recency
   probes that assess the recency of criteria for diagnosis of key syndromes. These
   recency probes allow the calculation of remission for various periods of time
   (syndrome present in the past 2 weeks, 4 weeks, 6 months or year). If remission
   occurred mote than a year previously, it is also possible to indicate at what age
   R last experienced the problem.
2. Measures of duration can be obtained by specific questions for some syndromes
   (e.g. depression, manina, GAD). Some authors have also used the time difference
   between recency and onset to derive a rather crude measure of duration. This
   measure merely indicates that the respective syndrome was at least present
   at age of onset and at age of recency. It does not necessarily indicate, however,
   whether it has been present during the full time interval.
3. Measures of help-seeking and impairment can be obtained for many symptoms
   and syndromes (e.g., anxiety, affective and psychotic disorders) using the probe
   flow chart. The CIDI allows a determination of whether the person sought professional help from medical doctors or other health professionals, took medication
   more than once or reported a lot of interference. This information, however, is
   not specifically dated and refers to liftime reports. By using the computerized version (CIDI-AUTO) it is also possible to print out this information for each individual symptom for which probe questions were used.
4. Measures of change cannot be derived directly from the CID Core due to the lack
   of any dimensional cross-section items. However, some research groups have used
   the CIDI in longitudinal studies by simply modifying the questions in the follow-
   up investigation to cover exclusively the follow-up period. By assessing at time

1 lifetime information and by focusing for example on a 1-year time frame in the case of a 1-year follow-up investigation, an indirect assessment of changes in diagnostic status can be done. The resulting measures are new diagnoses that occurred in the time interval between investigations. By using more sophisticated analytic procedures changes between subthreshold and threshold conditions based on the number of diagnostic criteria met can also be identified.

To summarize, the CIDI core version has not been constructed for outcome measurement; thus it is not surprising that only rather limited options are available.

The University of Michigan CIDI

Characteristics

This interview is a modified version of the CIDI (WHO, 1990), in which the CIDI diagnostic programs are used for generating DSM-III-R diagnoses. It has been modified to meet the needs of the US-NCS (Kessler et al., 1994), the first national study of mental disorders in the United States and also the first to examine the frequency, form and the implications of mental disorder comorbidity. The modifications include:

1. Deletion of some sections of the CIDI, such as the lengthy section on somatoform disorders.
2. Modification of some CIDI questions, such as breaking down long and complex questions into separate sub-questions, placing important explanations for words or concepts that are part of the CIDI Interviewer Manual directly into the interview, and adding clarifying probes in places where pilot tests showed that there was confusion in the original CIDI.
3. Rearrangement of the order in which CIDI questions are asked to improve comprehension and flow; for example many of the stem questions are moved to the beginning of the interview.
4. Streamlining of the probe flow chart used in the CIDI.
5. The use of visual symptom checklists and review cards to simplify the complex cognitive tasks required of respondents during the interview.
6. Implementation of a lifetime review section for diagnostic stem questions.

Mental Health Service and Outcome Measures

Although almost identical to the CIDI Core in most respects, the UM-CIDI incorporates a slightly wider range of measures, potentially relevant for mental health service and outcome research. For each diagnosis the UM-CIDI comprises a longer series of help-seeking questions, including separate questions for medical doctors, psychiatrists, other mental health specialists and other professionals. Separate questions are asked for each category about the age the R. first contacted those. Thus lifetime symptom information can be more accurately related to certain episodes. The standard questions regarding psychosocial impairment as well as some other symptoms were transformed into four-point ratings, with response options ranging from a lot of interference to none. Furthermore additional questions were added in most sections to assess the effect of prescribed medication on mental disorders (e.g., anxiety), remission from episodes (e.g., depression) and to determine the sequence in which psychopathological syndromes occurred. Similar to the CIDI Core, the focus is on the lifetime assessment and no current state information is assessed for any of these domains.

Primary Care Version of the CIDI

Characteristics

The CIDI-PMC (WHO 1992) was developed in the context of an international multi-center study (Üstün and Sartorius, 1995). Designed as a longitudinal study, specific emphasis was placed on modifications of the CID Core which would allow comparisons to be made over time and the quantification of change. Because mental disorders in primary care were believed to be frequently atypical subthreshold conditions as well as mixed anxiety disorders, modifications were made to allow the derivation of various new diagnoses, which were not originally covered in the CIDI Core (e.g., a combination of anxiety, depression and neurasthenia, generalized anxiety syndrome). The CIDI-PMC enables the researcher to code both information lifetime as well as symptoms which are currently present (past 4 weeks). This allows the calculation of current symptom scores for all major syndromes covered (somatoform and pain, generalized anxiety, depressive syndromes). It is important to note, however, that the CIDI-PMC covers only some of the standard CIDI diagnostic sections. There are no sections for substance use disorders (except alcohol), hypochondriasis, simple, social phobia and obsessive-compulsive disorder, mania and psychotic as well as eating disorders.

Mental Health Service and Outcome Measures

Unlike the previously discussed instruments the CIDI-PMC allows in addition to the above mentioned options of the CIDI Core:

1. The derivation of syndrome symptom counts that can be compared over time
2. The monitoring of changes in specific symptoms over time and of different assessment
3. The evaluation of subthreshold conditions as well as changes between subthreshold and threshold status.

Thus the researcher can directly compare changes in current symptoms between different examinations and monitor changes over time for each of the key syndromes. No corresponding changes were implemented for the CIDI psychosocial impairment questions, because this study used a specific generic dimensional disability measure, the Disability Assessment Schedule (Üstün and Sartorius, 1995).

The Munich CIDI

Characteristics

The M-CIDI is the latest step in the development of the CIDI family. It is also the only version covering DSM-IV criteria (APA, 1994) instead of DSM-III-R. By maintaining a basic comparability with the ICD-10 DCR of CIDI version 1.2, various procedural modifications were implemented such as:

1. The use of respondent lists to reduce administration time and to take advantage of cognitive probes (comparable to the UM-CIDI)
2. A dimensional lifetime version of the psychosocial impairment criteria for each diagnosis instead of the categorical original approach
3. A more specific current (four weeks) psychosocial impairment rating for each diagnosis which allows the rating of the degree of impairment with regard to work, household, study, leisure activities and interpersonal aspects
4. The possibility to directly relate the symtpom assessed to one specific episode in time, including current syndromes, which allows the determination of several course and severity specifiers for many key syndromes covered.

In addition, two compatible interview versions are offered, one for lifetime (M-CIDI-LT) and the other for the previous 12 months (M-CIDI-12 Month), which permits the computation of current diagnoses and symptom counts (see Table 2). Changes in the M-CIDI include coverage of DSM-IV criteria, a wider spectrum of diagnoses (post-traumatic stress disorder, subtypes of disorders, organic anxiety and depressive disorders) as well as various subthreshold conditions. By using the optional computerized interview versions, the researcher also has symptom specific impairment and help seeking data available.

Unlike to all previous CIDI versions, the M-CIDI is constructed in a modular way so that sections can be completely skipped and other scales and instruments that might be of interest for a specific research project can be added. This change was made in response to the fact that the vast majority of users in the past did not use the full CIDI Core, but rather restricted themselves for reasons of time and resources to certain sections. Since this module structure with all its options is rather complicated to use, it is highly recommended for ease of administration to use the CAPI version of the M-CIDI, which allows the interviewer and researcher to design the interview according to his or her needs. A computerized entry menu enables the interviewer to conveniently choose the required M-CIDI elements. The computer program then automatically configures the interview accordingly.

Mental Health Service and Outcome Measures

Both the lifetime and the 12-month version of the M-CIDI are more specifically designed for follow-up studies as well as to measure a change in status. In addition to all the above mentioned options (diagnoses, age of onset and finish, duration, frequency, impairment and help-seeking) the M-CIDI also includes the following features:

Table 2. Examples of questions from the Munich-Composite International Diagnostic Interview (M-CIDI)

Domains		Question examples
Lifetime or episode peak ratings for psychosocial impairments	C55A	If you think back on the worst time, how much, did these worries affect your life and your everyday activities? Would you say ... not at all, somewhat, a lot, very much?
	B	And in the last four weeks, how much did these worries affect ... 1. .. your work, homework or studies? 2. .. your leisure activities? 3. .. your social contacts with family, friends and colleagues?
Current symptom assessments	D	In the past twelve months during your attack(s) which of the following problems did you have? A. did your heart pound or race B. did you sweat? etc.
	D8	And how many attacks like that have you had in the last 4 weeks? Approximately how many in the past 12 months?
Questions on persistence	D40	In the last 12 months, how often has this fear or the wish to avoid such situations been present. Would you say ... most of the time, sometimes or only once?
	E14	You told me that in the last twelve weeks ... And when did this period of two weeks or more start? (code as accurately as possible). And when did it end?
	E42	Pleasure turn to the next page of your booklet. I would like to talk with you about the course of your mood difficulties in the past 12 months. Which of these profiles would you say best applies to you and your mood problems (code number of pattern)?

1. Measurement of cross-sectional symptom counts including severity for selected somatoform syndromes, panic, GAD, social and agoraphobia, PTSD, depressive and psychotic disorders as well as substance use disorders.
2. Assessment of current disorder-specific impairments related to each disorder dimension with one generic measure for the peak of illness severity as well as more specifically (work, household management, leisure time and social interaction) for the past 4 weeks.
3. Determination of the date of the episode peak for many conditions.
4. A description of the course of the disorder may be obtained by asking questions about onset and course; graphic course patterns may also be used.
5. Detection of syndrome changes over time for disorders and various subthreshold conditions.
6. A lay persons version of the Brief Psychiatric Rating Scale to measure the current severity of several psychopathological syndromes.

Furthermore it is noteworthy that the M-CIDI can be combined with questionnaires which are compatible with the interview. The following scales, which were developed from the M-CIDI methodological studies for screening purpose, are available: Social Phobia Questionnaire (Lepine et al., in preparation), Anxiety Screening Questionnaire (Wittchen et al., 1994) and Depression Screening Questionnaire (Wittchen et al., 1995). In addition a Stem question Screening Questionnaire is being tested, which can be used in an initial screening before starting the M-CIDI interview. This may shorten the average administration time of 65 minutes considerably.

Summary and Outlook

The various Composite International Diagnostic Interviews discussed above were not specifically designed for mental health outcome measurement. As a primarily epidemiological case finding (diagnostic) instrument, along the operationalised and explicit criteria of DSM and ICD its categorical structure still dominates the philosophy. The strength of the CIDI lies in its reliability and validity as a diagnostic instrument, and in its ease of administration even by trained non-clinicians. Although measurement of syndrome change is possible with this tool, it is not its main purpose. Hence, for the vast majority of researchers interested in outcome and mental health service evaluation more specific interview questions or questionnaires are needed to supplement the CIDI.

This overview described several useful and unique options in each of the CIDI variants. In particular the more recent modifications made in the PMC-CIDI and the new M-CIDI are a considerable improvement on the rather crude measurements which are possible with the CIDI Core.

The WHO advisory group which supervises and coordinates the CIDI development has recently acknowledged the emerging trend to favour cross-sectional and dimensional measures as well as the modular approach (CIDI tool box). The group is currently exploring various options for the development of these more complex tools. The CIDI 2.0 version for the assessment of DSM-IV criteria, which will hopefully be available at the end of 1996, does not, however, address these issues. Based on the experience with the more experimental M-CIDI, it is likely that CIDI 3.0 will have a modular structure, a more detailed disability module and dimensional ratings, focusing on the assessment of current symptomatology.

References

American Psychiatric Association (1987) Diagnostic and Statistical Manual of Mental Disorders (3rd rev. edn.). American Psychiatric Association, Washington DC
American Psychiatric Association (1994) Diagnostic and Statistical Manual of Mental Disorders (4th edn.). American Psychiatric Association, Washington
Andrews G, Morris-Yates A, Peters L, Teesson M (1993) CIDI-Auto. Administrator's guide and reference, Version 1.1. Available from: Training and Reference Center for WHO CIDI, Sidney
Kessler RC, McGonagle KA, Zhao S, Nelson CB, Hughes M, Esbleman S, Wittchen H-U, Kendler KS (1994) Lifetime and 12-month prevalence of DSM-III-R psychiatric disorders in the United States: Results from the National Comorbidity Survey. Arch Gen Psychiatry 51: 8–19
Kessler RC, Sonnega A, Bromet E, Nelson CB (1995) Postraumatic stress disorder in the National Comorbidity Survey. Arch Gen Psychiatry 52: 1048–1060
Robins LN, Helzer JE, Croughan J, Ratcliff KS (1981) National Institute of Mental Health Diagnostic Interview Schedule: its history, characteristics and validity. Arch Gen Psychiatry 38: 381–389

Robins LN, Locke BZ, Regier DA (1991) An overview of psychiatric disorders in America. In: Robins LN, Regier DA (eds) Psychiatric disorders in America. The Epidemiologic Catchment Area Study. Macmillan, New York, pp 328–366

Wing JK, Cooper JE, Sartorius N (1974) Measurement and classification of psychiatric symptoms: Cambridge University Press, Cambridge

Wittchen H-U (1994) Reliability and validity studies of the WHO-Composite International Diagnostic Interview (CIDI): A critical review. J Psychiatr Res 28 (1): 57–84

Wittchen H-U, Beloch E, Garzcynski E, Holly A, Lachner G, Perkonigg A, Pfütze E-M, Schuster P, Vodermaier A, Vossen A, Wunderlich U, Zieglgänsberger S (1995a) Münchener Composite International Diagnostic Interview (M-CIDI, Paper-pencil 2.2, 2/95). Max-Planck-Institut für Psychiatrie, Klinisches Institut, München

Wittchen H-U, Beloch E, Garzcynski E, Holly A, Lachner G, Perkonigg A, Pfütze E-M, Schuster P, Vodermaier A, Vossen A, Wunderlich U, Zieglgänsberger S (1995b) Manual zum Münchener Composite International Diagnostic Interview (M-CIDI, Paper-Pencil 2.0, 1/95). Max-Planck-Institut für Psychiatrie, Klinisches Institut, München

Wittchen H-U, Beloch E, Garzcynski E, Holly A, Lachner G, Perkonigg A, Pfütze E-M, Schuster P, Vodermaier A, Vossen A, Wunderlich U, Zieglgänsberger S (1995c). Listenheft zum Münchener Composite International Diagnostic Interview (M-CIDI, Paper-Pencil 2.2, 2/95). Max-Planck-Institut für Psychiatrie, Klinisches Institut, München

Wittchen H-U, Kessler RC (1994) Modification of the CIDI in the National Comorbidity Survey: The development of the UM-CIDI. NCS working paper #2. Ann Arbor: Institute of Social Research, The University of Michigan

World Health Organization (1990) Composite International Diagnostic Interview (CIDI) World Health Organisation, Division of Mental Health, Geneva

Üstün TB, Sartorius N (1995) The background and rationale of the WHO collaborative study on 'psychological problems in general health care'. Wiley, Chichester

CHAPTER 14

Assessment Instruments in Psychiatry: Description and Psychometric Properties

Luis Salvador-Carulla

Assessment Instruments: Basic Concepts

Assessment may be defined as the process of applying a systematic method to describe phenomena or objects. Its degree of systematization may vary widely, from merely assigning pre-established codes to algorithmic quantification systems. Assessment may be subjective or objective. Subjective assessment is characterized by the description of hypothetical or intangible elements (e.g., quality of life, depression) as opposed to the tangible entities described by the experimental sciences, such as weight or height, that is, objective assessment. In the health sciences, this differentiation is not always very clear since there is a great deal of individual discretion involved in the interpretation of complex complementary evidence (i.e. histology, imaging diagnosis, neurophysiology). This means that many quality norms are the same for objective and subjective instruments. Subjective assessment is less precie, and has been undervalued until very recently. The growing demand for intangible parameters – such as satisfaction, support, autonomy, quality of life or level of disability – dictates that the use of these instruments is currently essential in any health care field.

Assessment may also be descriptive or quantitative. A quantitative assessment consists of elaborating rules to assign numbers to a given phenomenon, with the aim of quantifying one or more of its attributes. These rules are a codified series of procedures for assigning numbers. When assessing a certain phenomenon, it is important to place it within a categorical or dimensional model, and in the latter case, to decide whether it is uni- or multidimensional. Assessment instruments comprise a variable number of items. An item is the basic information unit of an assessment instrument, and usually consists of a question – generally a closed question – and an answer, which can be assigned a code. The glossary is an additional list of explanatory notes regarding the precise definition of each item, and how to combine them in categories or dimensions (Stromgren 1988).

Basis for Description and Classification of Assessment Instruments

Bech et al. (1993) described assessment scales in terms of the scales' objectives and composition:

1. Assessment area: diagnostic, symptomatic and personality scales, and scales for other specific purposes

University of Cadiz, Edif. cycas 7D, Urb. el Bosque, Jerez de la frontera, E-11405, Cadiz, Spain

2. Type of administration: scales for the patient, the doctor or other health care staff
3. Retrospective time access: time frame of the assessment
4. Selection of items: distinguishes among first generation scales (based on clinical experience) and second generation scales (derived from the former)
5. Number of items on the scale
6. Definition of individual items. The work of other authors (such as Thompson 1989a; Wittchen and Essau 1991) has led to modifications of Bech's original proposal in order to permit a more complete description of the different instruments used in mental health. In general terms, this is based on their complexity, the purpose of the instrument (condition assessed, population of reference, assessment period, etc.) and construction (structure, composition of its items, and the measures taken to prevent potential bias in its completion). The changes in terminology with respect to that used by Bech are detailed in each section.

Complexity

Assessment instruments may be classified in a series of groupings, according to their complexity (Salvador-Carulla and Roca 1995). *Descriptive questionnaires* may be placed in the first group (e.g., socio-demographic questionnaires), as well as symptom inventories (e.g., inventory of adverse effects). The items of these instruments cannot be quantified, so they may be considered to be merely checklists.

On a second level are the *rating scales*. As their name indicates, their items can be accumulatively scaled, generating overall scores at the end of the assessment. They are composed of individual items, each one describing a well-defined characteristic of the phenomenon being assessed. Their accumulative nature differentiates them from data collection questionnaires and simple symptom inventories.

On a third level are the *standardized interviews*. These are classified according to their objectives (general or specific), and according to the level of training required for their administration. The latter depends on how structured they are as far as formulating the questions and codifying the answers is concerned (the more structured the interview, the less previous experience interviewers need in order to administer it). Standardized interviews may be accompanied by a computerized correction system for assigning diagnostic criteria.

Standardized diagnostic systems constitute a fourth level. They provide a codification of nosologic entities, with a detailed description of each one of them in a glossary, to make diagnosis easier. Diagnostic systems are called operational when they provide a series of rules for diagnosis based on inclusion criteria (presence of a minimum number of characteristics of the phenomenon for its diagnosis) and exclusion criteria (casting off other characteristics unrelated to the phenomenon). When the exclusion criteria refer to the presence of other syndrome-related entities, the system is considered hierarchical, since it imposes a hierarchical structure on the nosologic entities included in the system for their differential diagnosis. If the standardized diagnostic system also allows for the codification of various entities or aspects related in different axes, it is considered to be a multiaxial system. There are two principal systems of hierarchical and multiaxial operative diagnosis currently in use: the ICD-10 research system and the DSM-IV. According to some authors, dignostic systems should not be considered as assessment instruments. However, in their construction and use, diagnostic systems comply with the general rules of standardized subjective evaluation.

Composite assessment batteries may be placed on the next level. These are sets of different instruments (e. g., a data collection questionnaire, assessment scales incorporated into a battery, a standardized interview on past symptoms and/or current state, and a computerized system for multiple diagnosis, which allows diagnostic codification according to different systems). Examples of compound batteries are the SCAN, based on the PSE (Pull and Wittchen 1991; Vazquez-Barquero 1993), and the CASH battery for assessment of schizophrenia and mood disorders, developed from the SANS/SAPS for assessment of positive and negative symptoms in schizophrenia, among other instruments (Andreasen et al. 1992). *Clinical information systems* comprise a whole array of automated instruments designed for handling data bases (Mezzich 1986).

Purpose of a Scale

The purpose of a scale will determine the content of its items and different aspects related to its structure. A scale should always limit itself to the area for which it has been designed, at least until it can be standardized. The purpose is related to the dimension being assessed, the population under study, the assessment period and how the scale is filled out.

Area to be Assessed

The different psychosocial scales assess a wide range of areas, such as symptoms (clinical scales) personality social, family, sexual and vocational functioning or disability. Bech (1993) makes a distinction between two types of clinical scales: diagnostic and symptomatic. This distinction is conflictive, since there are symptomatic scales which have been used for diagnosis after calculating a cut-off point by means of a predictive validity study (see quality parameters of a scale), and vice versa.

Objective of the Study

It is important to differentiate between general scales (such as those for evaluating pychiatric caseness and specific scales (e. g., for evaluation of depression). Specific scales may therefore have different gradations (e. g., HDRS for the assessment of major depression, and the Newcastle scale for the assessment of endogenous depression). Wittchen and Essau (1991) distinguish between scales based on a "wide" or "restrictive" concept of mental disorder. The most restrictive instruments value specificity over sensitivity and vice versa (this factor is particularly important in the use of standardized diagnostic systems).

Time Frame

Based on the stability of the phenomenon under assessment, we can differentiate between *trait scales,* which assess phenomena that are relatively stable over time (e. g., personality test, locus of control), and *status scales,* which assess the subject's current situation (such as depression, or positive and negative symptoms), usually dur-

ing the previous month, the previous week or few weeks, or during the three days before the assessment ("here and now" scales). The time frame should be detailed in
the instructions for administering the scale.

In status scales, the assessment period differentiates *detection scales* (e.g., for
identifying psychiatric cases, such as the GHQ) from *follow-up scales*. Non-transitional follow-up scales assess change based on the difference in the score from one
assessment to another (e.g., HDRS); transitional follow-up scales directly assess the
degree of improvement or worsening experienced by the patient between both assessments (e.g., CGI change scale). When studying a follow-up scale, it is important
to know its sensitivity to change.

Type of Administration

Self-administered scales are designed to be filled out by the subject, or by an informant. Sometimes they include items to calibrate the validity of the answers based
on a tendency to dissimulate or simulate (e.g., Eysenck's EPQ). Bech et al. (1993)
calls this group of instruments "questionnaires"; however, this term is too general.

Interviewer-administered scales (which Bech termed "observer scales") are filled
out by an examiner. Such assessment instruments require different degrees of professional training for their use (this factor is particularly important in designing and
administering structured interviews). These scales require a previous standardization of raters by means of an analysis of their agreement with reference examiner
(see inter-rater reliability). Two extremes in the application of interviewer-administered scales have been pointed out: an *alpha situation* (expert rater who carries out
a closed interview and uses a scale with a few, well-defined items, which include criteria of improvement and health), and a *beta situation* (unskilled rater, who conducts
an open-ended interview, and uses a scale with many, poorly-defined items, and
without criteria of improvement and health) (Bech et al. 1993).

Some clinical assessment instruments are of a mixed type and include one section
for reported symptoms and another for symptoms observed during the interview.

Construction of Assessment Scales

As mentioned above, the item is the basic information unit of an assessment instrument, and generally consists of a closed question and its answer.

Number of Items

Scales may be divided into unitary or global scales, composed of a single item (e.g.,
CGI, GAS, analogue scales of pain or well-being) and multi-item scales. As a general
rule, it is agreed that a phenomenon should be assessed with a minimum of 6 items
(Bech et al. 1993). Scales generally consist of 10–90 items. Different scales are available in different versions: Goldberg's GHQ in versions with 60, 30, 28, and 12 items;
Hamilton's HDRS in versions with 21 or 17 items (in addition to other scales derived
from this test).

Content of the Items

Unidimensional and multidimensional scales are differentiated by their content. With a unidimensional scale, more than 80 % of the items evaluate a single dimension, in accordance with Israel's model (1983). For example McGill's pain questionnaire, evaluates the physical dimension (symptoms related to somatic or medical aspects), BDI evaluates psychic dimensions (cognitive aspects), and ADL evaluates social dimension. With multidimensional scales, the items assess two or three of these dimensions (e.g., GHQ, HDRS). With interviewer-administered scales, there is also a distinction made between the items reported by the patient and those observed by the interviewer.

The item bias or its orientation refers to the part of the syndrome which appears best reflected in the scale. This is represented by a percentage of the maximum theoretical score for each category of symptoms (Thompson 1989 a). For example, HDRS has an item bias for the somatic symptoms of depression.

Definition

The definition of each item should be exhaustive and mutually exclusive (Guilford's criteria; Bech et al. 1993). The following aspects should be considered when formulating the questions and alternative answers and when ordering the set of items which compose the scale:

1. *Comprehension:* The language and formulation of the questions and answers need to be adapted to the patient's socio-cultural environment. For example, comprehension of the use of linear analogues tends to be better in some cultural environments while the understanding of decimal numeric analogues is better in others. There are different indices for assessing the comprehensibleness of a text (e.g., Flesch's index for English; Thompson 1989 a). The problem of comprehension is extremely important in assessing specific populations, such as the mentally retarded. On the other hand, the translation and adaptation of a scale previously developed in another language, for another cultural context, should follow a specific procedure, including the process of back-translation. Recently, more complex systems have been applied, such as conceptual translation (see below).
2. *Acceptability:* It is fundamental that the items be acceptable to the subject under evaluation. Social desirability is a typs of potential bias which can alter the validity of the answers given (Wittchen and Essau 1991). This should be taken into account when formulating questions for certain items (this type of bvias is important in assessing attitudes regarding certain illnesses, such as AIDS or Mental Retardation, because the subject tends to give the most socially acceptable answers). It is also necessary to limit the number of items, to avoid fatigue and to encourage the subject's collaboration (this problem is evident with questionnaires or batteries with more than 100 items, such as the MMPI).
3. *Preventing bias in completion:* Aquiescence (the tendency to answer a question affirmatively) requires that alternate questions be formulated "positively" and "negatively". However, this may significantly diminish the patient's comprehension, and the reliability of the answers (for example, items such as: "It is untrue that Columbus discovered America – T/F" may easily confound patients with low attention span). Central tendency error refers to the reluctance to choose the ex-

treme alternatives in an item, giving preference to the central ones. This problem mainly affects verbal analogue scales with three or five alternatives (e.g., None, Some, A lot). Another type of bias is related to the tendency to answer with the alternatives situated to the right or to the left, and this bias increases when one of the two extremes always contains the "desirable" alternatives. This can be avoided by alternating which side the positive alternatives are on (first left, then right).

When an interviewer-administered scale is designed, different types of specific should be kept in mind. The *halo effect* refers to the tendency to make a judgment at the beginning of the interview (e.g., heuristic diagnosis), which influences how the following items are filled out. This can happen when completing the HDRS, which groups items directly related with depression and severity at the beginning of the interview. The halo effect is important in the assessment of co-morbidity with those instruments which use a single evaluator (Buchanan and Carpenter 1994). *Logical error* occurs if all those items which are apparently related are scored in a similar way. (Thus, it might be assumed that a patient with a high score on "suicidal ideation" will also have a high score on "hopelessness".) *Proximity error* leads the rater to score adjoining items in a similar way. Another source of error is *terminology variance,* and is due to the attribution of different meanings to the same term. This problem has a special impact on clinical scales, given the different interpretations of a term according to an evaluator's psychopathologic orientation or background knowledge. This bias can be avoided by including an appendix with a glossary (e.g., BPRS).

Selection, Analysis and Ordering of the Items

Meehl and Golden (1982) have described a series of principles or steps in the construction of a symptoms assessment scale:

1. Select the items based on their clinical relevance and validity.
2. Select the items based on their internal correlation when they are applied to a mixed group of patients (one which includes patients with and without the assessed symptom).
3. Select items with different hierarchical weights (describing different aspects of the phenomenon assessed); that is, they should not be redundant.
4. All things being equal, select items with the greatest potential for consensus.
5. Check the results of the group of items selected based on different external criteria (age, gender, etc.), in order to assess their transferability.
6. When steps 3, 4 and 5 cannot be carried out, repeat the analysis with modified items regarding definition or content.

Items can also be selected on the basis of their usefulness. This is assessed using three criteria (Thompson 1989b):

1. *Calibration:* sufficient frequency of replies on an individual item in the population being tested in order to guarantee its inclusion in the scale. Arbitrarily this can be fixed at 10%.

2. *Ascending monotonicity:* The item should show a significant correlation with the global assessment.
3. *Dispersion:* Low dispersion with regard to the line of regression of the above correlation.

There are various models for the psychometric analysis of items (Garcia-Cueto 1993; Martinez-Arias 1995). *Classical Test Theory* (CTT) is a psychometric model which describes the influence of measurement errors on the scores observed of an individual. The true score for a given variable is defined as that which really corresponds to an individual. However, when something is measured with any instrument, a measurement error always occurs, which gives rise to a difference between the true theoretical score and the observed score, obtained by direct observation using a measurement instrument. The CTT is based on a mathematically acceptable definition of the true score which is conceptually usable and makes certain basic suppositions which relate the true score to measurement error.

Item Response Theory (IRT), or latent trait theory, attempts to specify the relationship between a subject's "observable" score in a test, and the "latent traits" which it is assumed lie behind these scores. The models are uni- or multi-dimensional, depending on the set of latent traits which are necessary to explain the behavior under study. Although the IRT considers two more parameters to be kept in mind when studying the psychometric characteristics of a test, i.e., getting the right answer by chance and false positives, both are complementary for the analysis and construction of a test. The process of constructing an assessment scale composed of binary items may begin with the use of total-item correlation indices of the classic test model, followed by an analysis of its latent structure using Rasch's model. Thus it is possible to establish the relationship by means of manifest answers and the latent dimension (Andersen 1989).

Generalizability theory (GT) uses a set of techniques for studying the degree to which a series of measures from a group of subjects can be generalized and extended to a different group of subjects. GT takes into account the multiple factors which can produce variations in subject's scores by means of applying a multivariate design. This makes it possible to estimate the variance attributable to each one of them, as well as their interactions. By diversifying the measurement conditions, the representativeness (generalizability) of the results is increased. It also facilitates the design of measurement procedures in which the confounding factors are represented (Muñiz 1992).

Factor analysis enables investigators to check the uni- or multidimensional structure of an instrument. Its application to instruments which have already been constructed or to new versions of them means that it can be more adequately discussed in the consistency section.

Answer Codification Systems

Dichotomous categorical scale comprises a series of questions with two possible answers: Yes/No or True/False (e.g., personality tests such as the EPQ or the MMPI). *Analogues scales* can be differentiated on the basis of the analogue system used for the answer into five different types:

1. Linear-analogue scale: Ranking is done using a line of 7–10 cm (e.g., pain or well-being scales).

   Example:
   Not at all sad   ————————————————   As sad as I have ever been

2. Analogue-numerical scales: Ranking is similar to that of analogue scales except, that numbers are used (from 0 to 7 or 10). With thermometric unitary scales, the numbers are arranged vertically. These may be graded from 0–100 (e.g., GAF for assessment of general functioning). Sometimes visual and numerical analogues are combined to increase comprehension.

   Example:
   Not at all sad   0 1 2 3 4 5 6 7 8 9   As sad as I have ever been

3. Graphic scales: Ranking is done by means of drawings (e.g., Face scale for assessment of well-being). Some authors consider graphic scales to be linear.

4. Verbal-analogues scales: Ranking is done using previously calibrated verbal categories (e.g., by means of Guttman's escalation system). Generally, the response options range between 3 and 7. Likert considered 5 to be the optimal number of alternatives. Goldberg preferred to use four options to avoid central tendency bias. It is generally agreed that above 6 options, the level of reliability diminishes significantly. Severity scales use more degrees than detection scales (e.g., the CGI has 7, while the GHQ has 4). These scales are also called Likert scales in honor of the man who introduced them 60 years ago (Bech et al., 1986). However, a specific scoring system bears the same name, so this usage can be confusing.

   Example: No more   Somewhat less   Quite More   Much more
              than usual   than usual   than usual   than usual

5. Categorical-analogue scales: This group comprises a series of scales which combine numerical and verbal ranking (e.g., CGI, GAF; Bech et al. 1986). They are also known as Discretized Analogues Scales (DSICAN).

   Example: 1 2 3   4 5 6   7 8 9
     ·   No more   Somewhat less   Quite More
              than usual   than usual   than usual

Scoring the Items

The scoring system can vary substantially from one scale to another and even within the same scale in the case of verbal-analogue scales. Unitary scales of severity (non-transitional) tend to have a maximum score of 8 or 10 when dealing with verbal analogues or other combined forms (DISCAN). The GAF can be scored up to 99, but it really presents 10 degrees of response in decimals.

Unitary global scales of a transitional type are generally bipolar, allowing for a positive or negative score (from greater worsening to greater improvement). For technical reasons, they can also be scored from 1–7, although the scale's polarity may not be adequately reflected in this approach.

- Alternative A: -3/-2/-1/0/1/2/3
- Alternative B: 1/2/3/4/5/6/7

Multi-item verbal scales allow for different numerical assignations. Thus, Goldberg's GHQ permits three different scorings: two are based on the system originally proposed by Likert in the 1930s, and the other was proposed by Goldberg himself. The HDRS and the SANS/SAPS are scored in accordance with the system proposed by M. Hamilton, which differentiates between the options of absent (0), doubtful (1) and different degrees of intensity (from 2–4 or 5).

- Goldberg   0-0-2-2
- Likert I   0-1-2-3
- Likert II   0-0-1-2
- Hamilton   0-1-2-3-4

Quality Parameters of an Assessment Instrument

There are three basic parameters for assessing the quality of an assessment instrument: its consistency, its reliability and its validity. For follow-up scales, a fourth should be added, i.e., sensitivity to change. Other parameters to consider are redundancy and the "cost-utility" of using a certain instrument for the purpose of a study. Unfortunately, there is no consensus on a definition of these terms in epidemiology; their meaning varies according to the area of study and even between different authors within the same area. This problem is especially clear in the area of subjective assessment instruments.

Consistency (Internal Consistency)

Consistency comprises the psychometric solidity of a scale, its internal structure, the level to which its different items are interrelated and the possibility of adding them up to obtain overall scores. Some authors include consistency within the category of reliability or validity. According to Hernandez-Aguado et al. (1990), consistency is that "property which defines the level of agreement or conformity of a set of measurements among themselves". Unfortunately, this author does not provide an operative definition of the term. In this review, while stating in one paragraph that consistency is synonymous with reliability, he affirms the contrary in the next. Thompson (1989b) considers dispersion about the regression line with the global assessment to be a test of reliability. To avoid such terminological confusion, we distinguish here between the *internal consistency* and the *external reliability* of a test.

Some statistical methods, such as factor analysis, provide data on both the internal structure of a scale and on its relationship to external models. This is the case with scales for assessment of positive and negative symptoms of schizophrenia, a factor analysis of which can serve to validate, revise or even refute the models on which the construction of the instrument itself is based (Liddle, 1987; Buchanan and Carpenter, 1994). Many of the aspects related to consistency have been mentioned in the context of selecting items or the hierarchy of their order.

Homogeneity, which indicates the degree of agreement among the items on a scale, determines if they can be accumulated to generate an overall score. It can be obtained by studying the correlation of the items with the total (split-half, Corn-bach's alpha), by a factor analysis or by using Rasch's statistical objectivity models (1980). The split-half estimates the level of homogeneity on the basis of the correlation between two equivalent halves of the scale (e.g., items from the first half versus items from the second half, or odd-numbered items versus even ones). Cronbach's alpha coefficient indicates the degree to which different items exhibit a positive correlation (internal consistency above 0.7 is considered adequate; Bech et al. 1993). Another test for calculating internal consistency, which is less often used, is the Kuder-Richardson test. Homogeneity based on factor analysis (acceptability of the global score as the sum of that obtained for each item) is confirmed if a unidimensional structure is obtained, that is, if all the items show a positive load on the first factor (Thompson 1989b). In addition to exploratory factor techniques such as principal component analysis and principal factor analysis, the structure of a scale can be assessed using other techniques, such as the non-metric multidimensional scale or the structural equation analysis (Buchanan 1994). Rasch's unidimensional model considers a scale to be homogeneous when all of its items contribute independently to the total information contained in the scale. In latent trait theory, the nexus between manifest (clinical) answers and their latent (theoretical) dimension is defined by the requirement that the answers can be combined by adding them until a total score is reached (Andersen 1989). Rasch's model also makes it possible to study the internal hierarchy of a scale, classifying its homogenous items in a hierarchy ranging from the most inclusive (those which measure the dimension's most severe symptoms).

The reproducibility coefficient indicates to what degree the scale reflects all of the subject's response patterns regarding the parameter measured. Transferability refers to the degree to which the scale can be applied to different population groups which present the evaluated phenomenon, independent of their age, gender or other relevant external criteria (Bech et al. 1993).

Reliability (External Reliability)

Reliability indicates the degree to which the results of a test are reproducible. This measure depends on the stability of the test's measures, in spite of changes in different external parameters (that is, changes not inherent to the test). The study of external reliability will provide information about the reproducibility of the test's results in different situations. McDowel and Newell (1987) exemplify the difference between validity and reliability with an excellent simile, involving a marksman who has to learn to hit a target, and then do so consistently. Validity would be the shot's proximity to the bull's-eye, while authors prefer the term variability to describe the differences among results obtained under different assessment conditions (Hernandez-Aguado et al. 1990).

A study on the rebliability of a diagnostic test should include at least an analysis of the level of agreement obtained when the same sample is assessed under the same conditions by two different raters (inter-rater reliability). This has also been termed inter-observer reliability (Hernandez-Aguado et al. 1990). The importance of having evaluators with similar experience, as far as their training and use of the assessment instrument being analysed are concerned, has been pointed out. Andersen (1989) indicates other factors which differentiate between inter-observer and intra-observer reliability, such as their attitudes about assessment scales and therapeutic preferences.

A measure of a test's stability is obtained when the same sample is assessed by the same rater in two different situations (test-retest reliability or intraobserver reliability). In some cases (such as child psychiatry or mental handicaps) data is obtained from informants, making it necessary to analyse the agreement of the data obtained with the test using the same sample and the same evaluator, but collecting the data from two different informants (inter-informant reliability). The procedure for obtaining such information has been extensively reviewed by Costello (1994).

The statistical index used for evaluating concordance depends on the characteristics of the variables to be assessed. The use of Kendall's concordance coefficient (Siegel 1966) in various studies is open to discussion. In the case of dichotomous or binary variables, item-by-item concordance can be analyzed using percentage of agreement and unweighted kappa (Kramer and Feinstein 1981). The kappa concordance coefficient reveals the level of agreement obtained, once concordance which was produced by chance has been eliminated. This makes it more reliable than a simple percentage of agreement. However, the same kappa value can result from different response patterns. Therefore, it is also expedient to record the frequency of each item's appearance and its agreement percentage (Costello 1994) as well as the confidence interval. Feinstein (1985) proposes the scheme shown in Table 1 for analysing kappa results.

In the case of ordinal variables, analysis of item-by-item concordance can be conducted using the weighted agreement percentage and the weighted kappa. These are considered better than their unweighted analogues, since they give a more realistic measure of the level of agreement. This is achieved by weighting disagreement according to the number of degrees separating the score assigned by one evaluator from that assigned by another. Thus, the assigned weight can be "0" for complete agreement, "1" when there is one degree of difference, "2" when there are two, and so on (Kramer and Feinstein 1981).

The method for analysing the concordance of a test's overall scores is controversial. Usually correlation coefficients are used to determine the degree of agreement. These coefficients should not be used to analyse concordance between two evaluations: the tendency can be perfect, with a correlation coefficient of 1 (Feinstein 1985). In continuous measures, the coefficient of intraclass correlation (ICC) can be used (Bartko and Carpenter 1976). Bech et al. (1993) also proposed the use of the ICC to assess test-re-test reliability when the data are collected by different evalua-

Table 1. Analysis of kappa results

Kappa value	Level of agreement
< 0	Poor
0–0.20	Low
0.21–0.40	Fair
0.41–0.60	Moderate
0.61–0.80	Strong
0.81–1.0	Almost perfect

tors, although this is a debatable application. There is currently no general agreement on the sample size required for reliability studies of scales (Bech et al. 1993).

Validity

Validity is defined as the degree to which an instrument measures that which it is supposed to measure. Validity is present when the instrument predicts a criteria, or consistently fits a series of related constructs in an accepted theory. It indicates which proportion of information collected is relevant to the question being posed. There are multiple forms of validity; unfortunately some authors use the same term to define different concepts. *Face validity* reflects what experts consider significant measures. *Content validity* refers to the degree to which the set of items in a test adequately represents a domain. These are two obvious types of validity that cannot be tested (Thompson 1989 a). *Criterion validity* refers to the degree to which an instrument's scores correspond to external criteria, the so-called gold standard, and can be considered a substitute for it (Thiemann et al. 1987). *Construct validity* is calculated when no adequate gold standard is available (Martínez-Arias 1995). Psychological attributes and mental processes are intangible parameters which cannot be measured directly, like height or weight, therefore, they are hypothetical concepts or constructs. However, it is accepted that many psychiatric constructs are close to a gold standard (such as depression or anhedonia), while others cannot be compared with external criteria (e. g., quality of life or social integration). This leads to terminological confusion. Thus, concurrent and predictive validity are types of criterion validity for some authors (Strang et al. 1989; Martínez-Arias 1995), and types of construct validity for others (Thompson 1989 i). Whether these techniques provide construct or criterion validity depends on the degree to which the comparator can be considered a true gold-standard.

Factorial Validity

When the construct validity does not refer to a nosologic entity, but rather to an assessment instrument, the use of exploratory factor analysis is sometimes regarded as a construct validity method; in fact exploratory factor analysis is a sophisticated technique for analyzing internal structure or consistency. There is, however, a group of confirmatory factor analysis techniques whereby the investigator tries to verify an explicit hypothesis which serves as the "external" criterion, such as the structural equation models [e. g., LISREL-VII (Joreskog and Sorbom 1989)].

Concurrent Validity

This provides a measure of the association between the scores for different items and the overall scores for other scales of reference with an equivalent purpose and content. It is generally limited to the study of correlations between scores. Czobor (1991) suggests the use of canonical component analysis. This method can be considered an extension of factor analysis for two groups of variables.

Predictive Validity

Predictive observation validity refers to the probability that a scale gives a correct judgment of the observed phenomenon. By using Bayes' analysis makes it possible to determine the predictive validity of a test, its utility and its comparability, based on an analysis of the distribution of "cases" and "non-cases" in a given population, and its relationship with the results obtained on the test under study (positive or negative). A 2 × 2 contingency table expresses this relationship in true positives, true negatives, false positives and false negatives. The following predictive validity coefficients obtained with a contingency table are defined: sensitivity, specificity, positive predictive value and negative predictive value (Baldessarini et al. 1988; Strang et al. 1989). Other parameters which can be obtained by applying Bayes' theorem are the overall misclassification rate, (proportion of unproperly classified cases out of the total), bias (quotient between those assessed who were considered positive and negative) and efficiency (cases not detected by the test in relation to the total number of cases). These coefficients enable us to adjust the cut-off point with regard to the object of the study. If the study is aimed at conducting a two-stage sample study, it should seek the cut-off point which allows detection of the maximum number of cases, even though some may be false positives (acceptable specificity with optimal sensitivity). If, on the other hand, the aim is to find the probable morbidity of a population through is scores in the test, a cut-off point should be selected such that the highest number of "non-cases" is rejected, even if this results in the loss of some false negatives (acceptable sensitivity with optimal specificity).

On the other hand, the ideal cut-off point for a test can be calculated based on receiver operating characteristics analysis (ROC) (Strang et al. 1989). This technique was developed in the 1960s to assess the capacity of radar controllers to discriminate between signals. First, a graphic representation of the rate of true positives (sensitivity) and false positives (specificity) is obtained for each cut-off point. The calculation of the area beneath the resulting curve indicates the tests' discriminatory capacity throughout the spectrum of morbidity. When this diagonal line whose lower area is 0.5 (sensitivity equal to the rate of false positives). An ideal test would produce 100% ture positives before admitting a single false negative, so that the area below the curve obtained would be 1.0. In practice, the areas below the curve oscillate between 0.5 and 1.0, allowing for a graphic representation of the discriminatory capacity of different tests for the same dimension, the best one being that which corresponds to the curve farthest away from the diagonal.

The predictive validity of a self-administered test can be reduced due to an error in the reference criteria. This problem can be solved with factor analysis models, calculating factor validity.

Other Quality Parameters for Tests

In addition to confirming their consistency, reliability and validity, it is necessary to rule out the possibility that the scale is redundant, and sensitive to change, if response to treatment is going to be assessed.

External Redundancy

Generally, redundance or overlapping of the items on a scale is only assessed while the scale itself is being constructed (internal redundancy). However, it is also important to investigate the possible redundancy of the items and overalls scores with other, similar scales (external redundancy). This parameter is not equivalent to the association obtained in concurrent validity [e. g., in multivariate cases, it is possible to find near-zero redundancy even though there may be a perfect fit between the two tests (Czobor 1991)]. The use of equivalent scales with redundant items in similar populations does not increase the amount of information obtained; however, it does raise the possibility of completion errors (due to fatigue, transcription mistakes, etc.), increase type I and type II statistical errors, and diminish the cost-utility of administering the tests (Thiemann et al. 1987; Czobor et al. 1991). According to Wollenberg (1977), redundancy analysis can be considered an extension of factor analysis for two groups of separate variables. Factors are taken from a group of variables (e. g., test A) which explains the variance in another group of variables (e. g., test B). The derivation of linear criterion variates makes it possible to assess the importance of each variate in the redundancy relationship between two instruments (Johansson 1981). Thiemann et al. (1987) expressed the opinion that, in a way, redundancy is somewhat equivalent to the instrument's intertest reliability. In fact, redundancy has sometimes been assessed according to the kappa agreement of the items (Kibel et al. 1993; Fenton and McGlashan 1992).

Sensitivity to Change

Sensitivity to change can be examined with correlation studies and by analyzing the principal components at the baseline and after the assessment period (e. g., after treatment), comparing the factor structures at both points. For calculating sensitivity to change, it is useful to compare ratings with a transitional global measure (e. g., CGI to evaluate a well-being scale's sensitivity to change). In this case, a covariance analysis can be conducted on the score obtained after treatment, taking the baseline score as a covariable, regarding the factor of change in the severity determined by the variation in the other scale (Salvador-Carulla et al. 1996).

Selection of an Assessment Instrument

The appropriate selection of a subjective assessment instrument is essential for any clinical research in psychiatry. In light of this, the limited number of methodological reviews in this specific area is surprising. Bech et al. (1993) mention a series of key aspects to consider in a clinical trial:

1. Identify the motive: Why is it necessary to use an assessment scale in the study?
2. Identify the problem: What is being assessed?
3. Identify its importance: What is the relevance of scales in relation to the hypothesis being investigated?
4. Cost-utility evaluation: What is the utility of the information obtained by means of the instrument in relation to the cost of its use?

The last aspect is overlooked for too often in clinical research. In this case, cost-utility evluation considers the need for training and preparation before the scale can be used, taking into account the necessary time and requirements for statistical analysis. It is also necessary to evaluate whether the additonal information to be obtained justifies the higher costs and the time employed both in scoring the tests and analyzing the data. The possibility of increased bias with the addition of a supplementary instrument to an assessment battery should also be considered, whether due to interviewee fatigue or an increase in measure or type I or II errors when using redundant scales, such as jointly administering the BPRS and the SANS (Czobor et al. 1991; Thiemann et al. 1987).

Transcultural Use Criteria

The use of the same questionnaire in different cultures involves a series of exceedingly complex methodological problems, two of the most important being equivalence levels and translation systems.

Level of Transcultural Equivalence

The possibility of international use is a major aspect in the selection of assessment instruments. This involves a considerable number of problems, however, to the point that some authors feel it necessary to tackle this aspect in the construction of the questionnaire itself. This is really not very feasible, so other alternatives must be sought.

Flaherty (1988) has proposed five levels of transcultural equivalence:

1. Content equivalence: The content of each item on the instrument is relevant to the phenomenon in each culture.
2. Syntax equivalence: The meaning of each item is identical in each culture after its translation into the idiomatic language (written and oral) of each culture. There are a number of sources of variation, here (words, colloquialisms, register).
3. Technical equivalence: The assessment method (e. g., pencil and paper, interview) is comparable in each culture with regard to the data which it produces.
4. Conceptual equivalence: The instrument measures the same theoretical construct in each culture. Sometimes the translation of a word can be very close to the original, while being extremely different on a conceptual level in the two languages.

Translation Systems

The most widely used system is that of the back-translation. This is different from a direct translation, in that after a first translation by one or more translators, the instrument is then "retranslated" by another translator or team. Thus, both versions can be compared with the original. This system, however, is not ideal, and its results are often poor as far as conceptual equivalence is concerned (Brislin 1970). In mental health studies, investigators have tried to complement his system with techniques which enable them to turn a merely linguistic translation into a cultural one. Among these, some of the most striking are pretest techniques (based on the congruence of the answers obtained) and different forms of translating committees.

The recent translation of the SCAN into Spanish is a good example of the systematization of these processes in what has been called a conceptual translation (Vazquez-Barquero 1993). A conceptual translation is one in which the essence of the experience being assessed is clearly reflected in the version in a second language. Concept equivalence takes precedence over syntax. The preparation of such a version is considerably more complicated than the methods discussed above: first, a literal translation is prepared, on the basis of which two independent teams make conceptual translations. Next, these translations are verified to detect problematic terms and concepts, arriving at a consensus in accordance with the target environment's cultural reality. This version is then back-translated, and finally the head of the project evaluates the conceptual similarity of each item.

Other Tests for Transcultural Evaluation

There is no consensus regaring the psychometric tests required for an assessment instrument to be used in different cultures. Some authors consider that an instrument should go through the entire analytical process once again. However, this tends to be too expensive. The need to reassess reliability (Wittchen et al. 1991) and validity (above all in the case of screening instruments in which a cut-off point for detection has been established) is evident. The need for an exhaustive analysis of internal consistency is questionable.

Conclusion

The use of psychiatric assessment scales is well established in different areas, from clinical epidemiology to pharmacologic studies (the purpose for which many clinical follow-up scales were originally developed). However, given their number, diversity, and the fact that new ones are being developed all the time, computerized, systematic inventories are now more important than ever for the orientation of clinicians and investigators. One guide for their classification could be based on the following parameters: complexity, purpose, and design. Evaluation of the quality of each instrument can be based on a series of parameters related to its consistency, reliability, validity, and sensitivity to change. Lastly, it is necessary to consider cost-effectiveness aspects in the selection of an instrument and its relationship to other instruments used in the study (redundancy). An adequate adaptation and standardization should be performed in every different culture setting.

Acknowledgement. Supported in part by Grant FIS 95/1961 and BIOMED PL93/1304.

References

Andersen J, Larsen JK, Schultz V, Nielsen BM, Korner A, Behnke K et al (1989) The Brief Psychiatric Rating Scale: Dimension of schizophrenia-reliability and construct validity. Psychopathology, 22, 168–176
Andreasen NC, Flaum M, Arndt S (1992) The comprehensive assessment of symptoms and history (CASH): An instrument for assessing diagnosis and psychopathology. Archives of General Psychiatry, 49, 615–623
Baldessarini RJ, Finklestein S, Arana GW (1988) Predictive power of diagnostic tests. In: F Flasch (ed), "Psychobiology and Psychopharmacology", pp 175–189. New York: Norton & Company

Bartko JJ, Carpenter WT (1976) On the methods and theory of reliability. J Nerv Ment Dis 163: 307–317
Bech P, Kastrup M, Rafaelsen OJ (1986) Mini compendium of rating scales for states of anxiety, depression, mania, schizophrenia with corresponding DSM-III syndromes. Acta Psychiatr Scand, 73, Suppl 326, 1–37
Bech P, Malt UF, Dencker SJ, Ahlfors UG, Elgen K, Lewander T, Lundell A, Simpson GM, Lingjaerde O (eds) (1993) Scales for assessment of diagnosis and severity of mental disorders. Acta Psychiatrica Scandinavica, 87 (Suppl 372), 1–87
Brislin RW (1970) Back-translation for cross-cultural research. Journal of cross-cultural Psychology, 1(3), 185–216
Buchanan RW, Carpenter WT (1994) Domains of psychopathology. An approach to the reduction of heterogeneity in Schizophrenia. J Nerv Ment Dis, 182, 193–204
Costello CG (1994) Advantages of the symptom approach to schizophrenia. In CG Costello (ed) "Symptoms of schizophrenia", pp 1–26. New York: John Wiley & Sons
Czobor P, Bitter I, Volavka J (1991) Relationship between the Brief Psychiatric Rating Scale and the Scale for the Assessment of Negative Symptoms: A study of their correlation and redundancy. Psychiatry Research, 36, 129–139
Feinstein AR (1985) Clinical epidemiology. Philadelphia: WB Saunders
Fenton W, McGlashan TH (1991) Testing systems for assessment of negative symptoms in schizophrenia. Arch Gen Psychiatry, 49: 179–184
Flaherty JA, Gaviria FM, Pathak D, Mitchell T, Wintrob R, Richman JA, Birz S (1988) Developing instruments for cross-cultural psychiatric research. J Nerv Ment Dis, 176, 257–163
Garcia-Cueto E (1993) Introduccion a la psicometria. Madrid: Siglo XXI
Hernandez-Aguado I, Porta M, Miralles M, García-Benavides F, Bolúmar F (1990) La cuantificación de la variabilidad en las observaciones clínicas. Medicina Clínica (Barcelona), 95, 424–429
Israel L, Kozarevic D, Sartorius N (1984) Source book for the geriatric assessment: I. Evaluation in gerontology. World Health Organization, Basel: Karger, Basel
Joreskog KG, Sorbom D (1989) LISREL VII. User's reference guide. Mooresville: Scientific Software, Inc.
Kibel DA, Laffont I, Liddle PF (1993) The composition of the negative syndrome of chronic schizophrenia. British Journal of Psychiatry, 162, 744–750
Kind P (1990) Issues in the design and construction of a quality of life measure. In: S Baldwin, C Godfrey, C Popper, eds, "Quality of Life: Perspectives and Policies", pp 63–71. London: Routledge
Kramer MS, Feinstein AR (1981) Clinical biostatistics: LIV. The biostatistics of concordance. Clin Pharmacol Ther, 29, 111–123
Liddle PF (1987) Schizophrenic syndromes, cognitive performance and neurological dysfunction. Psychological Medicine, 17, 49–57
Likert R (1932) A technique for measurement of attitudes. Archives of Psychology, 140, 1–55
Martinez-Arias R (1995) Psicometria: Teoria de los tests psicologicos y educativos. Madrid: Editorial Síntesis
McDowell lI, Newell C (1987) Measuring health: A guide to rating scales and questionnaires. Oxford: Oxford University Press
Meehl P, Golden RR (1982) Taxonometric methods. In: PC Kendall, JN Butcher, eds., Handbook of research methodology in clinical psychology, pp 127–181, New York: Wiley & sons
Mezzich JE (ed) (1986) Clinical Care and Information Systems in Psychiatry. Washington: American Psychiatric Press
Muñiz J (1992) Teoría clasica de los test. Madrid: Ediciones Piramide
Pull BC, Wittchen HU (1991) The CIDI, SCAN, and IPDE: Structured diagnostic interviews for ICD-10 and DSM-III-R. European Pschiatry, 6, 227–285
Rasch G (1980) Probabilistic models for some intelligence and attainment tests. Chicago: University of Chicago Press
Salvador-Carulla L, Roca M (1995) "Instrumentos de evaluacíon subjectiva en Salud Mental". Actas Luso-Esp Neurol Psiquiatr, 23, 1–9
Salvador-Carulla L, Huete T, Hernan MA et al (1996) Validación del Indice de Bienestar General en pacientes con depresión mayor. In: M Gutierrez, J Ezcurra y P Pichot, eds, "Advances en trastornos afectivos". Barcelona: Ediciones en Neurociencias
Siegel S (1966) Non-parametric statistics for behavioral sciences. New York: McGraw-Hill
Strang J, Bradley B, Stockwell T (1989) Assessment of drug and alcohol use. In C Thompson, ed, "The instruments of psychiatric research", pp 211–232. Chichester: John Wiley & sons
Stromgren E (1988) The lexicon and issues in the relation of psychiatric concepts and terms. In: JE - Mezzich, M von Cranach, eds, "International classification in psychiatry", pp 175–179, Cambridge: Cambridge University Press

Tanaka Y (1972) Values in the subjective culture: A social psychological view. Journal of Cross-cultural Psychology, 3, 57–69
Thiemann S, Csernansky JG, Berger P (1987) Rating scales in research: The case of negative symptoms. Psychiatry Research, 20, 47–55
Thompson C (1989 i) Introduction. In: C Thompson, ed, "The instruments of psychiatric research", pp 1–17. Chichester: John Wiley & sons
Thompson C (1989) Affective disorders. In: C Thompson, ed, "The instruments of psychiatric research", pp 87–126. Chichester: John Wiley & sons
Vazquez-Barquero JL (1993) SCAN. Cuestionarios para la evaluación clínica en psiquiatría, Madrid: Meditor
Wittchen H-U, Essau CA (1990) Assessment of symptoms and psychosocial disabilities in primary care. In: N Sartorius, D Goldberg, G de Girolamo, J Costa e Silva, Y Lecrubier y U. Wittchen, eds, Psychological disorders in general medical settings, pp 111–136, Toronto: Hogrefe & Huber Publ
Wittchen H-U, Robins LN, Cottler LB, Sartorius N, Burke JD, Regier D et al (1991) Cross-cultural feasibility, reliability and sources of variance of the Composite International Diagnostic Interview (CIDI). British Journal of Psychiatry, 159, 645–653
van den Wollenberg AL (1977) Redundancy analysis: An alternative to canonical correlation analysis. Psychometrika, 42, 207–219

List of Scales Mentioned in the Text (see Bech et al. 1993)

ADL: Activity of Daily Living – Index (Katz 1976)

BDI: Beck Deprepression Inventory (Beck et al. 1961)

BPRS: Brief Psychiatric Rating Scale (Overll and Gorham 1962)

CASH: Comprehensive Assessment of History and Symptoms (Andreasen et al. 1992)

CGI: Clinical Global Impression (Guy 1976)

GAS: Global Assessment Scale (Endicott 1976)

EPQ: Eysenck Personality Questionnaire (Eysenck et al. 1975)

GHQ: General Health Questionnaire (Goldberg 1972)

HDRS: Hamilton Depression Rating Scale (Hamilton 1960)

MPQ: McGill Pain Questionnaire (Melzack 1980)

MMPI: Minnesota Multiphasic Personality Inventory (Hathaway and McKinley 1937)

NDS: Newcastle Depression Scale (Carney et al. 1965)

PSE: Present State Examination (Cooper et al. 1972)

SANS/SAPS: Scale for the Assessment of Negative Symptoms/Scale for the Assessment of Positive Symptoms (Andreasen 1981)

SCAN: Schedules for Clinical Assessment in Neuropsychiatry – Spanish ed. (Vazquez-Barquero 1993)

CHAPTER 15

Multi-dimensional Assessment of Outcome: The Analysis of Conditional Independence as an Integrated Statistical Tool to Model the Relationships Between Variables

ANNIBALE BIGGERI, PAOLA RUCCI, MIRELLA RUGGERI and MICHELE TANSELLA

The Need for Comprehensive Models to Assess Outcome

The impression of reductionism may overwhelm clinicians when reading scientific reports on the outcome of psychiatric care. What clinicians consider *reductionism* often corresponds to an attempt by researchers to *simplify* the complexity of the studies on outcome of care in psychiatry. Such an attitude is evident also in the choice of the indicators of outcome. Morbidity and mortality rates or data on service utilisation have almost exclusively been the indicators of choice for outcome studies, although their limits in reflecting the real outcome of psychiatric care have often been emphasized (Jenkins 1990; Mirin and Namerow 1991; Attkisson et al. 1992; Ruggeri and Tansella 1995, 1996; Tansella and Ruggeri 1996). The result of this tendency has been to enlarge the gap between research and clinical practice and to favour the widespread use of treatments of unproven efficacy.

In order to change this trend, psychiatric services should be flexible in their organization and able to modify their treatment strategies on the basis of the results of outcome studies. Furthermore, indicators of outcome should correspond to the needs and the complexity of routine clinical practice. It is now clear that, in order to be valid and useful for clinical practice, outcome studies should first of all be comprehensive and combine optimal measures at both the "service level" (Tansella 1989) and the "patient level" (Ruggeri and Tansella 1995). At the service level the use of process variables still seems to give useful information on the outcome of care, provided they are complemented by other indicators. At the patient level, indicators should explore the effect of an intervention on various *dimensions*, including clinical variables (the severity and course of symptoms), social variables (social functioning, social support, quality of life), and the user's interaction with the service (needs, burden, satisfaction). Moreover, the assessment should take into account various points of view or *axes* simultaneously. In psychiatric settings, professionals, paraprofessionals, patients and relatives are all involved in care and should be considered legitimate assessors of an intervention's effectiveness, albeit from different perspectives (Mayer and Rosenblatt 1974; Dowds and Fontana 1977; Gunkel and Priebe 1993, Andrews et al. 1986).

A. Biggeri
Dipartimento di Statistica, Università di Firenze, I-50134 Firenze, Italy

P. Rucci, M. Ruggeri and M. Tansella
Servizio di Psicologia Medica, Istituto di Psichiatria, Università di Verona, Ospedale Policlinico, I-37134 Verona, Italy

Thus, *multi-dimensionality* and *multi-axiality* are key components in the assessment of outcome. Another fundamental requirement is to perform these kinds of studies in "real-world services" according to a longitudinal design. An advantage of such an approach is that it provides a complete picture without preliminary assumptions about the relevance of one indicator, or perspective, with respect to the others: in the light of available knowledge, such assumptions could not in fact be fully legitimate. A drawback of the multi-dimensional and multi-axial approach is that it takes into account so many variables simultaneously that their mutual interaction may appear obscure without appropriate data analysis; common statistical techniques appear unsatisfactory for this purpose. To deal with this complexity, and to gain insight into the phenomena investigated, integrated methods for data representation and analysis are needed.

The aims of this chapter are to introduce an integrated statistical method, based on graphical modelling, for studying the relationship between variables, and to show its practical application with sets of data on the outcome of community psychiatric care. Data from a naturalistic longitudinal project, currently being conducted in South-Verona, which is based on a multi-dimensional and multi-axial assessment model will be used.

Statistical Methods to Analyse Complex Sets of Data

Regression Models

The approach to the study of the association between outcome (response) variables and one or more predictors (covariates) is based on multiple regression models. The need for mathematical and statistical modelling emerged when the researcher had to manage several quantitative and qualitative predictors and stratified analysis was not possible due to data sparseness.

Most of variables dealt with in epidemiology are categorical or measured on an ordinal scale. A great effort was therefore devoted in last twenty years to setting up suitable techniques to treat non-continuous data. In particular, the logistic regression model for dichotomous outcomes, such as the clinical hard outcomes mortality (dead/alive) and morbidity (ill/not-ill), became very popular among social scientists, and alternative multivariate techniques as discriminant analysis were almost abandoned (Greenland 1987). The reasons for this changing trend can be traced to the straightforward interpretation of the regression coefficients: in the logistic model they are log odds ratios and, depending on study design, can be read as the logarithm of relative risks, which is a sensitive measure of association between outcome and predictors. In contrast, other regression models for discrete data, based on trigonometric transformations of the response variable, lead to uninterpretable results. Moreover, the multivariate discriminant analysis relies on strong distributional assumptions about the set of covariates. In the field of epidemiology, the set of covariates is badly conditioned and depends on study design, since there is no easy way to reduce it to any sort of random sample. Parallel to these developments, covariance selection models were refined for continuous data (Dempster 1972).

When an association is found between two variables, it is good practice to check whether it is a spurious or indirect relationship. When potential confounders of the true association between two variables are too numerous or are mostly unknown, log-linear and regression models are needed to control for their effects. Graphical modelling (Lauritzen and Wermuth 1989, Whittaker 1990; Wermuth and Lauritzen 1990; Edwards 1995) takes advantage of these techniques by integrating them in a common framework. The suggestive idea behind it is that "any kind of relationship should be analysed as a *conditional* relationship" (Kreiner 1996); in other words a relationship between two variables exists if and only if it does not disappear when one controls for the effect of antecedent or intervening variables.

Graphical modelling yields undistorted estimates of the association between variables *independent* of the study design due to its capability to control for all confounding effects at the same time. Indeed it extends the familiar regression approach to more than one response and to more than one stage. We can imagine three sets of predictors: A contains the responses, B, the variables that affect the responses, and C, the variables that affect both A and B. At least three issues can be addressed: (1) the relationship between each predictor and each response, being fixed the other effects; (2) the pattern of associations among predictors; and (3) the reciprocal influence of the responses. The complex patterns of association like those emerging in a comprehensive assessment of outcome of psychiatric care require that all of these issues are dealt with. In community-based longitudinal studies, where random sampling can safely be assumed if representativeness of followed-up patients is ensured, graphical modelling can provide an interactive way to build up and test specific research hypotheses.

Graphical Models

The idea of representing a statistical model and causal relationships between variables graphically is an old one. Readers may be familiar with Path Analysis which some years ago gained popularity in psychological research (Fienberg 1980). Logistic and log-linear models were used to analyse contingency tables obtained cross-classifying the subjects by several discrete variables. They represent the expected frequencies of the table as a log-linear function of parameters which are interpretable as odds (main effects), odds ratios (first-order interactions), ratios of odds ratios (second-order interactions) and so on. The associations among discrete variables are then modelled in terms of odds ratios. As an example let us take the analysis of a $2 \times 2 \times 2$ contingency table obtained by classifying the subjects enrolled in a cross-sectional study by low/high score on psychopathology, using for instance the Brief Psychiatric Rating Scale (BPRS), by marital status (married/unmarried) and by education (low/high). Let us consider the log-linear model which specifies the following relationships between the three variables, X, Y and Z:

$$\log m(ijk) = 1 + \lambda(X) + \lambda(Y) + \lambda(Z) + \lambda(XZ) + \lambda(YZ) \tag{1}$$

where $m(ijk)$ denote the expected frequency for the cell (ijk) of the table. The parameters $\lambda(.)$ are log odds, and they are different from 0 if the distribution of values between the categories of the respective variable is asymmetrical. The first-order interaction terms, like $\lambda(XZ)$, are log odds ratios and denote an association between variables; the log odds ratio between X and Y is assumed to be zero. We can distinguish *crude* or *marginal* log odds ratios of the simpler model

$$\log m(ijk) = 1 + \lambda(X) + \lambda(Y) + \lambda(XY) \tag{2}$$

which have the same meaning as the correlation coefficient, from the log odds ratios of the previous models, which are adjusted for the third variable. The *adjusted* log odds ratios can be interpreted as partial correlation coefficients.

Restricting our attention to the relationship between high score on BPRS and marital status λ(XY), the crude odds ratios cannot be used for causal inference since they may depend on the unbalanced distribution by education. The adjusted odds ratios, in contrast, reflect the fact that X and Y are independent given the third variable. To correctly analyse the pattern of associations, we need to take all of the relevant variables into account. In the case of continuous variables, this means that we have to consider the partial correlation coefficients matrix.

A graph is a schematic picture of the conditional independence relationship between several variables, and consists of vertices and edges. Each vertex represents one variable; it is drawn as a circle if the variable is on a continuous scale, and as a point if it is discrete. Any edge between a pair of vertices denotes the presence of an association between the two variables, given all the other variables in the graph.

Two variables are said to be *conditionally independent* if there is no direct association between them and therefore there is no edge connecting the two respective vertices in the graph. This does not mean that the two variables are *marginally* independent. They may be dependent if the two vertices are connected indirectly by other vertices.

In the case of discrete variables, adjusted odds ratios substitute for the correlation coefficient; an odds ratio equal to 1 denotes the absence of association. In the previous example, X and Y are connected through Z, therefore λ(XY) in the simpler marginal model (Eq. 2) is different from zero.

The partial correlation matrix is used to obtain the association graph for continuous variables. For any pair of variables a 0 partial correlation coefficient means conditional independence and lack of a direct edge between the corresponding vertices in the graph. The statistical analysis aims to model the partial correlation matrix or its inverse. The association graph is drawn from estimated partial correlation matrices (for an example, see Fig. 1). With mixed data the partial correlation matrix is calculated separately for each level of the categorical variables.

The usefulness of graphic models is even more evident when we consider *directed graphs*. In these graphs an arrow between vertices (variables) shows associations which can be interpreted directionally (causally). Variables can be hierarchically ordered as responses (dependent) and potentially explanatory (independent) on the basis of previous knowledge. A trivial example is when variables are temporally ordered as in longitudinal studies, where subsequent assessments are scheduled. In this case, the associations between dependent and independent variables should be statistically evaluated, having been conditioned to all associations among the predictors.

Graphic chain models are especially suited to the analysis of complex sets of variables, some of which are responses, some are predictors and some are intermediate between them. The study of the undirected associations among such variables is conducted within each set. Directed causal association is then assessed conditionally to all the associations among predictors and intermediate variables.

In this chapter methods of estimation and fitting of graphic models are not discussed (for details see Whittaker 1990; Edwards 1995). Maximum likelihood estimates and likelihood ratios are used to compare nested models. For discrete data, the maximum likelihood equations are derived from the Poisson distribution or from multi-nomial sampling; for continuous data, these equations are derived from the multi-variate Gaussian. For recent developments regarding mixed data, see Lauritzen and Wermuth (1989). In earlier statistical literature log-linear modelling for discrete data and covariance selection models for continuous data were widely used. The novelty of the graphic approach resides in the treatment of mixed data and on the modelling strategy using conditional independence. Directed and chain graphs extend the cap-ability of such models to cover a wide range of substantive research hypotheses.

An Application of the Conditional Independence Model to the Multidimensional Assessment of Outcome

The South Verona Outcome Project

The South Verona Outcome Project (OUT-*pro*) is an attempt to standardize informa-tion that clinicians collect in their everyday clinical practice and during periodical reviews of cases in treatment. It also seeks to employ professionals involved in the clinical work for service evaluation. Most of the assessments are actually completed by the clinicians themselves, after a short training. Other assessments are made by the patient with the help of research workers. Standardized assessments encompass global functioning, psychopathology, social disability, needs for care, quality of life and satisfaction with services. They take place twice a year in the South Verona com-munity-based psychiatric service (CPS): the assessment from April to June is called wave A and that from October to December, wave B: during these periods, patients are assessed either the first time or, at the latest, the second time they are seen. In wave A the assessment is made only by the key professional (in most cases a psy-chiatrist or a clinical psychologist), and includes the Global Assessment of Function-ing Scale (GAF; Endicott and Spitzer 1976) the Brief Psychiatric Rating Scale (BPRS, expanded version, Lukoff et al. 1986), eight items from the Disability Assessment Scale (DAS-II; WHO 1988) and the Camberwell Assessment of Needs (CAN; Phelan et al. 1995). In wave B the assessment is made both by the key-professionals (again using GAF, BPRS and DAS) and the patients, who are requested to complete the Lan-cashire Quality of Life Profile (LQL; Oliver 1991) and the Verona Service Satisfaction Scale (VSSS; Ruggeri & DallÁgnola 1993; Ruggeri et al. 1994). Socio-demographic characteristics, psychiatric history of the patients and service utilization are routine-ly recorded in the South Verona Psychiatric Case Register (PCR) (Tansella 1991). All of these data are recorded and are available on line to clinicians.

The project started in 1994 and about 80 % of the patients in contact with the ser-vice in that year were assessed in both waves.

Graphical Representation of a Subset of Variables from the South Verona Outcome Project

Figure 1 shows a simplified independence graph depicting the relationships between eight variables from the south Verona OUT-pro assessments obtained in 1994; 194 patients completed both wave A and wave B assessments. The variables were mean BPRS (1 = symptom absent, 7 = extremely severe), DAS (0 = no dysfunction, 5 = maximum dysfunction), mean LQL (1 = couldn't be worse, 7 = couldn't be bet-

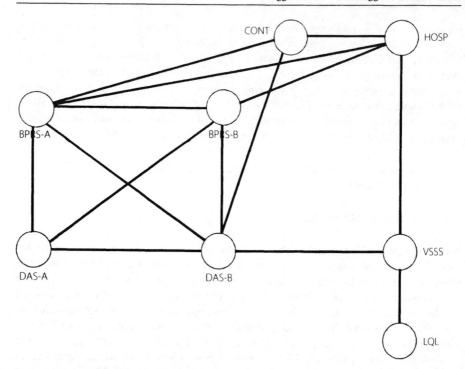

Fig. 1. Independence graph showing the relationships between variables in the South Verona Outcome Project. Data were collected in wave A and B in 1994 and apply to 194 patients. *Open circles* indicate variables; *edges* between adjacent variables indicate direct associations. The lack of an edge between non-adjacent variables indicates conditional independence. BPRS, Brief Psychiatric Rating
Scale; DAS, Disability Assessment Scale; LQL, Lancashire Quality of Life Profile; VSSS, Verona Service
Satisfaction Scale; CONT, number of contacts with the South Verona CPS; HOSP, days of hospitalization in the interval between wave A and wave B. Suffixes A and B indicate the wave of assessment

ter),[1] VSSS (1 = terrible, 5 = excellent), number of contacts with the South Verona
CPS (CONT) and days of hospitalization (HOSP) in the interval between wave A
and B (information on the last two variables was provided by the South Verona
PCR). For BPRS and DAS, global ratings were made on both occasions; for LQL
and VSSS, global ratings were made during wave B.

BPRS-B, DAS-B, LQL, VSSS and the afore-mentioned service utilization measures
can be considered response variables, while BPRS-A and DAS-A can be considered
explanatory variables. Here no distinction was made a priori between process and
outcome indicators. The aim in using a graphical model to analyse the present data
set was twofold: (a) to assess the influence of explanatory variables on the set of response variables; (b) to analyse the relationship between response variables. The latter is, in fact, most relevant to the study purpose.

The observed correlation and partial correlation coefficients are shown in Tables 1
and 2. Correlation coefficients should be read by taking into account the directional-
ity of the scales in the row data, where high scores on BPRS and DAS denote a poor

---

[1] Only LQL items on subjective perception of quality of life are considered here.

condition, while high scores on LQL and VSSS denote high quality of life and satisfaction. For instance, the partial correlation coefficients for VSSS show that the more satisfied patients have a slight trend towards a lower number of contacts and less disability but also towards more severe psychopathology and more days of hospitalization; a significant linear relationship is present between VSSS and LQL. Moderate positive correlations emerged between BPRS-A, DAS-A and DAS-B, between BPRS-A and days of hospitalization, and between LQL and VSSS. The partial correlations confirm these results, but the relationships between BPRS-B and DAS-A change in sign. It is difficult to obtain a clear pattern on the basis of the other correlation coefficients.

The procedure for modelling the partial correlation coefficients matrix obtained using the MIM program (Edwards 1987) consisted of the following steps:

1. An automatic search procedure (Edwards and Harvranek 1987) was first run. In the present example this procedure tested 187 out of 2^{28} (= 268 435 456) possible models, and selected four models which were most consistent with the data at the 0.05 significance level. The overall number of models to be tested illustrates the unfeasibility of any manual attempt to perform the same task.
2. Among the four models automatically selected by the program, the one with the lowest likelihood ratio (LR) was taken to build up a final model (LR = 12.96, df = 13, p = 0.45).
3. In addition to statistical criteria, the choice of the final model shown in the graph was also driven by the inherent temporal structure of the data: the relationships between the set of variables measured at wave A and those measured at wave B can only be regarded as asymmetrical, i.e. pointing from the antecedent to the

Table 1. Empirical correlation matrix

	CONT	HOSP	BPRS-A	BPRS-B	DAS-A	DAS-B	LQL	VSSS
CONT	1.000							
HOSP	0.424	1.000						
BPRS-A	0.440	0.493	1.000					
BPRS-B	0.372	0.444	0.649	1.000				
DAS-A	0.341	0.376	0.631	0.392	1.000			
DAS-B	0.429	0.329	0.544	0.710	0.571	1.000		
LQL	−0.138	0.010	−0.075	−0.100	−0.096	−0.138	1.000	
VSSS	−0.174	0.039	−0.087	−0.091	−0.209	−0.230	0.489	1.000

Table 2. Empirical partial correlation matrix

	CONT	HOSP	BPRS-A	BPRS-B	DAS-A	DAS-B	LQL	VSSS
CONT	1.000							
HOSP	0.279	1.000						
BPRS-A	0.177	0.133	1.000					
BPRS-B	−0.071	0.206	0.456	1.000				
DAS-A	−0.053	0.149	0.492	−0.301	1.000			
DAS-B	0.205	−0.114	−0.123	0.607	0.419	1.000		
LQL	−0.056	0.031	−0.009	−0.050	0.027	0.018	1.000	
VSSS	−0.097	0.119	0.057	0.045	−0.131	−0.117	0.465	1.000

consequent. The modelling strategy required therefore that we tested the conditional independence of one variable from variables measured at a previous time point, having specified all the relationships among its antecedent.

4. A backward stepwise procedure was performed to delete redundant associations (edges) between variables: only the edge connecting DAS-A and days of hospitalization was removed and a final model was obtained with LR = 14.66, df = 14 and p = 0.40.

The resulting fitted correlation and fitted partial correlation matrices are shown in Tables 3 and 4. Empirical correlations are nicely reproduced and partial correlations are considerably simplified. In the graph of Fig. 1 which depicts this model, a complete subgraph can be identified in which all four vertices corresponding to DAS-A and B and BPRS-A and B assessments are directly connected. LQL displays conditional independence from all variables given VSSS. Only one edge in fact connects it with VSSS while all other connections are missing. VSSS is also directly connected with DAS-B and days in hospital, both of which originate from BPRS-A.

Findings from this model can be summarised as follows:

1. Disability and psychopathology are intimately related; for both of them, wave A ratings affect those of wave B, as is obvious from the clinical point of view. Service utilization measurements are both directly dependent on psychopathology as measured during wave A; direct connections are also found with BPRS and DAS wave-B assessments.

Table 3. Fitted correlation matrix

	CONT	HOSP	BPRS-A	BPRS-B	DAS-A	DAS-B	LQL	VSSS
CONT	1.000							
HOSP	0.424	1.000						
BPRS-A	0.440	0.493	1.000					
BPRS-B	0.401	0.444	0.649	1.000				
DAS-A	0.333	0.314	0.631	0.392	1.000			
DAS-B	0.429	0.359	0.544	0.710	0.571	1.000		
LQL	−0.030	0.019	−0.041	−0.067	−0.057	−0.113	1.000	
VSSS	−0.061	0.039	−0.084	−0.137	−0.116	−0.230	0.489	1.000

Table 4. Fitted partial correlation[a] matrix

	CONT	HOSP	BPRS-A	BPRS-B	DAS-A	DAS-B	LQL	VSSS
CONT	1.000							
HOSP	0.239	1.000						
BPRS-A	0.138	0.208	1.000					
BPRS-B	−0.000	0.132	0.454	1.000				
DAS-A	−0.000	−0.000	0.509	−0.287	1.000			
DAS-B	0.170	0.000	−0.136	0.581	0.428	1.000		
LQL	−0.000	0.000	−0.000	0.000	−0.000	−0.000	1.000	
VSSS	0.000	0.105	−0.000	−0.000	0.000	−0.155	0.475	1.000

[a] Partial correlation coefficients equal to zero denote conditional independence.

2. The direct and positive association between length of hospitalization and increased service satisfaction seems to emphasize the powerful impact of hospitalization on the subjective perception of patients and the favourable impression that patients get from this experience in the South Verona system of care.

3. Besides being directly connected with days of hospitalization, self-reported satisfaction with services is also directly connected with DAS-B and LQL. The conditional independence of satisfaction from measures taken at wave A and the exclusive explanatory role it plays for LQL is an extremely interesting finding, suggestive of various research hypotheses which need to be fully tested.

4. Quality of life is completely external to the graph and its relationships with all the other variables are mediated by VSSS. A plausible interpretation of this finding could be that both satisfaction with services and quality of life reflect a subjective perception which may be based on a common attitude. Another possibility is that in psychiatric patients quality of life is strongly determined by satisfaction with care. These hypotheses need further investigation.

These preliminary findings are promising and show the enormous capability of this statistical tool to derive a simple model from a complex set of variables. However, caution should be exercised in interpreting the associations due to possible non-linear trends in the data. Before drawing any definite conclusion, suitable transformations of data should be therefore be considered (Edwards 1995; Cox and Wermuth 1994).

Conclusions

Bridging the gap between reductionism and over-complexity in evaluating the outcome of mental health services is a challenge for research in psychiatric epidemiology. This work will certainly require a large-scale application of comprehensive models of outcome assessment, and consequently, the capability to manage large sets of data and to understand complex relationships between variables. A necessary step in epidemiological research in this area is to accept that we are in a *hypothesis generating* and not in a *hypothesis testing* phase. The implication is that we have to proceed as far as possible without restrictive a priori assumptions on such data.

The multi-dimensional and multi-axial model that we proposed for the assessment of outcome, and its application to a naturalistic and longitudinal design which makes use of the information that clinicians collect and record in their everyday clinical practice, seems to be a good compromise between practicality and comprehensiveness. Graphical modelling and the strategy of conditional independence on which it relies represent a powerful tool in dealing with the complexities involved in assessing outcome. Moreover, they provide a sound statistical ground for both generating and testing hypotheses due to the possibility which they offer to interpret the undirected (non-causal) and directed (causal) relationships between variables.

References

Andrews S., Leavy A., DeChillo N. & Frances A. (1986) Patient – therapist mismatch: we would rather switch than fight. Hospital and Community Psychiatry 37, 918–922.
Attkisson C., Cook J., Karno M., Lehman A., et al. (1992) Clinical services research. Schizophrenia Bulletin, 18, 4, 627–668.

Box G. E. P. & Cox D. R. (1964) An analysis of transformations (with discussion). Journal of the Royal Statistical Society B, 26, 211–250.

Cox D. R. & Wermuth N. (1994) Tests of linearity, multivariate normality and the adequacy of linear scores. Applied Statistics, 43, 347–355.

Dempster D. P. (1972) Covariance selection models. Biometrics, 28, 157–175.

Dowds B. & Fontana A. (1977) Patients' and therapists' expectations and evaluations of hospital treatment. Comprehensive Psychiatry 18, 295–300.

Edwards D. (1995). Introduction to Graphical Modelling. Springer, Verlag, New York.

Edwards D. & Havranek T. (1987) A fast model selection for large families of models. Journal of the American Statistical Association, 82, 397, 205–213.

Endicott J. & Spitzer R. L. 1976) The Global Assessment Scale. A procedure for measuring overall severity of psychiatric disturbance. Archives of General Psychiatry, 33, 766–771.

Fienberg S. E. (1980) The Analysis of Cross-Classified Categorical Data, MIT Press, Cambridge.

Greenland S. (1987) Evolution of Epidemiologic Ideas, Epidemiology Research inc., Chestnut Hill.

Gunkel S. & Priebe S. (1993) Different perspectives of short-term changes in the rehabilitation of schizophrenic patients. Comprehensive Psychiatry 34, 352–359.

Jenkins R. (1990) Toward a system of outcome indicators for mental health care. British Journal of Psychiatry, 157, 500–514.

Knudsen H. C. & Thornicroft G. (eds) (1996) Mental Health Service Evaluation. Cambridge University Press: Cambridge.

Kreiner S. (1996) An informal introduction to graphical modelling. In: Mental Health Service Evaluation (eds. H. C. Knudsen and G. Tornicroft), pp. 156–175. Cambridge University Press: Cambridge.

Lauritzen S. L. & Wermuth N. (1989) Graphical models for associations between variables, some of which are qualitative and some quantitative, Annals of Statistics, 17, 31–54.

Lukoff D., Nuechterlein K. & Ventura J. (1986) Manual for expanded Brief Psychiatric Rating Scale (BPRS). Schizophrenia Bulletin, 4, 594–602.

Mayer J. & Rosenblatt A. (1974) Clash in perspective between mental patients and staff. American Journal of Orthopsychiatry, 44, 432–441.

Mirin S. M. & Namerow M. Jo (1991) Why study treatment outcome? Hospital and Community Psychiatry, 42, 1007–1013.

Oliver J. P. 1991) The social care directive: development of a quality of life profile for use in community services for the mentally ill. Social Work & Social Science Review, 3, 4–45.

Phelan M., Slade M., Thornicroft G., Dunn G., Holloway F., Wykes T., Strathdee G., Loftus L., McCrone P. & Hayward P. (1995) The Camberwell Assessment of Needs: the validity and reliability of an instrument to assess the needs of people with severe mental illness. British Journal of Psychiatry, 167, 589–595.

Ruggeri M. (1994) Patients' and relatives' satisfaction with psychiatric services: the state of the art of its measurement. Social Psychiatry and Psychiatric Epidemiology, 28, 212–227.

Ruggeri M. & Tansella M. (1995) Evaluating outcome in mental health care. Current Opinion in Psychiatry 8, 116–121.

Ruggeri M. & Tansella M. (1996) Individual patient outcomes. In: Mental Health Service Evaluation (eds. H. C. Knudsen and G. Thornicroft), pp. 281–295. Cambridge University Press: Cambridge.

Ruggeri M., Dall'Agnola R., Agostini C. & Bisoffi G. (1994) Acceptability, sensitivity and content validity of VECS and VSSS in measuring expectations and satisfaction in psychiatric patients and their relatives, Social Psychiatry and Psychiatric Epidemiology, 29, 265–276.

Schulberg H. C. & Bromet E. (1981) Strategies for evaluating the outcome of community services for the chronically mentally ill. American Journal of Psychiatry, 138, 930–935.

Tansella M. (ed) (1991) Community-Based Psychiatry. Long-Term Patterns of Care in South-Verona, Psychological Medicine Monograph Supplement 19, pp. 1–54. Cambridge University Press: Cambridge.

Tansella M. & Ruggeri M. (1996) Monitoring and evaluating a community-based mental health service: the epidemiological approach. In: The Scientific Basis of Health Services (eds. M. Peckham and R. Smith), pp. 160–169, British Medical Journal Publishing Group, London.

Wermuth N. & Lauritzen S. L. (1990) On Substantive Research Hypotheses, Conditional Independence Graphs and Graphical Chain Models, Journal of the Royal Statistical Society, Series B, 52, 21–50.

Whittaker J. (1990) Graphical Models in Applied Multivariate Statistics, Wiley, Chichester.

Wright R. G., Heiman J. R. Shupe J. & Olvera G. (1989) Defining and measuring stabilization of patients during 4 years of intensive community support. American Journal of Psychiatry, 146, 1293–1298.

CHAPTER 16

Assessing Needs for Mental Health Services

SONIA JOHNSON, GRAHAM THORNICROFT, MICHAEL PHELAN and MICHAEL SLADE

Introduction

If mental health services aim to meet needs both at the levels of the individual patient and of the whole population, then three key issues emerge: how can needs be
defined, who should assess them and how can this information be best used? This
chapter addresses these issues in three stages: by presenting definitions of need, by
reviewing methods of assessing individual needs for treatment, and by outlining
how needs for services at the population level can be measured.

Needs: The Problem of Definition

There is at present no consensus on how needs should be defined (Holloway 1994) or
who should define them (Ellis 1993; Slade 1994). The *Oxford English Dictionary* offers: "necessity, requirement and essential", and in a different sense: "destitution,
distress, indigence, poverty or want". These clusters of meanings overlap in so far
as they define 'need' as a vital element which is lacking, and this chapter will use
this sense as its point of departure. Need will therefore be used here to refer to significant essentials of life which are insufficient. The fact that a need is present does
not mean that it can be met. For example, some needs may remain unmet because
other problems take priority, because an effective method is not available locally, or
because the person in need refuses treatment.

    In psychological terms, Maslow (1968) has set out a hierarchy of five levels reflect-
ing, in sequence, needs for physiological functioning, safety, love, self-esteem and
self-actualization. Similarly, in a philosophical analysis of the field, Liss (1990) has
distinguished four elements of need. The first is the 'ill health' approach, which
equates need with a deficiency in health that requires medical care. In this model
the required intervention is simply the provision of the absent treatment. For Mallman and Marcus (1980), for example, need is "an objective requirement to avoid a
state of illness" (p.165). Second, Liss describes the 'supply notion', where the existence of a need presumes that an acceptable and effective treatment exists to offer re-
medy, and this is referred to by Stevens and Gabbay (1991) as 'the ability to benefit in
some way from health care'. Third, the 'normative notion' of need proposes that
need is a matter of opinion, and therefore a needs assessment has to be put in the
context of the beliefs of those involved, often referred to as "felt" or "perceived"
needs to distinguish them from needs that are considered to have a more objective

PRiSM, Institute of Psychiatry, De Crespigny Park, Denmark Hill, London SE5 8AF, UK basis. The view that "need is seen as a shortfall compared with a state of being which is generally acceptable" exemplifies this approach (Davies and Challis 1986, p. 562). Fourth, the 'instrumental view' of need is that health is required to reach a certain state or defined goal. For example, Tracy (1986) described a need as "a lack of a specific resource which is useful for or required by the purpose of [a living system]" (p. 212). In this view, the accuracy of the needs assessment and the effectiveness of the treatment intervention can therefore be gauded by the extent to which the instrumental goal is achieved. Need in this sense can be distinguished from demand (expressed wish) and supply (utilization).

Need, demand and supply are related to each other (Stevens and Gabbay 1991). A demand for care exists when an individual expresses a wish to receive it. In an alternative formulation, demand is what people would be willing to pay for in a market or might wish to use in a system of free health care (Stevens and Raftery 1994). Supply includes interventions, agents, and settings, whether or not they are used in any particular case. Care co-ordination entails providing such a pattern of service after initial assessment and then updating the assessment regularly to assess outcomes and to modify the care if needs remain unmet. Over-provision occurs when provision exceed need, while need in excess of provision is unmet need. A need may exist, as defined by a professional, even if the intervention is refused by a patient. At the same time, a proper needs assessment process should not lead to the imposition of expert solution upon patients. A professionally defined need may remain unmet and have to be replaced by one acceptable to the patients.

Another approach to defining need has been proposed by health economists. Their contributions include first the proposal that need refers both to the capacity to benefit from an intervention and the amount of expenditure required to reduce the capacity to benefit to zero; it is therefore a product of benefit and cost-effectiveness (Culyer and Wagstaff 1992). Second, health economists have proposed that diagnosis-related groups are notably irrelevant for mental health services (McCrone and Strathdee 1994) and, thirdly, that empirical data should guide operational needs definitions (Beecham et al. 1993).

In the particular case of mental health services, needs have been described in terms of the gaps between the service needs of patients and of populations and the services actually provided. Lehtinen et al. (1990) interpret needs as reflecting an inadequate level of service for the severity of the problem: patients with severe disorders who receive primary rather than specialized psychiatric care would therefore be rated as having unmet need. Similarly, for Shapiro et al. (1985), unmet needs are defined as the combination of definite morbidity and lack of mental health service utilization. A third view is that needs represent an insufficient supply of particular treatment interventions, and this approach is embodied in the three individual needs assessment instruments now described.

Needs at the Individual Level

Patients who suffer from severe mental illness have a range of needs which go far beyond the purely medical, as described in the National Institute of Mental Health's document

Toward a Model Plan for a Comprehensive Community-Based Mental Health System

(1987). The issue of how best to make a individual assessment of need has taxed both researchers and clinicians, not least because their requirements differ. An ideal assessment tool for use in a routine clinical setting would be one which is brief, easily learned, takes little time to administer, does not require the use of personnel in addition to the usual clinical team, is valid and reliable in different settings, and, above all, can be used as an integral part of routine clinical work. Macdonald (1991) suggests that in such a scale should also be sensitive to change, the potential inter-rater and test-rater reliability should be high, and it should logically inform clinical management (Hillier et al. 1991; Thornicroft and Bebbington 1996). The decision about which scale to use depends on whether the approach is to focus on particular diagnostic or care groups, on the balance to be struck between economy of time and inclusiveness of the ratings, and on the range of areas of clinical and social functioning to be assessed.

Camberwell Assessment of Need (CAN)

A clinically oriented and relatively brief instrument is the Camberwell Assessment of Need (CAN), which has been recently published by the PRiSM team at the Institute of Psychiatry (Phelan et al. 1995). It is intended both for research and for clinical use, especially in relation to the requirements of the NHS and Community Care Act (House of Commons 1990) to undertake needs assessments of people with severe mental health problems. It includes both patient and staff views, considers a comprehensive range of health and social needs, and assesses needs separately from interventions.

The principles which have guided the development of the CAN are that needs are universal, that many psychiatric patients have multiple needs, that need assessment should be an integral part of clinical practice, and that the process should involve ratings by both staff and patients. In the construction of the scale the authors aimed to establish that it had adequate psychometric properties, could be completed within 30 min, was comprehensive, was usable by wide range of staff, could record help from informal carers and staff, and would be suitable for both research and clinical use.

The 22 areas assessed are basic needs (accommodation, food and occupation), health needs (physical health, psychotic and neurotic symptoms, drugs and alcohol, safety to self and others), social needs (company, intimate relationship and sexual expression), everyday functioning (household skills, self-care and childcare, basic education, budgeting), and service receipt (information, telephone, transport and welfare benefits).

The psychometric properties of the scale have now been established both in terms of validity (face, consensual, content, criterion and construct) and reliability (Phelan et al. 1995) and the results are acceptable (Table 1). It was striking that in a survey of severely disabled psychiatric patients in south London, the mean number of problems identified by staff was 7.5 (95% CI, 6.7–8.4), and by patients was 7.9 (6.8–8.9). When examined in detail, however, the degree of agreement by staff and patients for individual items was rather poor, so that the hypothesis that staff and pa-

Table 1. Camberwell Assessment of Needs: summary of reliability scores

	r	Significance level
Inter-rater		
Staff	0.99	$p < 0.001$
Patient	0.98	$p < 0.001$
Test – re-test		
Staff	0.78	$p < 0.001$
Patient	0.71	$p < 0.001$

tients would rate problems similarly was rejected (Slade et al. 1994). The CAN is now being introduced to field trials in routine clinical settings, is being translated into 14 European languages, and is being published in an electronic PC version (called PELiCAN)

MRC Needs for Care Assessment

The Medical Research Council (MRC) Needs for Care schedule (Brewin 1992) is based on the following formal definitions: (a) a need is present when a patient's functioning (social disablement) falls below or threatens to fall below some minimum specified level, and this is due to a remediable, or potentially remediable, cause; (b) a need is met if it has attracted some at least partly effective item of care, and if no other items of care of greater potential effectiveness exist; and (c) a need is unmet when it has attracted an only partly effective or no item of care and when other items of care of greater potential effectiveness exist.

In this schedule "needs for care" have been defined as requirements for specific activities or interventions that have the potential to ameliorate disabling symptoms or reactions. In contrast, "needs for services" reflect institutional requirements and are defined as needs for specific agents or agencies to deliver those interventions (Brewin et al. 1987). Mangen and Brewin (1996) outline a procedure for deriving estimates of needs for services from individuals' needs for specific items of care. Substantial data have now been presented on individual needs assessments using this instrument (Brewin et al. 1988; Brewin et al. 1990; Lesage et al. 1991; Pryce et al. 1993; Van Haaster et al. 1994) along with a detailed critique of this approach (Hogg and Marshall 1992; Brewin and Wing 1993).

Cardinal Needs Schedule

A third approach to individual needs assessment is that of Marshall (1994), who is developing the Cardinal Needs Schedule. This is a modification of the MRC Needs for Care approach and identifies cardinal problems as those which satisfy three criteria: (1) the 'co-operation criterion' (the patient is willing to accept help for the problem); (2) the 'carer stress criterion' (the problem causes considerable anxiety, frustration or inconvenience to people caring for the patient); and (3) the 'severity criterion' (the problem endangers the health or safety of the patient or the safety of other people).

To rate this schedule, data is collected using the Manchester Scale for mental state assessment, the REHAB scale and a specially developed additional information questionnaire. A computerized version (Autoneed) has also been developed. Patients' views are rated using the Client Opinion Interview and the Carer Stress Interview, which includes carers' ratings. Marshall is also undertaking both inter-rater and test-retest reliability studies.

Population – Based Needs Assessment

The ideal method for the development of comprehensive and appropriate local services is the use of a standardized method such as those discussed above for individual assessment of the needs of all those identified as mentally ill within the catchment area. Services should then be developed so that they fit the aggregated needs of this population as closely as possible. However, direct data on service needs are often absent or of very poor quality, so that local planners need methods of estimating the extent of local needs for services from widely available demographic and service use data. A number of proxies for more comprehensive needs assessment have been developed, each with their own limitations (Shapiro et al. 1985). First, local need may be estimated on the basis of epidemiological studies which provide figures for the national prevalence of the disorders and which may bring individuals into contact with the psychiatric services. Second, data about national and international patterns of service utilization provision may be extrapolated to give expected levels of service use by the local population. Third, current local services may be compared with expert views on desirable levels of services. Fourth, the validity of these various types of estimate may be increased by using a deprivation weighted approach. Estimates of service need may be adjusted on the basis of knowledge about relationships of psychiatric disorders to age, sex, ethnic group, marital status, economic status and other social variables. Finally, geographical distribution of mental health facilities should also be considered: services should be accessible to all, and their availability in parts of the catchment area where need is likely to be highest should be a particular consideration. Each of these methods is summarized below, and illustrations of how population need may be estimated for a catchment area are provided by Johnson et al. (1996).

Estimating Local Needs from Epidemiological Data

Taking the first of the approaches, a simple estimate of local morbidity may be derived from epidemiological studies of the prevalence of psychiatric disorders carried out elsewhere. The strength of prevalence data from community surveys is that they allow estimates to be made of the total levels of need existing in the population. However, this method does not identify the types of services likely to be needed to meet these needs. This is problematic for disorders such as depression or anxiety, where most symptomatic individuals will not require referral to specialist mental health services. However, such community prevalence data are more useful for schizophrenia and other psychoses, as it is reasonable to assume that the majority of people with such illnesses will require some form of long-term contact with secondary services.

Service Utilization as a Proxy for Service Need

The work of Goldberg and Huxley (1980, 1992) may be used as a basis for comparing local service use with national and international data on service utilization. For example, their calculations suggest that in an average area, 2.4% of the adult population are expected to have contact with specialist mental health services in any 1 year and 0.6% will be admitted to a psychiatric hospital. Other sources of data on service utilization include statistics on admissions collected nationally, such as the Hospital Episode Statistics in the UK, and data from local case registers, which have the advantage that they are likely to provide more accurate data than national statistics, particularly for outpatient and community services (Glover 1991).

Service utilization data of this kind may be used to calculate the levels of service use which would be expected for a local catchment area population. This does not, of course, allow a normative assessment of the services which an area *should* ideally have. However, service planners may find it useful to have some idea of whether current numbers of contacts with particular components of their local services are relatively large or small compared with patterns elsewhere.

Comparing Local Services with Desirable Levels of Service Provision

There is considerable debate about optimal numbers of psychiatric treatment and care places required to meet local needs (Wing 1971, 1989; Thornicroft and Strathdee 1994). In the UK, a Royal College of Psychiatrists working party estimated an acute requirement of 44 beds per 100 000 population (Hirsch 1988) Strathdee and Thornicroft (1992) have set out targets for service provision based on epidemiological findings regarding the prevalence of psychiatric disorder and on a Delphi method of summerizing expert opinion. The targets assume that as far as possible services should be community based, with community residential and day places taking the place of institutional care. Wing (1992) has made a similar set of estimates of targets for general adult residential services. These estimates are shown in Table 2: they provide a basis for comparing actual local service provision with desirable levels of places of various types.

A Deprivation-Weighted Approach to Estimating Population Needs

The approaches delineated so far do not provide a way of taking into account the particular sociodemographic characteristics of the local catchment area. This is unsatisfactory, as the evidence for a close association between social and demographic factors and measured rates of psychiatric disorder is strong. For example, in the UK, the Jarman combined index of social deprivation has been shown to be highly correlated with psychiatric admission rates (Jarman 1983, 1984; Hirsch 1988; Thornicroft 1991; Thornicroft et al. 1993). It therefore seems reasonable to use overall deprivation scores such as the Jarman index to make weighted estimates of likely local needs for services. For example, if an area has a level of deprivation in the upper 10% of the national range, one would estimate that numbers of acute beds and residential places needed to meet local needs will also be in the upper 10% of ranges such as those shown in Table 2.

Table 2. Estimated need for general adult residential provision per 250 000 population (Wing 1992; Strathdee and Thornicroft 1992)

Type of accommodation	Wing (1990)		Strathdee and Thornicroft (1992)	
	Midpoint number of places	Range	Midpoint number of places	Range
Staff awake at night				
Acute and crisis care	100	50–150	95	50–150
Intensive care unit	10	5–15	8	5–10
Regional Secure Unit and Special Hospital	4	1–10	5	1–10
Hostel wards	50	25–75		
Other staffed housing				
High-staffed hostel	75	40–110	95	40–150
Day-staffed hostel	50	25–75	75	30–120
Group homes (visited)	45	20–70	64	48–80
Respite facilities			3	0–5
No specialist staff				
Supported bed-sits	30	–		
Direct access	30	–		
Adult placement schemes			8	0–15
Total per 250 000	394	226–585	357	174–540

Taking overall social deprivation into account is a helpful beginning in making epidemilogically based estimates of needs for services. Such estimates will be further improved by taking into account a number of local factors with specific implications for needs for mental health services. Ethnicity is particularly important: ethnic minority populations have been found to have different patterns of service use from others in their communities, and both the effects of local minority populations on numbers of places requires and their particular needs for culturally and linguistically appropriate services should be taken into account (Fernando 1991; McGovern and Cope 1991; King et al. 1994). Any groups of recently arrived refugees living locally are likely to be experiencing high levels of deprivation and of post-traumatic disorders. The extent of the local homeless population should also be considered, as the homeless have high rates of psychiatric disorder and may not be reached by conventional psychiatric services (Timms and Fry 1989, Marshall 1989). Local rates of unemployment should also be considered, as this is associated with poor mental health (Warr et al. 1988).

Service Needs from a Geographical Perspective

Meeting needs across a catchment area requires not only the provision of adequate numbers of places in a range of forms of care, but also the location of services so that they are accessible to those who need them. Not only the overall characteristics but also the detailed geography of a catchment area thus need to be considered. Sectorization is now regarded in many European countries as an essential prerequisite to the development of effective community services (Johnson and Thornicroft 1993). Such a division of larger catchment areas into smaller geographically defined sectors, with services for each area located centrally within it, is an important principle in ensuring that services are accessible to people throughout the catchment area. It is also important for service planners to examine public transport routes to ensure local bases can be reached reasonably quickly from each part of each sector. A further important principle in considering the geography of the catchment area is that particular attention should be paid to service provision in those areas where the greatest levels of needs may be expected, as in areas where there is severe poverty or where homeless people tend to congregate.

Conclusion

There is now widespread agreement on the principle that the needs of the local population of people with mental illnesses should guide the development and provision of community mental health services. No consensus exists as yet on how to define such needs, either at an individual or a population level. However, some methodologies are now available both for needs assessment at an individual level and for estimating the likely aggregate needs of populations. While these methods are still at an early stage of development, their wider application in service planning and provision promises to promote the development of services which are more appropriate for mentally ill individuals. They also make available a means of assessing the current extent of unmet needs and the degree to which services may currently lack enough finding to be capable of meeting needs through their catchment area populations.

References

Beecham J., Knapp M. and Fenyo A. (1993) Costs, Needs and Outcomes in Community Mental Health Care. In Costing Community Care. Edited by Netten A, Beecham J. Aldershot: Aldgate.

Brewin C., Veltro F., Wing J., et al. (1990) The assessment of psychiatric disability in the community: A comparison of clinical, staff, and family interviews. British Journal of Psychiatry, 157, 671–674.

Brewin C. (1992) Measuring individual needs for care and services. In: Tornicroft G., Brewin C.R., & Wing J. (1992) Measuring Mental Health Needs. Gaskell and Royal College of Psychiatrists: London.

Brewin C., Wing J., Mangen S., et al. (1988) Needs for care among the long-term mentally ill: A report from the Camberwell High Contact Survey. Psychological Medicine, 18, 457–468.

Brewin C., Wing J.K., Mangen S.P., Brugha T.S. & MacCarthy B. (1987) Principles and practice of measuring needs in the long-term mentally ill: the MRC Needs for Care Assessment. Psychological Medicine 17, 971–982.

Brewin C., Wing J. (1993) The MRC Needs for Care Assessment: progress and controversies. Psychological Medicine, 23, 837–841.

Culyer A., Wagstaff A. (1992) Need, equity and equality in health and health care. Centre for Health Economics, Health Economics Consortium, University of York, York.

Davies B., Challis D. (1986) Matching Resources to Needs in Community Care. London: Gower.

Ellis K. (1993) Squaring the circle: User and carer participation in needs assessment. York: Joseph Rowntree Foundation.

Fernando S. (1991) Mental health, race and culture. London: MIND/Macmillan.

Glover G. (1991) The official data available on mental health. In Jenkins R and Griffiths S (eds) Indicators for Mental Health in the Population. London: HMSO.

Goldberg D., Huxley P. (1992) Common Mental Disorders. A Bio-Social Model. Routledge, London.

Goldberg D., Huxley P. (1980) Mental Illness in the Community. London: Tavistock.

Hillier W, Zaudig M. & Mobour W. (1991) Development of diagnostic checklists for use in routine clinical care. Archives of General Psychiatry 47, 782–784.

Hirsch S (1988) Psychiatric beds and resources: Factors influencing bed use and service planning. London: Gaskell (Royal College of Psychiatrists).

Hogg L., Marshall M. (1992) Can we measure need in the homeless mentally ill? Using the MRC Needs for Care Assessment in hostels for the homeless. Psychological Medicine, 22, 1027–1034.

Holloway F. (1994) Need in community psychiatry: a consensus is required. Psychiatric Bulletin 18, 321–323.

House of Commons (1990) The National Health Service and Community Care Act. London: HMSO.

Jarman B. (1984) Underprivileged areas: validation and distribution of scores. British Medical Journal, 289, 1587–1592.

Jarman B. (1983) Identification of underprivileged areas. British Medical Journal, 286, 1705–1709.

Johnson S., Thornicroft G. (1993) The sectorisation of psychiatric services in England and Wales. Social Psychiatry and Psychiatric Epidemiology, 28, 45–47.

Johnson S., Thornicroft G. and Strathdee S. (1996) Population-based assessment of needs for services. In Strathdee S. and Thornicroft G. (eds) Commissioning Mental Health Services. London: HMSO (In press)

King M., Coker E, Leavey G., Hoare A. and Johnson-Sabine E. (1994) Incidence of psychotic illness in London: a comparison of ethnic groups. British Medical Journal 309: 1115–1119.

Lesage A. D., Mignolli G., Faccincani C. et al. (1991) Standardised assessment of the needs for care in a cohort of patients with schizophrenic psychoses. In Community-based Psychiatry: Long-term Patterns of Care in South-Verona (ed M. Tansella), pp. 27–33. Psychological Medicine Monograph Supplement 19.

Liss P. (1990) Health Care Need: Meaning and Measurement. Studies in arts and Science, Linkoping.

MacDonald A. (1991) How can we measure mental health? In Indicators for Mental Health in the Population. (ed. R. Jenkins and S. Griffiths). London: HMSO.

McGovern D. and Cope R. (1991) Second generation Afro-Caribbeans and young Whites with a first admission diagnosis of schizophrenia. Social Psychiatry and Psychiatric Epidemiology 26: 95–99

Mallman C. A., Marcus S. (1980) Logical clarifications in the study of needs. In Human Needs (ed. K. Lederer), pp. 163–185. Cambridge, MA: Oelgeschlager, Gunn, & Hain.

Mangen S., Brewin C. R. (in press) The measurement of need. In Social psychiatry: Theory, methodology and practice (ed. P. E. Bebbington). Transaction Press.

Marshall M. (1989) Collected and neglected: are Oxford hostels filling up with disabled psychiatric patients. British Medical Journal 299, 706–709

Marshall M. (1994) How should we measure need? Phisolophy, Psychiatry & Psychology, 1, 27–36.

Maslow A. (1968) Towards a Psychology of Being, 2nd ed. D. van Nostrand, New York.

McCrone P., Strathdee G. (1994) Needs not diagnosis: towards a more rational approach to community mental health resourcing in Great Britain. International Journal of Social Psychiatry.

National Institute of Mental Health (1987) Toward a Model Plan for a Comprehensive Community-Based Mental Health System. Washington DC: NIMH.

Phclan M., Slade M., Thornicroft G., Dunn D., Holloway F., Wykes T., Strathdee G., Loftus L., McCrone P., & Hayward P. (1995) The Camberwell Assessment of Need (CAN): the validity and reliability of an instrument to assess the needs of people with severe mental illness. British Journal of Psychiatry.

Prycc I., Griffiths R., Gentry R., Hughes I., Montaguss L., Watkins S., Champney-Smith J., McLackland B. (1993) How important is the Assessment of Social Skills in a Long-Stay Psychiatric In-patients? British Journal of Psychiatry, 163, 498–502.

Shapiro S., Skinner E. A., Kramer M., et al. (1985) Measuring need for mental health services in a general population. Medical Care, 23, 1033–1043.

Slade M. (1994) Needs assessment: who needs to assess? British Journal of Psychiatry, 165, 287–292.

Slade M., Phelan M., Thornicroft G. and Parkman S. (1996) The Camberwell Assessment of Need: comparison of assessments by staff and patients of the needs of the severely mentally ill. Social Psychiatry and Psychiatric Epidemiology (in press).

Stevens A., Raftery J. (1994) Introduction. In Stevens A. & Raftery J. Health Care Needs Assessment. Radcliffe Medical Press, Oxford, pp 11–30.

Stevens A., Gabbay J. (1991) Needs assessment needs assessment. Health Trends 23, 20–23.

Strathdee G., and Thornicroft G. (1992) Community Sectors for Needs-Led Mental Health Services. In Measuring Mental Health Needs. (Thornicroft G., Brewin C. & Wing J. K. eds). Royal College of Psychiatrists, Gaskell Press, Chapter 8.

Thornicroft G. and Bebbington P. (1996) Quantitative methods in the Evaluation of Community Mental Health Services in Breakey W. (ed). Modern Community Psychiatry. Cambridge University Press, Cambridge.

Thornicroft G. (1991) Social deprivation and rates of treated mental disorder: developing statistical models to predict psychiatric service utilisation. British Journal of Psychiatry 1991; 158: 475–484.

Thornicroft G. and Strathdee G. (1994) How Many Psychiatric Beds? British Medical Journal: 309, 970–971.

Thornicroft G., De Salvia G., Tansella M. (1993) Urban-rural differences in the associations between social deprivation and psychiatric service utilisation in schizophrenia and all diagnoses: a case-register study in Northern Italy. Psychological Medicine 1993, 23: 487–469.

Timms P. and Fry A. (1989) Homelessness and mental illness. Health Trends 21, 70–71.

Tracy L. (1986) Toward an improved need theory: In response to legitimate criticism. Behavioural Science, 31, 205–218.

van Haaster I., Lesage A, Cyr M., Toupin J. (1994) Problems and needs for care of patients suffering from severe mental illness. Social Psychiatry & Psychiatric Epidemiology, 29, 141–148.

Warr P., Jackson P. and Banks M.H. (1988) Unemployment and mental health: some British studies. Journal of Social Issues 44, 47–68.

Wing J. (1971) How many psychiatric beds? Psychological Medicine 1, 189–190.

Wing J. (1989) Editor. Health Services Planning and Research. Contributions from Psychiatric Case Registers. London: Gaskell, 1989.

Wing J.K. (1992) Epidemiologically-Based-Needs-Assessments. Review of Research on Psychiatric Disorders. Department of Health: London.

CHAPTER 17

Measuring Outcomes in Mental Health: Implications for Policy

RACHEL JENKINS

The activities and purposes of mental health services can be described under three headings: inputs, processes, and outcomes. Until recently the focus of service description and evaluation has been largely on input and process variables. The strength of this book is that it illuminates the increasing number of possibilities to use outcome indicators as the main point of reference for measuring cost effectiveness.

The approach that uses inputs of service adequacy has historically focused on the numbers of beds available, the type and ranges of buildings and places that are provided, the numbers of staff of different disciplines and their levels of training and the amount of money injected into the service system. Although this information is vital for assessing the performance of a mental health service system, it is, however, a one sided approach. Such information may be entirely misleading if the investment in a service, described in these terms, produces no actual benefits to patients. The input approach on its own, although frequently used and administratively convenient, can give no indication about whether services are actually achieving their goals.

The second and most common approach to assessing mental health system performance is to use process measures. Examples of this approach are the determination of length of stay in hospital, bed occupancy rates, staffing levels, staff turnover rates, and the number and duration of community contacts for home treatment services. Again this information is vital for understanding the dynamic way in which a variety of services operates, how the physical and human resource infrastructures are deployed in practice, and the distribution of these resources in different geographical and administrative sectors. This approach is the focus of performance management which is increasingly emphasized as health services are run more and more along corporate lines. However, this can be compared to a detailed description of the functioning of an ocean liner without any reference as to whether the ship is sailing in the right direction. Auditing provides service process information, and service purchasing, and a middle management service provider decisions are often based upon such process information. As with input information, however, such process measures alone cannot shed any light on whether the intended aims of the service, both as a whole and in its components, are realised in practice.

The third approach, that of measuring outcome variables, is therefore the most important. The contributions in this book indicates that substantial technical progress has been made in developing and standardising measurement methods across a broad range of outcome domains. In terms of individual patient functioning, mea-

Department of Health, MHCC2, Wellington House, 133–155 Waterloo Road, London SE1 9RT, UK.

sures for symptoms, disability, quality of life, need, satisfaction, global functioning, and carer burden are now well developed, and have been translated into a large number of languages. During the last 5 years such scales have become more valid, reliable, sensitive, specific, and usable. It is likely that the criteria of adequacy set out in the chapter by Salvador will be increasingly used as bench marks in assessing the quality of such measures. In terms of evaluation of the service level, the contributions by Dunn, and Tansella and colleagues demonstrate that multivariate models of higher complexity will be required to analyse data in an attempt to identify the effective components of individual treatment programmes or service systems which improve patient outcomes. It is likely that such statistical sophistication will soon become a routine feature of mental health service evaluation.

We can view the development of mental health outcome measures in terms of four stages. In the first stage, outcome measures are used as single indices of health gain for individual patients and patient groups. This is the "Health Gain" approach in which health inputs are expected to improve the patient's status with respect to specific targed outcome domains. An example of this is the Health of the Nation Outcome Scales (HONOS). This was commissioned for England in order to measure the outcome of the health of the nation target, which is to improve the health and social functioning of people with mental illness. It is possible to use this approach in each of the subsequent stages.

In the second stage, the addition of cost information allows the calculation of cost effectiveness ratios so that different treatments can be compared in terms of their relative value for money. The limitation of this approach, which applies particularly to people with severe mental illnesses, is that symptoms and disability may not be entirely curable. In such cases the maintenance of a patient at a given level of functioning may in itself be the desirable outcome.

The third stage of outcome measure development is the use of cost effectiveness data in relation to the expected course and outcome for a particular diagnosis-related or outcome-related group. Although this has rarely been put into practice, such course and outcome expectations could be developed by using a consensus conference/delphi model. In this approach, experts and stakeholders estimate a set of reasonable expectations for the clinical course of patients with and without treatment. In effect, this is a process of calibration in which input data, output data, and the expected effects of treatments are combined in order to establish the relationship between clinical and social functioning, and service inputs and investments.

The fourth stage, not yet reached in practice, would be to combine such calibrated and consensual cost effectiveness outcomes with a wider view of which patient groups should receive priority for investment by health and social services. All political, policy, and planning decisions would be based on these priority decisions. The health of the nation targets in the area of mental health, established within Britain over the last 5 years, were not influenced by calibrated cost effectiveness data which would be available from stage three.

The challenge for clinical practice now is to include outcome information in assessing the value of clinical work. The challenge for mental health service research will be to proceed from stage 1 to stage 4, as discussed above, in order to gain a complete and detailed understanding of how services can best help people who suffer from mental illnesses.

Subject Index

Springer-Verlag
and the Environment

We at Springer-Verlag firmly believe that an international science publisher has a special obligation to the environment, and our corporate policies consistently reflect this conviction.

We also expect our business partners – paper mills, printers, packaging manufacturers, etc. – to commit themselves to using environmentally friendly materials and production processes.

The paper in this book is made from low- or no-chlorine pulp and is acid free, in conformance with international standards for paper permanency.

CPSIA information can be obtained at www.ICGtesting.com
Printed in the USA
LVOW070400110912

298287LV00002B/15/P